Mastering Emergency Medicine
A practical guide

Mastering Emergency Medicine
A practical guide

Edited by

Chetan R Trivedy BDS FDS RCS(Eng) MBBS PhD FRSH MCEM

Specialist Registrar in Emergency Medicine,
South East Thames, London Deanery, London, UK

Mathew Hall BMBCh PhD MCEM

Senior Clinical Fellow in Emergency Medicine,
Princess Royal University Hospital, Kent, UK

Andrew Parfitt MAEd FRCS FCEM

Associate Medical Director and Clinical Director of Acute Medicine
and Gastrointestinal Surgery,
Guy's and St Thomas' NHS Trust, London, UK

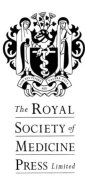

The ROYAL
SOCIETY *of*
MEDICINE
PRESS *Limited*

© 2010 Royal Society of Medicine Ltd

Published by the Royal Society of Medicine Press Ltd
1 Wimpole Street, London W1G OAE, UK
Tel: +44 (0)20 7290 2921
Fax: +44 (0)20 7290 2929
E-mail: publishing@rsmpress.co.uk

British Library Cataloguing in Publication Data
A catalogue record for this book is available from the British Library

ISBN: 978-1-85315-744-8

Distribution in Europe and Rest of the World:
Marston Book Services Ltd
PO Box 269
Abingdon
Oxon OX14 4YN, UK
Tel: +44 (0)1235 465500
Fax: +44 (0)1235 465555
Email: direct.order@marston.co.uk

Distribution in USA and Canada:
Royal Society of Medicine Press Ltd
c/o BookMasters Inc
30 Amberwood Parkway
Ashland, OH 44805, USA
Tel: +1 800 247 6553/ +1 800 266 5564
Fax: +1 410 281 6883
Email: order@bookmasters.com

Distribution in Australia and New Zealand:
Elsevier Australia
30–52 Smidmore Street
Marrickville NSW 2204, Australia
Tel: +61 2 9517 8999
Fax: +61 2 9517 2249
Email: service@elsevier.com.au

Typeset by Phoenix Photosetting, Chatham, Kent, UK
Printed by Bell & Bain Ltd., Glasgow

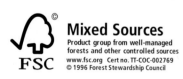

CONTENTS

CONTRIBUTORS

Harith Al-Rawi MBChB MRCS(Ed) FRCS(A&E) DCH FCEM Consultant in Adult and Paediatric Emergency Medicine, St Thomas' Hospital, London, UK

Russell Barber MBBS Anaesthetic Registrar, East Surrey Hospital, Surrey & Sussex Healthcare NHS Trust, Redhill, UK

Duncan Bootland MBBS BSc MCEM Specialist Registrar in Emergency Medicine, KSS Postgraduate Deanery, London, UK

Beth Christian MBBS FACEM FCEM Consultant in Emergency Medicine, Guy's and St Thomas' NHS Trust, London UK

Simon FJ Clarke MBChB DA FRCSEd FCEM Consultant Emergency Physician, Frimley Park NHS Foundation Trust, Frimley, UK; Honorary Consultant in Emergency Response and Medical Toxicology, Chemical Hazards and Poisons Division, Health Protection Agency, London, UK

Evan Coughlan MBBCh NUI MCEM DSEM Speciality Registrar in Emergency Medicine, London Deanery, London, UK

Bethany Davies MBBS MA MRCP MSc Specialist Registrar in Infectious Diseases and Medical Microbiology/Virology, London Deanery, London, UK

Shumontha Dev BSc(Hons) MBBS MRCS(Ed) FCEM Consultant in Emergency Medicine, St Thomas' Hospital, London, UK

Nicola Drake MB ChB FRCSEd(A&E) FCEM Consultant in Emergency Medicine, St Thomas' Hospital, London, UK

Francesca Garnham MBBS FRCS(Ed) FCEM Consultant in Emergency Medicine, Guy's and St Thomas' NHS Trust, London, UK

Mathew Hall BMBCh PhD MCEM Senior Clinical Fellow in Emergency Medicine, Princess Royal University Hospital, Kent, UK

Katherine IM Henderson MBBChir MSc MRCP FCEM Consultant in Emergency Medicine, Guy's and St Thomas' NHS Trust, London, UK

Peter Jaye BSc MRCP FCEM Consultant in Emergency Medicine, Guy's and St Thomas' NHS Trust, London, UK

Amit KJ Mandal MBBS(Lond) MRCP(UK) MRCP(Ed) Senior Specialist Registrar in Acute and General Internal Medicine with a specialist interest in Cardiology, Mersey and London Deaneries, Liverpool and London, UK

Zulfiquar Mirza MBChB DCH DRCOG MRCGP MRCP FFAEM Consultant in Emergency Medicine, West Middlesex University Hospital, Isleworth, UK; President Emergency Medicine Section Royal Society of Medicine, London, UK

Alastair Newton MBChB DA(UK) FRCS FCEM Consultant in Emergency Medicine, Royal Alexandra Hospital, Paisley, UK; Consultant in Retrieval Medicine, Emergency Medical Retrieval Service, Glasgow, UK

Savvas Pappasavvas FFEM FRCS MMSci Consultant Emergency Medicine, Guy's and St Thomas NHS Trust, London, UK

Andrew Parfitt MAEd FRCS FCEM Associate Medical Director and Clinical Director of Acute Medicine and Gastrointestinal Surgery, Guy's and St Thomas' NHS Trust, London, UK

Nick Payne MBBS DipMedTox FRCSEd(A&E) FCEM Consultant Emergency Physician, Frimley Park NHS Foundation Trust, Frimley, UK

David Roe FRCS FCEM Consultant in Emergency Medicine, Whiston Hospital, Liverpool, UK

Joban S Sehmi BSc MBBS MRCP Registrar in Cardiology Reseach, National Heart and Lung Institute, Imperial College London, UK

Natalie S Shenker BA(Hons) BMBCh(Oxon) MRCS(Eng) Specialist Trainee in Paediatric Surgery, London Deanery, London, UK

Chetan R Trivedy BDS FDS RCS(Eng) MBBS PhD FRSH MCEM Specialist Registrar in Emergency Medicine, South East Thames, London Deanery, London, UK

Charles Young MBBS BSc MRCP Editor in Chief, *Best Practice* and *BMJ Point of Care*; Editor, *Clinical Evidence*; Emergency Physician, St Thomas' Hospital, London, UK

FOREWORD

It is an absolute pleasure to welcome this new book and to congratulate the editors on providing an excellent addition to the emergency medicine library.

The College of Emergency Medicine (CEM) examinations, both membership and fellowship, are rigorous and demanding. This is absolutely essential to ensure that the doctors who successfully pass these examinations are of a high calibre who will then deliver the highest standard of care to their patients. Setting the bar at this very high level also allows the quality and safety agenda to be comprehensively addressed by specialists in emergency medicine.

From the candidates' perspective, the examinations can appear somewhat daunting, even for the most talented and well prepared. The editors have assembled an outstanding group of contributors, who provide comprehensive coverage of the CEM syllabus. This book has been written by trainees who have successfully negotiated all the hurdles and crossed the finishing line, and as such they have a huge insight into the knowledge and approach required to be successful in the examinations.

The main focus of the book is the OSCE component of the CEM examinations. This is, of course, a great opportunity for candidates to demonstrate their clinical skills and competencies, which will subsequently be provided for patients in their care. The assessments in the OSCEs are therefore very realistic and relevant to day-to-day patient care.

This important link to everyday patient care means that the content of this book is also useful in a non-examination setting, as it discusses optimal approaches to a wide range of emergency department clinical scenarios appropriate for trainees in emergency medicine and adjacent specialties.

Many congratulations to the editors and contributors of this book, which will have an invaluable role for all emergency medicine trainees preparing for their CEM examinations.

Good luck!

JOHN HEYWORTH
President, College of Emergency Medicine

PREFACE

The great challenge of emergency medicine is in the immense breadth of knowledge and clinical skills required for competent practice: knowledge and skills that overlap and incorporate aspects of virtually every medical specialty adapted for the emergency room environment.

In 2003, the newly formed College of Emergency Medicine (CEM) launched its own membership examination, the Membership of the College of Emergency Medicine (MCEM). This examination tests candidates' knowledge of basic sciences in Part A, clinical data interpretation in Part B, and clinical skills using Objective Structured Clinical Examinations (OSCEs) in Part C. Since its inception, the new MCEM examination has set a high standard and the gruelling OSCE circuit in particular has proved to be a real challenge for many aspiring emergency medicine trainees.

Unlike other postgraduate examinations, there are few resources for the emergency medicine trainee sitting the OSCE component of the CEM examinations. This book aims to fill that void by providing a comprehensive yet practical approach to the Part C examination, and in addition contains useful content for the OSCE component of the FCEM examination. We have included a breakdown of the CEM curriculum into core topics and examples of past OSCE stations, with the text guiding the reader through over a 100 practice OSCEs and providing essential background information, suggested approaches, revision checklists and sample score sheets. As such, this is a unique and essential revision aid to the MCEM Part C examination and beyond. Trainees in other acute medical specialties will also find this a useful hands-on guide for managing patients in the emergency department.

In putting this book together we have drawn on the experience of a wide range of contributors from the field of emergency medicine whose remit was to write each chapter with a strong focus on the attitudes, knowledge and clinical skills expected of a higher trainee in emergency medicine.

We hope that you will find this book useful both in revising for the MCEM and FCEM exams, but also as a useful resource to improve and consolidate your clinical skills in emergency medicine.

CT, MH, AP

1
Surviving the CEM Examination
CHETAN R TRIVEDY AND ANDREW PARFITT

The objective structured clinical examination (OSCE) has become the standard form of assessment for the majority of undergraduate and postgraduate examinations. Many candidates find the prospect of performing simulated scenarios under the pressures of time and examination conditions quite stressful.

The aim of this book is to give the prospective candidate a structured approach to the OSCE component of the College of Emergency Medicine (CEM) examinations. The content of the book is based on the CEM syllabus, and the sample OSCE scenarios are representative of the core skills that can be examined at both Membership and Fellowship levels.

The CEM OSCE has been described as 'a bad day at the office', and this is a pretty accurate description, since the scenarios typify cases that the candidate is likely to come across on a daily basis. The only difference is the pressure of time and the added stress of examination conditions.

PREPARATION TIPS

The importance of preparation cannot be overstated, and, unlike written examinations, cramming is not a realistic option for the OSCE assessment. Ideally, you should leave aside at least three months to prepare for the examination, of which the first month should involve developing an OSCE study group.

Unlike other types of examinations, preparation for which is usually self-directed, OSCEs should be tackled using a team approach. Setting up an OSCE study group is an essential part of the revision process and should be done early, since it often takes a few weeks for the team to gel together. The emergency department provides round-the-clock access to potential revision scenarios, and you should try to allocate as much time as you can spare around each shift to practise your clinical examination and history-taking skills.

You should take every opportunity to be observed by senior colleagues when you examine a patient, and should try to utilize other members of the emergency department team, who can provide constructive criticism on your verbal and non-verbal communication skills.

The vast majority of practical skills can be perfected within the emergency department, although it is often useful to practise in the skill laboratory or the resuscitation-training centre.

It is essential that you be familiar with the latest resuscitation guidelines, since you are almost certain to be faced with an OSCE based on the latest advanced life support (ALS), advanced trauma life support (ATLS) or advanced paediatric life support (APLS) guidelines.

Over the last few years, there has been an increase in the number of dedicated OSCE revision courses that allow the candidate to practise realistic OSCE scenarios under the scrutiny of the examiners. However, they are usually oversubscribed and often quite expensive, and so you should organize your study leave and budget as soon as you can.

THE OSCE EXAMINATION

At present, the MCEM OSCE assessment consists of 18 stations and a number of rest stations. There are no sudden-death stations and you have to pass 15/18 stations to pass the examination. Each station is 7 minutes in duration and you will be directed through the OSCE circuit.

As the format of the examination may undergo modification, you should visit the CEM website for up-to-date information on the structure of the OSCE assessment. The site also provides sample OSCE mark schemes and advice on all components of the CEM examination.

THE TEN GOLDEN OSCE RULES

1. Dress appropriately and be presentable – first impressions do count! It is acceptable to wear scrubs or smart attire. However, it is not acceptable to wear polo shirts and trousers in the examination.
2. **READ THE INSTRUCTIONS.** This cannot be overstressed, since many candidates will either misread or misinterpret the instructions. The marks are fixed and you can only score marks for what you are asked to do. If you are asked to examine the cardiovascular system, you will not get any marks for taking a cardiac history and you will waste valuable time.
3. If you are unsure about the instructions, ask the examiner to clarify them. If in doubt, reread the instructions.
4. Introduce yourself appropriately and confidently. Be yourself and pretend that this is just another patient in the emergency department. Always remember to decontaminate your hands with alcohol gel on entering and leaving each station.
5. Keep calm and collected at all times. You may be faced with an aggressive or difficult colleague or patient. The actors will have been primed to respond to your body language. You should not get aggressive or defensive and you should remain courteous at all times.
6. Talk through what you are doing unless the examiner asks you to present at the end of the OSCE. This also gives you the opportunity to talk through things that you would do in a real-life situation.
7. Engage your patient and develop a rapport with them. Ensuring their comfort and explaining what you are going to do before you do it will go a long way to enhancing your global score. A patient who is in pain should be offered analgesia.
8. There are no sudden-death stations. However, some candidates have a tendency to panic when things do not go to plan. This is very dangerous, since there is real risk of meltdown if you take your perceived poor performance and frustration from one station to the next. Do not assume failure, since it is very difficult to predict your performance for any given station; remember that you can fail three of the stations and still pass the examination.
9. Always conclude your station by ensuring that your patient has either follow-up or a management plan (if appropriate for the scenario).
10. Do not try to memorize mark sheets that you may have seen in books or courses. These are for revision purposes only and are likely to differ from the actual mark sheet.

THE 'TRIP' AND 'FALL' PRINCIPLES IN THE OSCE

Experience has led us to believe that success in the OSCE is not wholly related to clinical knowledge or the ability to perform clinical skills. The ability to respond to both verbal and non-verbal cues is often underrated by many candidates. The use of technical jargon, mannerisms, poor eye contact, and lack of empathy or rapport with the patient often results in the candidate not communicating effectively, and we have coined the term TRIP to exemplify this:

Technical jargon
Reduced rapport with the patient
Incoherency in communication
Patronizing

This term represents potential factors that may impair success in a history-taking or communication skill station.

Alternatively, the candidate may also FALL:

Failure to recognize non-verbal cues from the patient
Assuming failure
Lack of clinical knowledge
Lack of empathy with the patient

TRIP and FALL are important factors resulting in the candidate failing the OSCE station.

NON-VERBAL COMMUNICATION

It is important that you listen carefully to your patient and ask open questions. Some patients may have hidden concerns that may not be obvious at first but that you should try to explore. Pay attention to the patient's body language as well as your own. If a patient is aggressive, there is usually a good reason, and you should pick up on their verbal and non-verbal cues.

USEFUL RESOURCES

Recently, there has been an increase in the amount of Internet resources available for those sitting the MCEM/ FCEM examination. The CEM website has some sample OSCE scenarios. In addition, there are web resources that give advice and useful revision tips. Examples of OSCE scenarios that have appeared before are listed at the end of this chapter. They should be used purely as a guide and not as an exhaustive list of OSCEs.

OSCE TYPES

The OSCE scenarios can be divided into five broad categories; this list is likely to grow as examiners try to create more sophisticated OSCE scenarios.

The clinical examination OSCE

This type of OSCE requires a well-rehearsed examination of a system, and it is essential that you practise examining all of the major systems. As this is a Membership examination, you should have a slick and systematic approach to your clinical examination. You should present your findings as you proceed and remember to leave enough time in your routine to summarize your findings as well outline your differential diagnosis, investigations and management. You should pay close attention to the instructions to ensure that you are performing the correct examination as opposed to what you have revised. Most of the clinical examinations will be on either actors or patients; therefore be courteous and watchful of their dignity, try not to cause any pain or discomfort while examining them, and ensure that you have decontaminated your hands before and after the examination. You will not be expected to perform an intimate examination on a real patient, but it is essential that you address the actor linked with the model as if they were the patient. Ask for a chaperone where appropriate and get consent to examine a child. These points may seem obvious, but they can significantly influence your global score.

The skills OSCE

This type of OSCE involves performing a practical procedure in a very short time frame in what may seem to be a very artificial and surreal scenario. Nowhere else would you be expected to suture a wound or place a chest drain in less than 7 minutes. It is therefore crucial that you not only practise the common skills but also get into the habit of talking through a skill as you are performing it. Although the majority of the marks are for performing the skill, do not forget to interact with the actor or manikin as if they were the patient, since there will also be marks for obtaining consent and outlining follow-up. Some candidates find this type of station difficult because very little time is allowed. The CEM syllabus lists the practical procedures that you need to be aware of; we have summarized these in Chapter 31.

The teaching OSCE

The CEM examinations test not only your clinical skills as an emergency physician but also your ability to teach students or junior colleagues. This may seem a daunting prospect, since you not only have to know the subject matter but also have to pass on this knowledge in a constructive, non-judgemental and educationally approved manner. Whether you are asked to teach a medical student how to examine the ear or teach a patient how to use an inhaler, the principles are more or less the same. It is important that you appreciate that this type of OSCE is not just about how much you know of the subject matter but also about how you impart that knowledge; Table 1.1 outlines a generic approach to this type of OSCE.

Table 1.1 A generic approach to the teaching OSCE

Teaching a junior colleague	Teaching a patient
Find out how much they know about the particular skill	Review what the patient knows or has been told about their condition
Set the objectives for the teaching session clearly	Set the learning objectives
Demonstrate the skill in stages	Demonstrate and explain the skill, bearing in mind that you may be teaching a layperson
Stop after each stage and review that the student has understood what you have told them	Check that the patient has understood
If there is any misunderstanding, review the previous steps	Repeat steps for clarification
Ask the student to perform the skill	Ask the patient to perform the skill
Review the skill and provide feedback	Review and provide feedback
Encourage questions	Encourage questions
After dealing with any queries, plan for the next session	Arrange follow-up for the patient
Try to give pointers for resources that the student can use to prepare for the next session	Give an advice leaflet or written instructions
It is important that you are not judgemental or patronizing and that you do not spend your valuable minutes quizzing or berating the student	It is important that you are not judgemental or patronizing and that the patient is happy with your management

The communication skills OSCE

Good communication skills are essential in emergency medicine, and several stations in the CEM will be specifically designed to test your ability to communicate with a patient, colleague or other members of the multidisciplinary team. In addition, these stations also test your negotiation and diplomacy skills.

- Break bad news to a patient or family member.
- Explain a proposed treatment or condition.
- Make a difficult referral.
- Deal with a complaint.
- Deal with a failing colleague.
- Negotiate a management plan with a patient.
- Deal with a confidentiality/consent issue.

It is difficult to learn communication skills from a book, and the easiest way is to get a colleague to observe you and provide feedback. You should pay particular attention to your body language, since this is an important form of non-verbal communication. Silence is also an effective means of communication, and it is important that you give the patient ample opportunity to talk without interruption. Try to summarize what the patient has said to you back to them to ensure that your facts are accurate.

The history-taking OSCE

Taking a concise and accurate medical history is integral to success in the CEM examinations. As there is pressure of time in the examination, your questioning should be focused while not appearing to be an inquisition for the patient. Remember that, in addition to marks for asking clinical questions, there will also be marks from the patient/role player for your communication skills.

HOW TO USE THIS BOOK

As with all examination preparation texts, this book is only a guide to the type of OSCEs that may appear in the CEM examinations. Although it is primarily aimed at those sitting the MCEM examination, it should be also be a useful base for those preparing for the FCEM, since there is a significant overlap in the type of OSCEs. The CEM syllabus is extremely diverse and is continually remodelled, and so it is essential that you be aware of any additions or amendments.

It is also important to point out that this book does not prepare you with the core clinical knowledge required to pass the examination and is specifically aimed at providing the candidate with a number of mock OSCE scenarios to practice. Useful facts and guidelines have been included where possible, but, given the breadth of knowledge covered in the syllabus, it is impossible to provide essential facts for every topic or to cover every scenario. There are several core texts in emergency medicine, which should be used in conjunction with this OSCE-based revision guide.

The scope of this book is to give the candidate a broad overview of the potential OSCE scenarios that may be tested in the examination and a guide on how to approach these OSCEs. Do not make the mistake of rote-learning the mark sheets, since they are only guides and not validated mark sheets.

Marks are given for specific points/areas that you address appropriately. In addition, the actor/patient/student can give a score, usually out of 5, and the examiner can give a global score out of 5.

The scoring for each section of the mark sheet is as follows:
0 = inadequate/not done
1 = adequate
2 = good

It is crucial to appreciate that this is an arbitrary marking system that is a rough guide to your performance and does not in any way represent the official college score sheets. You should use the marks to see how your performance progresses as you step up your revision.

The key is to use this book as a template on which to base your revision and not as a substitute for seeing as many patients as possible in the emergency department.

PAST OSCE SCENARIOS

Chapter 2: Resuscitation

- Airway management
- Advanced life support (ALS) management – patient in systole
- ALS management – 34-week pregnant patient, involved in a motor vehicle collision
- ALS management – defibrillation technique and safety
- ALS management – pulseless electrical activity (PEA)
- ALS management – postresuscitation care
- ALS management – pulseless ventricular tachycardia (VT)
- ALS management – tricyclic antidepressant overdose and ventricular fibrillation
- ALS management – ventricular fibrillation
- Basic and advanced airway management (including endotracheal intubation)
- Transfer a patient with a head injury and reduced consciousness for a CT scan

Chapter 4: Wound management

- Suturing a laceration wound using the 'no-touch' technique
- Handwashing scenario

Chapter 5: Major trauma

- Advanced trauma life support (ATLS) scenario
- Clinical examination of an immobilized patient with a potential cervical spine injury
- Demonstrate a log-roll and spinal examination in a trauma scenario
- Manage a patient with a haemothorax following a motor vehicle collision
- Place and suture a chest drain

Chapter 6: Musculoskeletal emergencies

- Focused upper limb examination to assess nerves, vascular supply and tendons following a laceration injury
- Hand examination (neurovascular plus tendons)
- History, examination and management of a shoulder injury
- Knee joint examination and management
- Plaster cast application for a Colles fracture

Chapter 8: Abdominal emergencies

- Focused gastrointestinal history and general systems enquiry
- Focused history and management of a rectal bleed
- Traveller's diarrhoea – history and advice
- Cirrhosis of liver – history and management

Chapter 9: Genitourinary system

- Genitourinary history, clinical diagnosis and management
- Haematuria assessment

Chapter 10: Ophthalmology

- Acute red eye assessment and management
- Perform fundoscopy and make a clinical diagnosis
- Teaching a medical student to use an ophthalmoscope
- Examine a patient with an ocular injury

Chapter 11: ENT conditions

- Perform otoscopy and make a clinical diagnosis in a child or adult

Chapter 12: Maxillofacial emergencies

- Assault with facial injuries – examination
- Facial fractures examination

Chapter 13: Obstetrics and gynaecology

- 15-year-old girl requesting 'morning-after' emergency contraceptive pill
- Bimanual pelvic examination in female patient
- Management of a lost/split condom in a female
- Pelvic inflammatory disease history (sexual history)

Chapter 14: Respiratory emergencies

- Haemoptysis – take a history
- Mild asthma management and demonstration of inhaler technique
- Respiratory system examination and management of a patient with chronic obstructive pulmonary disease (COPD)

Chapter 15: Cardiological emergencies

- Assessment and management of chest pain (history consistent with acute myocardial infarction)
- Cardiovascular examination
- Interpretation of an ECG
- Teach a student how to interpret an ECG
- Full cardiovascular examination and clinical diagnosis

Chapter 16: Neurological emergencies

- Acute onset of severe headache
- Cranial nerve examination for new-onset left-sided weakness
- Assessment of a patient presenting with foot drop
- History and management of subarachnoid haemorrhage
- Perform a mental state examination
- Patient presenting with sciatica – examination of lower back and appropriate neurological testing
- Traumatic neck pain – examine peripheral neurology and give management plan

Chapter 18: Toxicological emergencies

- History and management of a patient with acute confusion (recreational drugs)
- Management of deliberate overdose of paracetamol

Chapter 19: Renal emergencies

- Renal colic – take a history

Chapter 20: Endocrine emergencies

- Explain diabetes to a patient
- Thyroid examination and endocrine assessment
- Take a history of a patient with thyrotoxicosis

Chapter 22: Infectious diseases

- Needlestick injury involving a 'high-risk' patient
- Needlestick injury involving a 'low-risk' patient

Chapter 23: Dermatology

- Scabies – diagnosis and management

Chapter 24: Oncological emergencies

- Terminal illness – discussion and management with the family

Chapter 25: Rheumatological emergencies

- Acute painful and hot knee joint (history and clinical diagnosis)

Chapter 26: Paediatrics

- Advanced paediatric life support (APLS) scenario – 18-month-old child with supraventricular tachycardia
- APLS scenario – meningococcal septicaemia
- APLS scenario – obstructed airway
- APLS scenario – trauma
- Limping child – take an appropriate history
- Non-accidental history (communication)
- Explain inhaler technique to a parent

Chapter 27: Psychiatric emergencies

- Acute confusional state
- Assessment of suicide risk (and appropriate referral/follow-up plan)
- Psychiatric history and mental state assessment
- History from a confused patient and further management decisions
- History from a manic patient

Chapter 30: Communication skills

- Communication – investigate polypharmacy in an elderly man
- Communication – no neurosurgical intervention recommended for a comatose patient
- Communication – the orthopaedic registrar refuses to see a patient with a cervical spine injury
- Communication – unwell patient with advanced cancer and ascites refusing further treatment
- Communication (to the patient's relative) – withdrawal of treatment
- Counsel a patient with missed fracture, recalled by letter (the patient may be very angry)

- Counselling parent – reasons for not prescribing antibiotics for upper respiratory tract infection (URTI) in a 3-year-old
- Refusal of blood transfusion – Jehovah's Witness (consent issue)
- *N*-Acetylcysteine in a paracetamol overdose – explain indications and its action to a nurse

Chapter 31: Practical skills for the emergency department

- Aspiration of simple pneumothorax
- Femoral nerve block
- Insertion of an internal jugular central venous catheter
- Insertion of urinary catheter for acute urinary retention
- Intraosseous needle insertion in a young child
- Safely secure a correctly inserted chest drain (and appropriate advice to ward staff)
- Spontaneous pneumothorax and method of chest drain insertion

Chapter 32: Management skills

- Clinical decision unit patient selection and management plans – paper exercise
- Performing a clinical board round
- Triage process and methodology

Acknowledgement

We would like to acknowledge Paul Hunt for his permission to reproduce these past OSCE scenarios from the MCEM website.

USEFUL WEBLINKS

- College of Emergency Medicine website: www.collemergencymed.ac.uk
- MCEM website: www.mcem.org.uk

2
Resuscitation
CHETAN R TRIVEDY AND RUSSELL BARBER

CORE TOPICS

- Airway management
- Cardiac arrest/peri-arrest
- Shock
- Coma

Resuscitation is clearly an important topic as far as the practice of emergency medicine and the CEM examinations is concerned. There are likely to be a number of advanced life support (ALS), advanced paediatric life support (APLS) and advanced trauma life support (ATLS) scenarios in the examination.

To cover the whole breadth of potential scenarios is outside the scope of this book, and you are strongly advised to be familiar with the latest resuscitation guidelines. It is also useful to speak to your local resuscitation training officer regarding training before the OSCE.

The scenarios presented in this chapter will attempt to highlight some of the approaches to tackling a resuscitation-type OSCE.

SCENARIO 2.1: MAINTAINING AN AIRWAY

A 20-year-old woman known to have epilepsy has been brought into the resuscitation department following a prolonged seizure. She has been given 10 mg of diazepam rectally.

Initial observations are:

BP 116/78 mmHg
Pulse 90 bpm regular
Pulse oximetry 94% on 15 L of O_2 via a non-rebreath mask
Temperature 38.1 °C
GCS 9

Using the manikin provided, demonstrate how you would initially manage this patient. You will be assessed predominantly on your airway skills, although you will not be expected to perform endotracheal intubation. You have an ALS-trained nurse to assist you.

SUGGESTED APPROACH

When there is time for preparation, effort should be made to assemble and utilize the available staff and subspecialties. You should ask for the emergency airway trolley, and all equipment should be checked and drugs prepared. In this scenario, an ALS-trained nurse is available. Do not fail to delegate tasks appropriately. Likewise remember to gather information from the ambulance crew.

The airway is the first step in every primary survey within the hospital setting, and this essential skill should be well rehearsed and fluent.

The mnemonic 'HATS' is a useful guide to prioritize the methods used to secure the airway; you should move down the list sequentially:

Hands (jaw thrust/chin lift)
Airway adjuncts (oropharyngeal/nasopharyngeal airway)
Tracheal intubation (gold standard)
Surgical airway (failed intubation)

Step 1: Examination of the oropharynx (with clearance if necessary)

Look into the oropharynx to reveal any removable obstruction such as vomitus, blood clot or food bolus. The airway should be cleared by suctioning vomitus from the airway using wall-mounted suction, a wide-bore catheter and direct vision. Magill's forceps can be employed to remove large food boluses; however, the finger sweep is not recommended, since it may further compromise the airway through trauma or by compaction of any foreign body, not to mention the risk of entrapping your fingers between clenched teeth! It is important to bear in mind that opening the airway before clearing it can lead to migration of contaminants further along the respiratory tract. Each manoeuvre should be followed by reevaluation for evidence of improved airway patency.

Step 2: Assessment of the degree of airway patency

Assess the degree of airway patency by listening for signs of airway obstruction and feeling for expiration against the side of your cheek. These can be done simultaneously.

Obstruction may be partial or complete and may arise from either the upper or lower airway (Table 2.1). In an unconscious or postictal patient, such as in this scenario, obstruction is most likely to arise from the pharynx. As a result of loss of muscle tone, and exacerbated by the supine position, the tongue and jaw slide backwards, obstructing the airway at the level of the pharynx.

Step 3: Manual airway opening (and application of oxygen)

The simplest and most readily available equipment to open an obstructed upper airway is your hands. Either a head-tilt chin lift or jaw thrust manoeuvre can be employed instantly. A head-tilt chin lift should be avoided in cases of C-spine injury.

After every intervention, the airway should be re-evaluated. In most cases, such manoeuvres will improve or at least convert a complete obstruction to a partial obstruction.

Step 4: Manual airway opening using simple adjuncts

Initial techniques may not be effective. In such cases, an oropharyngeal airway or nasopharyngeal tube should be inserted (Figures 2.1 and 2.2). In this scenario, where the patient is at risk of further seizures and clenching their teeth, a nasopharyngeal tube may be more appropriate. It is less likely to be expelled during moments of improved GCS and is well tolerated even in the awake patient. Placement of an oropharyngeal airway in a patient with an intact gag reflex may induce vomiting.

Table 2.1 Partial and complete airway obstruction

Examination	Partial	Complete
'Looking at the chest'	Respiratory excursion of the chest	Paradoxical ('see-saw') movement of the chest and abdomen
		Indrawing at the chest and neck due to negative pressure distal to the obstruction
'Listening'	Stridor	Silent
	Snoring (pharyngeal occlusion by the soft palate or tongue)	Silent
	Gurgling	Silent
'Feeling'	Movement of respiratory gases felt on expiration	No movement of respiratory gases felt

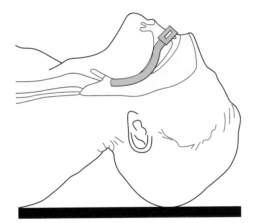

Figure 2.1 Oropharyngeal airway.

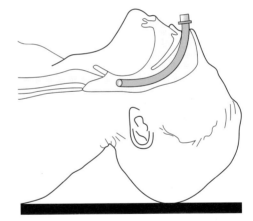

Figure 2.2 Nasopharyngeal airway.

The oropharyngeal airway is sized by estimating the distance from the upper central incisors to the angle of the jaw. In adults, it is inserted upside down into the roof of the mouth. It is rotated through 180° around the back of the tongue, following the curvature of the palate until the flange is in line with the anterior aspect of the teeth.

The size of the nasopharyngeal tube can be estimated as the diameter of the patient's little finger; however, this may be unreliable, and as a rule a size of 6–7 mm is suitable for most adults. A safety pin is placed through the flange to prevent unwanted proximal migration along the nasopharynx. Lubrication of the tube aids insertion, which should be through a patent nasal orifice. The tube is guided bevel end down along the floor of the nose. Gentle rotation of the tube is often useful. A correctly sized nasopharyngeal tube is less likely to stimulate vomiting. Airway patency should then be re-evaluated following insertion.

Step 5: Left lateral position

Utilization of the left lateral position aids in expelling vomit and secretions, as well as facilitating airway patency and maintenance. If active vomiting occurs, the bed can also be positioned head down to further prevent bronchial aspiration.

It is important to note that, although the simple airway manoeuvres and adjuncts described above can maintain the airway, they do not protect it – the ultimate means for doing this is a cuffed endotracheal tube passed beyond the vocal cords.

Although this OSCE has been designed to test your ability to manage a compromised airway, you would continue with your evaluation of breathing, circulation and disability. Complete the station by suggesting further investigations into the aetiology of seizures, and transfer for imaging or to a more appropriate place.

If the patient needs to be transferred for a CT scan of the head, they may need to be electively intubated to protect the airway while they are supine and isolated within the scanner. Likewise, intubation is needed if the patient's condition deteriorates or there is inadequate ventilation or oxygenation, and you should ask for anaesthetic back-up in the event that rapid sequence induction (RSI) becomes necessary.

It is worth mentioning the role of a laryngeal mask airway (LMA) in airway management. Although this is an option, it is of limited use in this scenario. While an LMA causes less stomach insufflation compared with a bag–valve mask, it provides no protection from aspiration and may direct vomit from the oesophagus into the airway. Successful placement is unlikely in this patient with some pharyngeal tone, and attempting to place an LMA in the presence of an intact gag reflex will provoke vomiting.

Scoring Scenario 2.1: Maintaining an airway

	Inadequate/ not done	Adequate	Good
Carries out an equipment check and asks for the airway trolley	0	1	2
Delegates roles	0	1	—

Makes a rapid assessment of the airway:
 1. Looks into the orpharynx:
   • removes foreign body or vomitus lying in the airway
 2. Listens for signs of partial or complete obstruction:
   • stridor
   • snoring
   • gurgling
   • movement of air
 3. Looks at the chest for:
   • paradoxical chest excursion
   • indrawing of the chest
	0	1	2

Immediate management (can ask assistant): 1. Places the patient on high-flow oxygen 2. Suctions airway 3. Organizes monitoring (ECG, oximetry and blood pressure) 4. Secures IV access and takes bloods 5. Draw up 2–4 mg of IV lorazepam 6. Sets up airway trolley	0	1	2
Places patient in left lateral position with or without head-down tilt	0	1	—
Demonstrates jaw thrust	0	1	2
Demonstrates chin lift	0	1	2
Correctly sizes and demonstrates the insertion of an oropharyngeal airway	0	1	—
Correctly sizes and demonstrates the insertion of a nasopharyngeal airway (being aware of contraindications)	0	1	—
Demonstrates the bag-and-valve mask technique (one- or two-handed technique)	0	1	2
Discusses use of LMA	0	1	—
Calls for anaesthetic back-up for RSI if airway deteriorates	0	1	—
Reassesses the airway for signs of obstruction	0	1	2
Global score from examiner	/5		
Total score	/25		

SCENARIO 2.2: EMERGENCY INTUBATION

A 68-year-old man is blue-lighted to the emergency department after having collapsed in the street. He is making a poor respiratory effort. He is currently being oxygenated via a bag–valve mask with an oropharyngeal airway in situ. His observations recorded by the ambulance crew are:

BP 80/60 mmHg
Pulse 120 bpm
Oxygen saturation is unrecordable on 15 L of O_2, and he is cyanosed
He has a GCS of 6

Make an assessment of this patient's airway and demonstrate how you would perform an endotracheal intubation on the manikin. You have an ALS-trained nurse to assist you.

SUGGESTED APPROACH

The situation that you are presented with – a patient with a GCS of 6 who is being oxygenated with a bag–valve mask and has undetectable saturations on 15 L of O_2 – is suggestive of imminent full respiratory arrest. You should identify this and call for help (invariably in the examination, the anaesthetist will be unavailable). Ask the nurse to apply monitoring.

Do not assume that the airway is patent because there is an oropharyngeal airway already in situ and ongoing bag–valve ventilation. Assess the airway for obstruction, confirm that the oropharyngeal airway is the appropriate size, and confirm successful ventilation with bag–valve ventilation (a two-person technique may be needed). The use of an LMA is an option. In this scenario, the bag–valve mask continues to be inadequate and intubation should be considered. Ventilation should continue, since some degree of oxygenation may be occurring while you prepare for intubation, but you should be aware of gastric insufflation.

Equipment

- Size 3 or 4 Macintosh laryngoscope (curved blade)
- Cuffed endotracheal tubes (sizes 7 and 8)
- Wide-bore suction and tilting bed
- 10 mL syringe for inflating the cuff
- Gum elastic bougie and stylet
- Aqueous gel lubricant
- Pillow
- Magill's forceps
- Ribbon or tape to secure the endotracheal (ET) tube
- Colorimetric end-tidal CO_2 monitor
- Anaesthetic drugs
- Emergency drugs (adrenaline and atropine)
- Difficult-airway set

Before you commence intubation, you should already have a back-up plan (plan B) in the event that you cannot intubate and cannot ventilate the patient. It is crucial that your team members be aware of this plan and so can prepare accordingly.

The three major situations encountered in the emergency department are:

1. A rapid sequence induction (RSI) where the patient is awake and unstarved (a full stomach). Measures are made to reduce the risk of aspiration, with a minimum delay between the patient being awake and asleep with cuffed tube in trachea.
2. Intubation where the patient is obtunded or is suspended. In these circumstances, the patient will not need to be sedated or paralysed.
3. Failed intubation where the patient cannot be ventilated or intubated.

The emergency intubation

It is worth being aware of the '10 Ps' of ET intubation before you plan your procedure:

1. **P**reparation
2. **P**lan for failure (failed intubation drill)
3. **P**ositioning the head
4. **P**re-oxygenation
5. **P**re-treatment
6. **P**rotection from aspiration (cricoid pressure)
7. **P**aralysis with induction
8. **P**lacement of the ET tube
9. **P**roof of correct ET tube placement
10. **P**ost-intubation placement

Preparation

It is essential that you have the right equipment and staff for the planned procedure. You should:

- Have a back-up plan if you run into difficulties.
- Have the patient on full monitoring (ECG/BP/pulse oximetry).
- Check all of the equipment (suction/laryngoscope/ET tube cuff).
- Ensure that there is intravenous access and the cannula is patent.
- Ensure that the emergency drugs are drawn up and labelled.
- Ensure that you have a trained assistant.

Plan for failure

The importance of having a back-up plan in the event that you cannot intubate the patient cannot be overstressed. If you are not comfortable in executing your back-up plans B, C or even D then you should really question whether you are the right person to be intubating the patient.

The failed-airway algorithm according to the Difficult Airway Society guidelines is shown in Figure 2.3. This algorithm is primarily intended for anaesthetists performing elective intubation, but suitably adopted it is also a useful drill for managing a difficult airway in the emergency department.

Positioning the head

The goal of positioning the head is to have the oral, pharyngeal and laryngeal inlets positioned in a straight line facilitating direct laryngoscopy. The ideal position is achieved by placing a pillow under the patient's head and extending the head on the neck in a 'sniffing the morning air' position (Figure 2.4). This is the optimum position for intubation; however, a neutral position and in-line immobilization must be maintained when you suspect a C-spine injury.

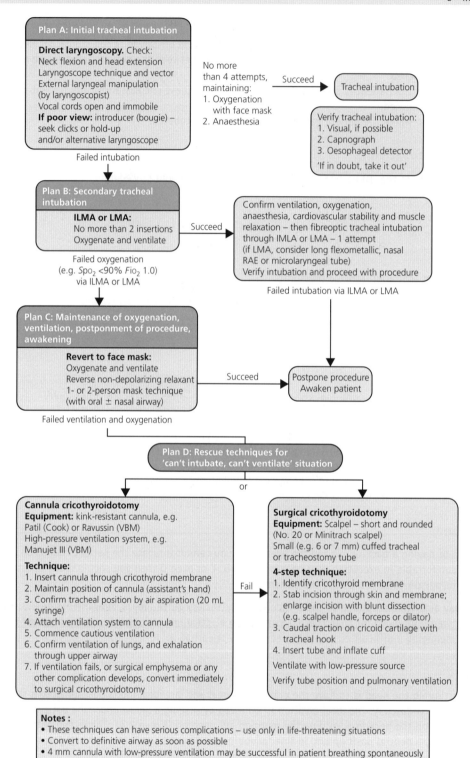

Figure 2.3 Failed-airway algorithm. LMA, laryngeal mask airway; ILMA, intubating LMA.

Reproduced with kind permission from Difficult Airway Society. *Difficult Airway Society Guidelines. Strategy for intubation by direct laryngoscopy, no predicted airway problem, no risk of regurgitation*. Reading: Difficult Airway Society, 2004 and Difficult Airway Society. *Failed Ventilation*. Reading: Difficult Airway Society, 2004.

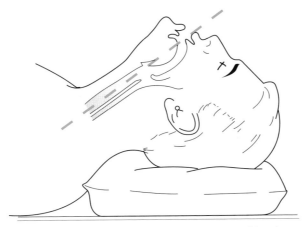

Figure 2.4 'Sniffing the morning air' position of head.

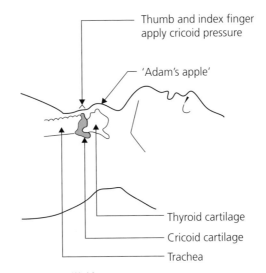

Figure 2.5 Sellick's manoeuvre.

Pre-oxygenation

Pre-oxygenation is performed with the patient breathing 100% oxygen through a tight-fitting non-rebreathing facemask for 3 minutes. This allows replacement of nitrogen-containing air with oxygen, and acts as an oxygen reservoir delaying the onset of hypoxia in cases of prolonged apnoea or difficult intubation. After each failed attempt at intubation, the patient should be pre-oxygenated.

In this scenario, pre-oxygenation is not possible, since there is failure to oxygenate despite mechanical ventilation.

Pre-treatment

Some situations require medications to attenuate the hypertensive response to larygnoscopy:

- lidocaine 1.5 mg kg^{-1}
- opioids (e.g. fentanyl or alfentanil)

These are not normally given in a crash induction, where the priority is securing the airway quickly and safely.

Protection of the airway

Protection of the airway from aspiration of gastric contents is only achieved when a tube is positioned within the trachea, with no leakage of air around the cuff. However, before the tube can be placed within the trachea, cricoid pressure must be applied to reduce the occurrence of passive regurgitation. Cricoid pressure (Sellick's manoeuvre, Figure 2.5) should be applied by a trained assistant using anteroposterior pressure on the cricoid cartilage at the onset of induction. The full 44 newtons of force should be applied when neuromuscular blocking agents are administered or when the patient is obtunded.

The complete circumferential ring of the cricoid compresses the lumen of the oesophagus against the sixth cervical vertebra. It does not prevent active vomiting, and continued application in such circumstances can result in oesophageal rupture. This is the only situation in which it should be released prematurely, and the bed tilted head down with the patient on the left lateral position to reduce aspiration. Otherwise, the cricoid should only be released after confirmed correct tube placement and adequate cuff inflation.

Paralysis with induction

- Only those trained in RSI and who routinely perform these techniques should administer muscle relaxants and anaesthetic agents, owing to contraindications and adverse complications associated with their use in the emergency setting.
- Give an appropriate intravenous induction agent: thiopental or propofol. These both cause hypnosis and amnesia.
- To ease laryngeal intubation, high-speed muscle relaxation is important. The drug of choice in most circumstances is suxamethonium, although you should be aware of its contraindications. Suxamethonium is a depolarizing muscle relaxant and causes muscle fasciculation before muscle relaxation.

Placement of the ET tube

You will be asked to demonstrate this on the manikin.

- Stand behind the patient.
- Hold the laryngoscope with your left hand and insert it into the mouth over the right side of the tongue.
- Sweep the tongue from right to left and push it upwards so that the tip of the epiglottis comes into view.
- Make sure that you do not use the teeth as a fulcrum and that the lower lip does not get caught between the blade of the laryngoscope and the teeth.
- Advance the tip of the laryngoscope into the valecula between the epiglottis and the tongue.
- To visualize the vocal cords, lift the contents of the oropharynx by moving the laryngoscope along the central axis of the handle.
- If you have a good view of the cords, you should insert the ET tube with your right hand so that it passes between the vocal cords into the trachea, ensuring that the cuff has passed beyond the vocal cords.
- In most adults, the tube will usually lie between 22 and 24 cm at the level of the incisors.
- Stabilize the tube until it is taped or tied in place.
- Connect the tube via a catheter mount and ventilate the patient with 12–15 L of oxygen.
- The cuff should be inflated until no audible leak of ventilation gases is heard to pass around the cuff.

Proof of correct ET tube placement

It is imperative that you ensure that the ET tube is in the correct place and at the correct depth, by (in chronological order):

- direct visualization of the tube passing through the cords
- compliance of the reservoir bag on manual ventilation and fogging of the tube
- symmetrical expansion of the chest wall
- auscultation of the chest bilaterally for breath sounds and auscultation over the epigastrium to exclude oesophageal intubation
- attachment of an end-tidal CO_2 monitor (capnograph or calometric)
- obtaining a chest X-ray to ensure placement of the tube above the carina and below the level of the cords

Complications

- Aspiration of gastric content – the risk is higher if:
  - there has been recent ingestion
  - gastric emptying is delayed secondary to trauma, pain, diabetes or opioids
  - the lower oesophageal sphincter is incompetent owing to obesity, pregnancy or hiatus hernia
  - the patient has been manually ventilated for a long time before performing the RSI, since this inflates the stomach
  - the appropriate cricoid pressure has not been applied
- Inability to intubate, exacerbated by trauma from repeated attempted intubations.
- Intubation of the oesophagus.
- Dislodgement of the tube.
- Bronchial intubation: commonly a tube inserted too far will occlude the right upper main bronchus, resulting in collapse of the lung section. If placed further, the entire left main bronchus may not be ventilated, leading to collapse of the lung and a higher risk of pneumothorax.
- Tracheal stenosis – prolonged intubation, especially with an inflated cuff, and more common in children who have soft, more easily damaged tracheas.
- Severe hypoxia if prolonged attempts are undertaken.
- Chipping, loosening or dislodgement of teeth.

Post tube placement

The tube should be secured and the level at the central incisors noted in case of tube migration. The patient should be carefully monitored, and, once they have been stabilized, a portable chest X-ray should be performed to ensure that the main bronchus has not been inadvertently intubated.

The above description should allow you deal with an OSCE scenario where you are asked to secure an airway in the emergency department.

Scoring Scenario 2.2: Emergency intubation

	Inadequate/ not done	Adequate	Good
Appropriate induction	0	1	—
Assigns roles to team members	0	1	—
Asks for the airway trolley to be set up	0	1	—
Appreciates that patient is in extremis and asks for the on-call anaesthetist	0	1	—

Makes a rapid assessment of the airway:
1. Looks for:
    • foreign body in the airway
    • central cyanosis
    • paradoxical chest excursion
2. Listens for signs of obstruction
3. Auscultates chest bilaterally
4. Checks chest expansion
	0	1	2

Asks for an experienced assistant	0	1	—
Immediate management (can ask assistant): 1. Places patient on high-flow oxygen 2. Suctions airway 3. Sets up monitoring (cardiac/sats probe and BP) 4. Secures IV access and takes bloods; checks blood sugar 5. Sets up airway trolley 6. Prepares difficult airway kit (LMA/surgical airway)	0	1	2
Checks equipment (laryngoscope/suction/ET tube)	0	1	—
Positions patient's head appropriately, 'sniffing the morning air' (pillow under head)	0	1	—
Holds the laryngoscope correctly with the left hand	0	1	—
Suctions airway	0	1	—
Avoids trauma to lips and teeth	0	1	—
Mentions use of bougie or stylet if the vocal cords are difficult to visualize	0	1	—
Places ET tube correctly beyond the vocal cords (22–24 cm at the level of the anterior teeth)	0	1	—
Inflates the cuff with air	0	1	—
Checks position of the ET tube (needs 3/5): 1. Equal chest expansion during ventilation 2. Auscultates the chest bilaterally 3. Fogging of the ET tube 4. CO_2 capnography 5. Chest X-ray	0	1	2
Discusses failed intubation drill (senior help/LMA/intubating LMA (ILMA)/ surgical airway) if unsuccessful	0	1	2
Global score from examiner	**/5**		
Total score	**/26**		

SCENARIO 2.3: CARDIAC ARREST

A 30-year-old man is brought to the emergency department with a displaced fracture of his left femur following a motor vehicle collision. Your consultant has just performed a femoral nerve block with bupivicaine to ease the pain. As you are writing up your notes, you notice that the patient has become unconscious. Your F2 and ALS-trained nurse are at hand to assist you.

Manage the resuscitation of this patient.

SUGGESTED APPROACH

This OSCE tests your ability to effectively run a cardiac arrest. The following may have contributed to the arrest:

- hypovolaemia (splenic tear or fractured pelvis)
- fat embolism arising as a result of the fractured femur
- cardiac tamponade following blunt chest trauma
- bupivicaine toxicity
- anaphylactic reaction to the local anaesthetic

It is essential that you be aware of the latest ALS resuscitation guidelines; these are available on the Resuscitation Council (UK) website (www.resus.org.uk/pages/mediMain.htm).

- After checking that it is safe to approach, you should check if the patient is responsive by employing the shake-and-shout regime: gently shake the patient by the shoulders and ask loudly if they are OK.
- If there is no response, shout for help and put the patient on their back.
- At the same time, open the airway and look for the presence of any foreign bodies.
- You should spend no more than 10 seconds looking, listening and feeling for any signs of life:
    - Look for chest wall movement.
    - Listen for breathing.
    - Feel for air on your cheek.
    - The carotid pulse can be checked at the same time as the chin lift manoeuvre.

If there is no sign of life, you should start cardiopulmonary resuscitation (CPR) immediately. Ask one of your team to put out a crash call by dialling 2222 and clearly indicating to the operator that you would like an adult cardiac arrest team to your location. However, some emergency departments have a policy of managing their own arrest calls and you should be aware of your local policy.

Ask your nurse to start CPR with 30 chest compressions followed by 2 breaths. The chest compressions should be carried out by placing your hands on the lower half of the sternum in the midline. You should aim at a rate of 100 compressions a minute and compress the chest by 4–5 cm.

Meanwhile you should insert an oropharyngeal airway and ventilate, ideally with a bag–valve mask and 100% oxygen. You should ask for an intubation trolley to be set up as soon as help arrives so that the airway can be secured.

While CPR is in progress, ask one of your team to attach the defibrillator pads to the chest and if possible secure a large-bore intravenous cannula. The standard positions for the placement of the pads are as follows:

- One pad is placed under the right clavicle on the chest and the second is placed at the site of the left mid-axillary line at the level of the fifth intercostal space.
- Alternatively the pads can be placed in an anteroposterior position over the left precordium and on the back just below the left scapula.

Bloods should be taken:

- full blood count (FBC)
- urea and electrolytes (U&E)
- bone profile
- coagulation screen
- glucose
- group and save

An arterial blood gas (ABG) is also useful in the immediate assessment of any electrolyte and metabolic disturbances. This should not interfere with CPR.

After the defibrillator pads have been attached to the chest, pause momentarily to check the rhythm, which can be either shockable or non-shockable:

shockable:
- ventricular fibrillation (VF) (Figure 2.6)
- ventricular tachycardia (VT) (Figure 2.7)
- pulseless VT
- torsades de pointes

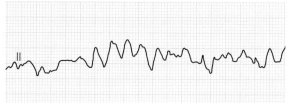

Figure 2.6 Ventricular fibrillation.

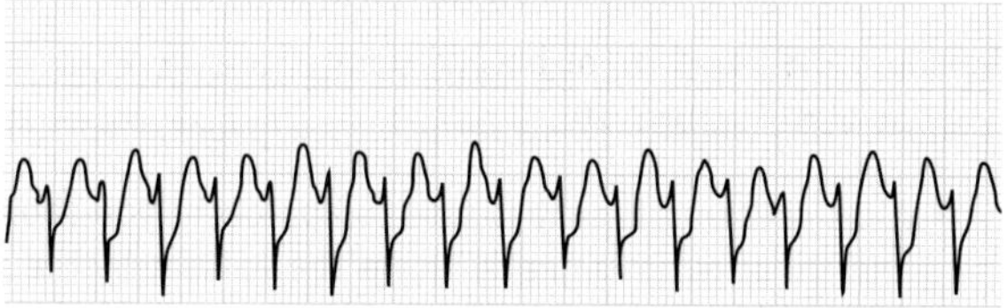

Figure 2.7 Ventricular tachycardia.

non-shockable:
- asystole (Figure 2.8)
- pulseless electrical activity (PEA) (Figure 2.9)

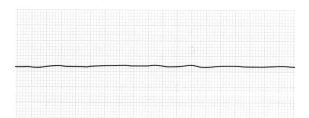

Figure 2.8 Asystole.

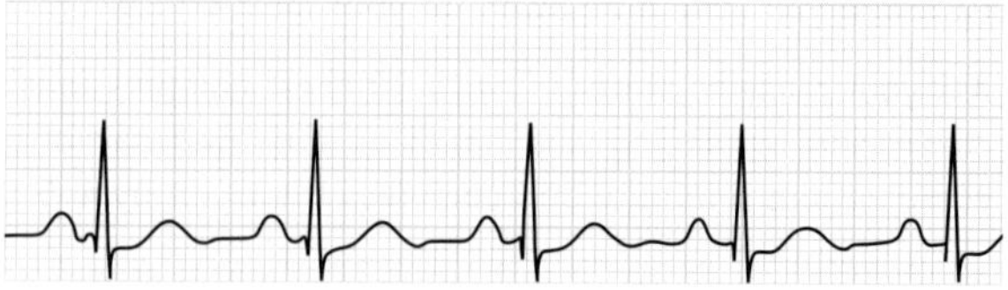

Figure 2.9 Pulseless electrical activity.

Shockable rhythms

As the name suggests, these rhythms may respond to electrical cardioversion, and successful defibrillation is defined as termination of the rhythm 5 seconds after delivery of the shock, accompanied by the return of spontaneous circulation.

As soon as you confirm a shockable rhythm on the monitor, you should give a single shock of 150–360 J biphasic (360 J monophasic). You should then resume chest compressions without checking the pulse or rhythm and continue CPR for another 2 minutes before checking the monitor. The first dose of adrenaline is given after you have diagnosed a shockable rhythm and just before the third shock. It is important to remember the sequence:
1. Drug
2. Shock
3. CPR
4. Check rhythm.

You will be assessed on your ability to defibrillate safely, and so you should know how to use the defibrillator and know the safety precautions:

- Ensure that your team know that you are going to shock the patient.
- Ask the oxygen to be moved away from the patient and ask everyone to stand well clear from the patient and the trolley **(WARNING 1)**.
- After selecting the energy level, you should warn those around you that you are **'Charging!' (WARNING 2)** as you charge the machine.
- Make a concerted effort to look around you to make sure that the field is clear and even say 'Top clear', 'Bottom clear', 'I'm clear', **'Shocking!' (WARNING 3)** just before you deliver the shock.
- As soon you have delivered the shock, commence CPR immediately (30 : 2) without looking for the monitor or feeling for a pulse.

The adult ALS protocol for both shockable and non-shockable rhythms from the Resuscitation Council (UK) is reproduced in Figure 2.10.

Non-shockable rhythms

These rhythms are managed with a combination of CPR and pharmacological agents. Give 1 mg of adrenaline (10 mL of 1:10 000 adrenaline solution) as soon as you have confirmed the rhythm and you have secured intravenous access.

Complete 2 minutes of CPR and then check the rhythm. If there is no change in the rhythm, commence the second cycle of CPR. Give 1 mg of adrenaline at the end of the second cycle; adrenaline should continue to be given every 3–5 minutes, assuming that there is no change in the rhythm. CPR should be continued until the airway is secured, following which you should perform continuous compressions.

If you are confronted with a non-shockable arrest, you must exclude reversible causes, which include the following ('4H and 4T'):

- **H**ypovolaemia
- **H**ypoxia
- **H**ypothermia
- **H**ypo/hyperkalaemia (metabolic disturbances)

- **T**hromboembolism
- **T**amponade
- **T**oxins
- **T**ension pneumothorax

If the patient is in asystole, check the gain function on the defibrillator followed by the leads to ensure that the trace is not a result of an artefact; also look carefully for P waves, since this may be ventricular standstill, which may respond to cardiac pacing.

Furthermore, if the patient goes into VF while you are in the middle of a compression, do not stop to defibrillate – finish the cycle and prepare to defibrillate as described.

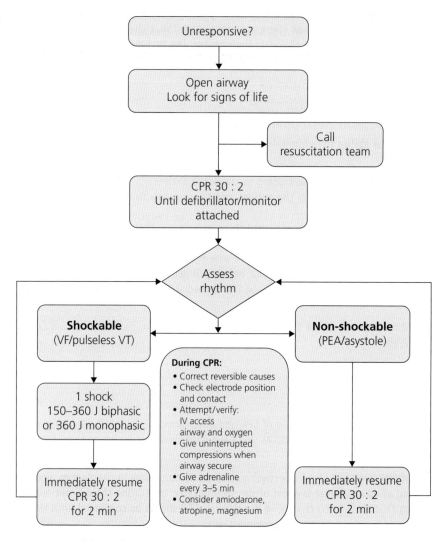

Figure 2.10 Adult advanced life support protocol.

Reproduced with kind permission from Resuscitation Council (UK). *Algorithms in Resuscitation Guidelines 2005*. London: Resuscitation Council (UK), 2005.

Special circumstances

You may be asked to resuscitate a patient under special circumstances where the resuscitation protocol may have to be amended. There will usually be a clue in the history, and you should read the details of the scenario carefully.

In this case, you are told that the patient has just been given a femoral nerve block with bupivicaine, which is a potentially cardiotoxic local anaesthetic agent. An overdose of local anaesthetic or intravascular injection may precipitate cardiac arrest.

The Association of Anaesthetists of Great Britain and Ireland (AGBI) guidelines for the management of severe local anaesthetic toxicity (available at: www.aagbi.org/publications/guidelines.htm) suggest that:

- Prolonged resuscitation may be required, since treatment of local-anaesthetic-induced cardiac arrest may take more than 1 hour.
- Cardiopulmonary bypass should be considered.
- Arrhythmias may be very refractory to treatment.

As local anaesthetics are lipophilic, the guidelines suggest treatment with lipid emulsion (20% Intralipid). This should be given initially as a bolus of 1.5 mL kg^{-1} over 1 minute and then continued as an infusion of 0.25 mL kg^{-1} min^{-1} over 20 minutes. Further doses should be given if output has not returned.

The guidelines also suggest that Intralipid should be available whenever procedures involving potentially cardiotoxic doses of local anaesthetic are performed.

Other arrest scenarios with special circumstances that you should be aware of are summarized in Table 2.2.

Table 2.2 Cardiac arrest scenarios with special circumstances

Special circumstance	Modification in ALS protocol in a cardiac arrest
Hyperkalaemia	• Treat the hyperkalaemia with 10 mL of 10% calcium chloride • 50 mmol of sodium bicarbonate • 50 mL of 50% glucose and 10 units of short-acting insulin • Haemodialysis
Hypokalaemia	• Replace potassium (2 mmol min^{-1} over 10 min, followed by 10 mmol min^{-1} over 10 min)
Hypercalcaemia	• Fluid replacement • Diuresis with furosemide 1 mg kg^{-1} • Haemodialysis
Hypocalcaemia	• 10–40 mL of 10% calcium chloride
Opioid overdose	• Naloxone 400–800 mg IV or 1–2 mg via the ET tube
Tricyclic antidepressant overdose	• Sodium bicarbonate or hypertonic saline
Hypothermia	• Active warming • Withhold adrenaline until core temperature > 30 °C. Double the time interval between doses in the temperature range 30–35 °C. Follow the normal protocol once temperature > 35 °C • Arrhythmias may not respond to shocks until core temperature > 30 °C • Consider cardiopulmonary bypass • Consider prolonged resuscitation until core temperature > 30 °C
Penetrating chest trauma	• Resuscitative thoracotomy may be performed following penetrating trauma if it can be done within 10 min of loss of cardiac output • The success rates for blunt trauma are poor, and thoracotomy can attempted if the patient arrests in the emergency department following blunt trauma to the chest
Pregnancy	• Tilt the patient on her left side by 15° • Ask for an urgent obstetric opinion and consider performing an emergency caesarean section. This should only considered if the fetus is believed to be viable

Scoring Scenario 2.3: Cardiac arrest

	Inadequate/ not done	Adequate	Good
Safe approach	0	1	—
Confirms cardiac arrest: 1. Shake and shout 2. Shouts for help 3. Performs chin lift 4. Assesses airway 5. Checks airway (10 s) and pulse simultaneously	0	1	2
Confirms cardiac arrest and calls crash team; knows number 2222	0	1	—
Starts CPR with 30 : 2; demonstrates correct landmarks for compressions as well as correct rate and depth	0	1	2
Uses airway adjunct and bag–valve mask to ventilate patient	0	1	—
Asks for cardiac, oxygen monitoring	0	1	—
Ask for defibrillator pads to be attached to the chest; demonstrates position	0	1	—
Asks assistant to secure IV access and take bloods and an ABG (does not interrupt CPR)	0	1	—
Correctly identifies rhythm: either VF or VT	0	1	—
Excludes the reversible causes ('4H and 4T')	0	1	2
Follows shockable rhythm algorithm	0	1	2
Defibrillation with single shock (150–200 J) with biphasic machine; must demonstrate safe technique	0	1	2
Continues chest compressions instantly	0	1	—
Reviews monitor after 2 min of CPR; if still in VF/VT gives second shock (150–360 J)	0	1	—
Gives adrenaline before third shock and then on alternate cycles (drug–shock–CPR–check)	0	1	2
Is aware that local anaesthetic toxicity may be responsible for cardiac arrest	0	1	—
Suggests prolonged resuscitation Use of Intralipid Cardiopulmonary bypass	0	1	2
Confirms return of output	0	1	—
Arranges for ITU review	0	1	—
Plans post-resuscitation care: 1. Intubation 2. Bedside echocardiography 3. Central venous catheter 4. Arterial line 5. Hypothermic resuscitation	0	1	2
Runs resuscitation effectively, engaging team members	0	1	2
Global score from examiner	**/5**		
Total score	**/35**		

SCENARIO 2.4: HEAD INJURY

You are asked to attend a trauma call. A 30-year-old unrestrained passenger has been ejected from a motor vehicle involved in a head-on collision. He is brought in by a paramedic crew; he is intubated and ventilated and his C-spine is immobilized. He has obvious facial lacerations and a frontal haematoma.

His observations are:

BP 85/50 mmHg
Pulse 95 bpm
Saturation 96% on 100% oxygen
GCS E1 M3 V1
Temperature 37.6 °C
Pupils are equally size 3

Carry out a focused assessment of the patient and outline how you would manage him in order to optimize his cerebral perfusion. You have an ALS-trained F2 to assist you.

SUGGESTED APPROACH

This man has a serious head injury; however, this should not distract attention from any of the other major systems. Some of his management has already begun, but the approach to the patient should not deviate from the usual systematic ABCDE approach.

Aggressive management of his traumatic brain injury is essential in preventing secondary brain injury through regional or global ischaemia. This involves:

1. Maximizing blood oxygen content
2. Maintaining cerebral blood delivery (cerebral blood flow) by:
   (a) maintaining the driving mean arterial pressure (MAP)
   (b) facilitating venous drainage from the head to prevent a rise in intracranial pressure (ICP)

Assessment of the airway and C-spine and prevention of hypoxia

- Confirm tracheal intubation, since tube displacement often occurs during transfer.
- Ensure that the ET tube is sufficiently inflated to prevent gastric aspiration.
- Deliver high-flow inspired oxygen and aim for a saturation of >95% or >13 kPa.
- Secure the ET tube using tape rather than a tie. Venous drainage above the head and neck can be restricted by using a constricting ribbon tie.
- Check that the C-spine is adequately immobilized as the patient is intubated and that it cannot be clinically cleared; the patient may require suitable imaging (CT neck).

Assessment of breathing and prevention of hypoxia

- Examine the chest for any evidence of an endobronchial intubation or other chest injury such as a pneumothorax. These should be treated immediately.
- Normocapnia should be the goal in order to maintain cerebral blood flow, and you should avoid hypoventilating or hyperventilating the patient. Arterial blood gas (ABG) and capnography should be used to adjust the respiratory rate and tidal volume on the ventilator.

Assessment of circulation and maintenance of cerebral blood flow

- Hypovolaemia should be corrected and you should aim for MAP > 90 mmHg. Hypotension will significantly impair cerebral perfusion. You should avoid fluids containing glucose unless the patient is hypoglycaemic.
- Correct anaemia: you should aim for a target haemaglobin of 8–10 g dL^{-1} and a haematocrit of 0.30. This is a compromise between maximizing blood oxygen content and maintaining blood flow by reducing blood viscosity.
- Cushing's sign (raised blood pressure with bradycardia) is a poor prognostic indicator.
- Invasive monitoring should be performed using central venous access and an arterial line.

Assessment of disability and prevention of a rise in ICP

- Ideally, the bed should be tilted in a head-up position 15–30° (with the head in the neutral position) in order to facilitate venous return.
- The patient should be prevented from coughing or straining while intubated, since this will raise the ICP. This can be achieved by the use of hypnotics and analgesics, and occasionally paralysis may be helpful. Hypnotics also reduce cerebral oxygen requirements, but at the expense of MAP.
- The pupils should be assessed for size and reactivity to light. With the patient sedated, the neurological examination is often difficult.

Control the environment

- Avoid hyperthermia, since this increases the cerebral metabolic rate: for every 1 °C rise in temperature, there is a 9% increase in the metabolic rate. You should aim for a core temperature of 36 °C.
- Aim for tight glycaemic control.
- The patient should be catheterized.
- The patient should be turned regularly to prevent pressure sores.

Scoring Scenario 2.4: Head injury

	Inadequate/ not done	Adequate	Good
Puts out a trauma call	0	1	—
Checks the airway and ET tube placement and that the cuff is blown up	0	1	2
Ensures that the C-spine is immobilized and cannot be clinically cleared	0	1	2
Places patient on high-flow oxygen and full monitoring	0	1	2
Checks chest for air entry and other chest injuries: • haemothorax • pneumothorax • flail chest	0	1	2
Asks to perform an ABG to check $P\text{co}_2$ (aim for normocapnia)	0	1	—
Obtains IV access, and obtains routine bloods and checks blood sugar	0	1	2
Corrects hypotension and anaemia	0	1	—
Suggests invasive monitoring with central venous line and arterial line	0	1	2
Is aware of Cushing's sign as a poor prognostic indicator	0	1	—
Examines pupils and observes for abnormal posturing: 1. Decorticate 2. Decerebrate posture	0	1	2
Performs a detailed secondary survey	0	1	2
Suggests tilting the head of the bed up at 15–30°	0	1	—
Nurses patient at 36 °C	0	1	—
Suggests tight glycaemic control	0	1	—
Places a urinary catheter	0	1	—
Arranges for an urgent CT scan of head and C-spine	0	1	—
Asks for anaesthetic assistance for transfer to CT	0	1	—
Requests neurosurgical review for patient	0	1	—
Global score from examiner	/5		
Total score	/32		

3
Anaesthetics and Pain Relief
PETER JAYE, RUSSELL BARBER AND CHETAN R TRIVEDY

CORE TOPICS

- Pain relief
- Local anaesthetic techniques
- Concious sedation

The curriculum for this subject contains a number of topics that are amenable to testing using OSCEs. We have selected five scenarios, with accompanying reviews of the responses. These OSCEs all include more than just a pure clinical assessment; it is in these additional sections of the OSCE that the differentiating marks lie. The pass/fail distinction is often based on the scoring in these areas.

SCENARIO 3.1: ANALGESIA AND CONFLICT RESOLUTION

You have been asked to review a 39-year-old man who tripped and fell over. He has been in the department for approximately 45 minutes. The triage nurse did not feel that there was any bony injury, but asked the F2 to organize an ankle X-ray as a precaution. You have reviewed his films and have found that he has an undisplaced fracture of the fibula.

The F2 has already placed a cannula in the right antecubital fossa and there is 1 L crystalloid running over 6 hours.

The patient's pulse is 100 bpm, BP 140/90 mmHg and O_2 saturation 100% on a non-rebreath mask. His partner is upset about the time delay in dealing with his pain, and demands that he needs morphine and should be seen privately since the NHS is not managing him adequately.

Take a focused history from the patient and outline your management plan. You do not have to examine the patient.

SUGGESTED APPROACH

This OSCE neatly illustrates the assessment of clinical skills alongside the management of conflict. The clinical skills in this OSCE are those required of a good F2, but in the presence of conflict these simple skills become significantly more difficult to complete. This reflects your actual clinical practice and therefore adds validity to the use of this technique to assess performance.

Clinically, an understanding of the analgesic ladder is required, alongside alternatives to analgesics for pain relief.

The more complex aspect of this OSCE is dealing with conflict. As with many other OSCEs in this book, there are certain key attributes or behaviours that will allow the candidate to score highly. This particular scenario tests the candidate's ability to deal with an angry relative and a patient in pain, as well as the clinical aspects of pain management.

Objectives

- To deliver pain relief in a safe and effective way to this patient with a fibular fracture.
- To understand the analgesic ladder (Figure 3.1).
- To demonstrate an understanding of additional techniques such as splinting and the use of nitrous oxide in providing pain relief.
- To resolve conflict effectively in a non-judgemental way.

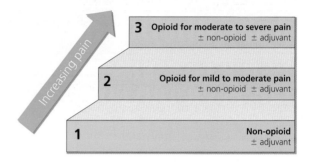

Figure 3.1 The WHO pain ladder.

Start the OSCE by trying to provide the patient with suitable analgesia, since this is the only thing that is likely to settle him so that you can get an adequate history. Make an assessment of the pain score – most patients understand the simple 0–10 scale. This should be recorded on the observation chart to assess the efficacy of the analgesia that you give.

Begin with simple analgesia, as well as adjuvant treatment measures such as splinting the leg. The patient can be given nitrous oxide/oxygen (Entonox) to facilitate splinting. You may find that this does not improve the situation and you may resort to opiates; it would not be unreasonable to give morphine. However, you should take a focused medical history to ensure that there are no contraindications for prescribing opiates. You may be pressurized by the partner, who insists that morphine be prescribed from the outset. You should try to explain to them that the patient will not be denied morphine but that you would like to try other measures to control the pain as well.

You should inform the examiner that, once the pain has eased, you would like to make a detailed assessment of the injury. Although you are not expected to examine the patient in this scenario, you should at least state your intention to do so.

It is likely that you will be met with aggression when you explain that there is a fracture on the X-ray, since the patient was told at triage that there was no fracture. It is imperative that you weather the storm and absorb their anger and frustration. The use of silence is helpful, and you should wait for the patient/partner to pause before you explain the nature of the injury and outline your management plan.

It is important that you show empathy and do not underplay the patient's symptoms. You should try to explain how different painkillers work and offer appropriate analgesia. You should also discuss adjuvant treatment, such as splinting the leg in a below-knee plaster of Paris back slab in an attempt to increase comfort.

If you manage successfully to address the patient's pain, the request for a private referral may be withdrawn. However, if it is still requested, you should offer to look into it and discuss it with the orthopaedic team on call. The key is to engage the partner as well the patient and not to be distracted by the partner's anger and insistence on intravenous opiates.

Scoring Scenario 3.1: Analgesia and conflict resolution

	Inadequate/ not done	Adequate	Good
Confirms patient's identity and introduces self	0	1	—
Confirms relative's relationship to patient	0	1	—
Confirms patient's consent to discuss case with partner	0	1	—
Makes quick assessment of injury	0	1	—
Asks about level of pain	0	1	—
Deals with patient's concerns appropriately	0	1	2
Deals with partner's concerns appropriately	0	1	2
Asks about previous medical history	0	1	—
Asks about drug history	0	1	—
Asks about allergies	0	1	—
Asks about alcohol and illicit drug use	0	1	—
Utilizes nitrous oxide	0	1	—
Utilizes splinting	0	1	—
Requests opiate analgesia	0	1	—
Gives opiate analgesia in an appropriate fashion	0	1	—
Responds appropriately to patient's requests for further pain relief	0	1	2
Deals appropriately with partner's requests for private intervention	0	1	2
Deals with conflict regarding pain relief in a non-judgemental way	0	1	2
Gives oral analgesia as follow-up	0	1	—
Provides appropriate management plan	0	1	2
Score from patient	/5		
Global score from examiner	/5		
Total score	/36		

SCENARIO 3.2 TEACHING LOCAL ANAESTHESIA

You have been asked by your consultant to describe the risks of local anaesthesia and the techniques to avoid them to a fourth-year medical student. You will not have to demonstrate any techniques.

SUGGESTED APPROACH

This is a teaching OSCE, where some of the marks are for imparting your knowledge of the adverse effects of local anaesthesia in a structured manner. You should start by ascertaining how much the student knows about local anaesthesia and whether they have seen it used before. You should then proceed to identify the objectives of your teaching session.

Objectives

- Demonstrate an understanding of the indications for the use of local anaesthesia.
- Demonstrate an understanding of the complications of local anaesthesia.
- Demonstrate an understanding of the toxicity of local anaesthetic agents (lidocaine).
- Demonstrate an understanding of the management of lidocaine toxicity.

After going through the objectives and reviewing areas that the student should know, you should complete the OSCE by proving the student with a reference or resource to do more reading on local anaesthesia and make a plan to meet up again.

You should encourage questions as you go along; you may be prompted by the student with the following questions:

- What are the indications for the use of local anaesthesia?
- Are there any complications?
- How do you treat the complications?
- What are the correct doses of the anaesthetic?
- Are they different for children?

Complications of local anaesthesia

Technique-related

- Direct nerve trauma
- Bleeding
- Haematoma
- Infection
- Intravascular injection
- Damage to surrounding structures (tendons, pneumothorax)

Drug-related

- Anaphylactoid
- Methaemoglobinuria (prilocaine)
- Toxicity by intravascular injection
- Toxicity by overdose and systemic absorption

Systemic toxicity

Systemic effects usually occur when blood concentrations of local anaesthetic increase to toxic levels. Adding a vasoconstrictor (e.g. adrenaline) can reduce the systemic absorption of an anaesthetic, thus increasing the maximum safe dosage

For lidocaine, the maximum safe dose is 3 mg per kg of body weight; 7 mg kg^{-1} can be used if the solution has adrenaline added.

Signs and symptoms of systemic toxicity

The progression of lidocaine toxicity correlates well with ascending serum levels, with initial benign symptoms developing at 5 µg mL^{-1}, deteriorating into life-threatening cardiac arrest at levels above 25 µg mL^{-1} (Table 3.1). Therefore the development of tinnitus, light-headedness, circumoral numbness, diplopia and a metallic taste in the mouth indicate the onset of toxicity and possible impending development of severe symptoms.

Table 3.1 The systemic effects of lidocaine toxicity

Dose of lidocaine ($\mu g\ mL^{-1}$)	Presenting symptom
5	• Light-headedness • Circumoral paraesthesia • Slurred speech • Tinnitus
10	• Convulsions • Loss of consciousness
15	• Coma • Myocardial depression
20	• Respiratory arrest • Cardiac arrhythmia
>25	• Cardiac arrest

Treatment of lidocaine toxicity

- Stop the injection of local anaesthetic.
- Apply appropriate airway manoeuvres and give oxygen.
- Support respiratory failure with mild hyperventilation. Respiratory acidosis exacerbates local anaesthetic toxicity.
- With severe lidocaine toxicity, intubation does not require anaesthetic drugs.
- Treat convulsions with benzodiazepines.
- Treat hypotension with fluids and inotropes such as adrenaline.
- Treat ventricular arrhythmias with amiodarone.
- Treat bradycardia with atropine or glycopyrrolate.
- Ensure effective CPR.
- CPR should be prolonged, because full recovery has occurred after local anaesthetic toxicity.
- Consider the use of Intralipid in local-anaesthetic-induced cardiac arrest or circulatory failure that is unresponsive to standard therapy.

Avoiding toxicity

- Use the correct dosage.
- Use the aspiration technique.
- Regional nerve blocks can be used to anaesthetize large areas with relatively little local anaesthetic.
- The appropriate use of adrenaline as a vasoconstrictor can reduce the overall dose of lidocaine.
- Use ultrasound.

Avoiding local effects

- A slow injection will reduce the pain.
- The use of a fine needle will minimize the risk of soft tissue trauma as well as reducing the pain during infiltration.

Scoring Scenario 3.2: Teaching local anaesthesia

	Inadequate/ not done	Adequate	Good
Appropriate introduction	0	1	—
Checks student's level of knowledge	0	1	—
Outlines objectives of the session	0	1	2
Discusses indications for local anaesthesia	0	1	
Mentions local side-effects, including: • Pain • Local infection • Nerve trauma • Haematoma/ecchymosis • Local irritation • Tendon injury	0	1	2
Outlines strategies to minimize pain (slow infiltration) and tissue irritation (buffered pH)	0	1	—
Mentions signs of nerve laceration (paraesthesias, shooting or sharp stinging sensations, and excessive pain during needle insertion)	0	1	2
Discusses management and prognosis of nerve laceration (withdraw needle)	0	1	—
Mentions mild CNS signs of toxicity (tinnitus, light-headedness, circumoral numbness, diplopia, metallic taste in the mouth, nausea and vomiting) (at least 3)	0	1	2
Mentions moderate CNS signs of toxicity (nystagmus, slurred speech, localized muscle twitching or fine tremors, hallucinations) (at least 3)	0	1	2
Mentions severe CNS signs of toxicity (seizure activity, respiratory depression, coma) (at least 3)	0	1	2
Mentions cardiovascular signs of toxicity (myocardial depression and peripheral vasodilation)	0	1	2
Mentions maximum doses of lidocaine: *Adult* • 3 mg kg^{-1} • 7 mg kg^{-1} with adrenaline *Child* • 1.5–2.5 mg kg^{-1} • 3–4 mg kg^{-1} with adrenaline	0	1	2
Adequately describes the appropriate management of toxicity (airway, oxygen, management of seizures and arrhythmias)	0	1	—
Reviews information given and allows questions	0	1	—
Provides the student with learning resources and arranges next teaching session	0	1	—

Continued

Scoring Scenario 3.2 *Continued*

	Inadequate/ not done	Adequate	Good
Provides clear and effective teaching; is not judgemental or patronizing	0	1	—
Score from role player		/5	
Global score from examiner		/5	
Total score		/35	

SCENARIO 3.3: FEMORAL NERVE BLOCK

A 34-year-man presents with a fracture of the shaft of the right femur. He has been given some opiate analgesia, but you feel that a femoral nerve block will be beneficial. An F2 asks if they can watch. Perform a femoral nerve block on the manikin, teaching the F2 what you are doing.

SUGGESTED APPROACH

Of note in this OSCE is the relatively small number of marks available for knowing how to perform a femoral nerve block. This OSCE marking scheme is easily adapted to various practical procedures. If the examiner wished to assess a digital nerve block for instance, there would be almost no change to this marking scheme. The only things that would need to be adapted are the instructions to the actor and candidate. In view of this, it is appropriate to focus on the generic aspects of the OSCE, these being primarily patient-focused. Check the patient's understanding and consent, and respond appropriately to their questions.

The second generic aspect to this OSCE involves the teaching component. This is often used in OSCEs for two main reasons. It allows a technique that is technically difficult to simulate to be tested. It facilitates the marking process, since it gets the candidate to vocalize their technique throughout the OSCE. With some simple techniques, it is relatively easy to score marks, even if your knowledge is poor.

Primarily use an open, questioning technique with your student. Remember that, in this artificial format, the student will have a very good idea what is expected of him, as he has tested this station a number of times before. So ask 'What do you know about this technique?', 'Do you know of any complications associated with this procedure?', 'What approach would you use?', etc. Your student may well have been primed to respond as little as possible, but remember that you might be the first to try this technique – and even if you are not, it is very difficult for the student to remain monosyllabic throughout.

Although the instructions ask you to explain the procedure to the F2, do not forget the patient or the manikin (which should be treated as if it were the patient). You should explain to the patient what the procedure involves and gain consent not only for the procedure but also for you to talk through the process with your junior colleague. This should be done before you launch into the finer points of the femoral nerve block with the F2. You should also ensure that you retain your rapport with the patient as you proceed.

Single-shot femoral nerve blockade

Indications

As a sole nerve block, it provides analgesia for a fractured femoral shaft.

Contraindications

- Patient non-compliance.
- Allergy to local anaesthetic.
- Suspected neurological deficit of the injured limb, where the nerve block may interfere with clinical assessment.

Preparation

Sterile drape, gloves and skin preparation. The patient should have a working venous cannula in situ and adequate monitoring.

Position

The patient lies on their back with legs flat but ankles spread slightly apart. The foot of the leg to be anaesthetized should be slightly externally rotated; however, the patient may find this uncomfortable.

Puncture site (after intradermal local anaesthetic)

This should be 2 cm distal and 1 cm lateral to the arterial pulsation, approximately in the region of the inguinal fold (Figure 3.2). The needle should be angulated 30° cephalad. Distal to this point, the femoral nerve divides into anterior and posterior branches: the anterior (superficial) branch supplies sensation to the skin of the anterior and medial thigh; the posterior (deep) branch supplies the quadriceps muscles, the medial knee joint, and the skin on the medial side of the calf and foot (via the saphenous nerve).

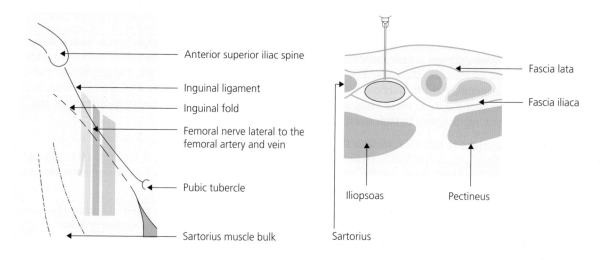

Figure 3.2 Surface anatomy for a femoral nerve block.

Figure 3.3 Anatomical layers and neighbouring structures.

Precision

Gentle advancement of the needle should produce two distinct fascial 'pops' as the needle penetrates the fascia lata and fascia iliaca (Figure 3.3).

A negative aspiration helps exclude vascular cannulation.

Gently inject a volume of 15–30 mL of bupivicaine or laevobupivicaine (maximum 2 mg per kg body weight).

- Stop injecting if there is resistance, since this suggests intraneural injection.
- Stop injecting if severe sharp pain is felt, since this may indicate intra-sensory-nerve injection. The absence of pain does not exclude intra-motor-nerve injection.

The use of a nerve stimulator has been associated with a higher success rate, better quality of blockade and lower incidence of nerve injury. This technique requires the use of an insulated needle, nerve stimulator and electrode to provide a stimulating current; the electrical current required to trigger muscle contractions correlates with the distance of the needle tip from the nerve. Close proximity to the femoral nerve will cause contraction of the quadriceps muscle group, and the patella will 'dance' at 1 mA. The current should be reduced in a stepwise manner, with needle reorientation if patella dance is lost. When contractions are still visible at 0.3–0.5 mA, the needle should be sufficiently close to the nerve. To exclude intraneural injection, contractions should not occur at less than 0.3 mA. Without movement of the needle, contractions should be recommenced with a current of 0.3–0.5 mA. After a negative aspiration, local anaesthetic can be administered. Contractions are lost after 1 mL of local anaesthetic has been injected.

Scoring Scenario 3.3: Femoral nerve block

	Inadequate/ not done	Adequate	Good
Introduces self to patient	0	1	—
Checks patient understanding	0	1	—
Gains consent for procedure	0	1	2
Checks consent for teaching	0	1	—
Outlines the objectives for the session	0	1	2
Explains indications for nerve block to F2	0	1	—
Explains contraindications to F2	0	1	—
Asks patient about any allergies and explains signs of lidocaine toxicity to patient	0	1	2
Positions patient appropriately and places them on monitoring; ensures that there is intravenous access	0	1	—
Uses appropriate aseptic technique (handwashing/sterile pack)	0	1	—
Uses universal precautions	0	1	—
Uses appropriate equipment (selects appropriate local anaesthetic, knows the safe dose, checks expiry date)	0	1	—
Describes anatomy correctly	0	1	2
Describes appropriate position for injection	0	1	—
Describes appropriate technique for injection	0	1	—
Uses appropriate teaching technique	0	1	2
Maintains verbal contact with patient throughout procedure	0	1	—
Deals with patient's questions appropriately	0	1	—
Comments on patient's prognosis	0	1	—
Gives the student learning resources and arranges further teaching opportunities	0	1	—
Score from student/patient	/5		
Global score from examiner	/5		
Total score	/35		

is hypotension, explained partially by histamine release. Administering the medication slowly can minimize this effect. Respiratory suppression can also occur, and its risk increases with coadministration of sedative agents.

Fentanyl

Fentanyl is a very potent synthetic opioid, and one of the commonly used analgesic adjuncts in the emergency department. It crosses the blood–brain barrier rapidly and thus has a rapid onset of analgesia (<90 s). However, the serum levels decline rapidly owing to tissue redistribution, making the duration of action about 30–40 minutes. Fentanyl has minimal cardiovascular effects such as hypotension. Respiratory depression is uncommon, but is potentiated when fentanyl is used in combination with benzodiazepines. The intravenous dose is 2–3 µg kg^{-1} (50–200 µg in adults), titrated in 50–100 µg increments. Fentanyl is the preferred drug for analgesia in short procedures and in cases of trauma with potential hemodynamic compromise.

Monitoring

A suitably trained individual, present throughout the procedure, must have a defined responsibility for monitoring patient safety and making a written record. This individual may not be present as you enter an OSCE, but you should still say that this is what you require for safe sedation. If this individual is not available because there are insufficient actors/examiners, you will be told that that person exists, and you will have scored points. This is true for any OSCE for which you feel you need extra staff. Remember to request their presence and do not just make do. Once told that they are 'virtually' there, however, you should proceed with the OSCE.

A pulse oximeter should be attached to the patient until discharge from the unit is contemplated. Monitoring of blood pressure and the ECG may not be necessary in young healthy patients, but is essential in older patients, especially if there are any cardiovascular problems. However, for the purposes of the examination, all patients should be fully monitored.

Oxygen therapy

While in reality some make an argument for applying oxygen only when required, in sedation for the purposes of the examination apply it to all patients, according to the recent British Thoracic Society guidelines (see Chapter 14).

It is useful to have a working knowledge of the American Society of Anesthesiologists (ASA) physical status classification system to risk-stratify patients receiving sedation for surgical procedures:

- class 1: a normal healthy patient
- class 2: a patient with mild disease
- class 3: a patient with severe disease
- class 4: a patient with severe disease that is a constant threat to life
- class 5: a moribund patient who is not expected to survive without the operation

ASA class 3 or more has been proved to be an independent risk factor for adverse outcome in patients undergoing general anaesthesia, and it is not our practice to attempt conscious sedation of these patients within the emergency department.

Postoperative monitoring

It is essential that you tell the examiner that the patient will have to be suitably monitored following the completion of the procedure. They should ideally be discharged into the care of another adult and be advised not to drive or operate machinery. The patient should be given written instructions.

Scoring Scenario 3.4: Conscious sedation

	Inadequate/ not done	Adequate	Good
Introduces self to patient	0	1	—
Reviews X-ray	0	1	—
Suggests transfer to resuscitation to perform sedation	0	1	—
Asks for additional doctor to assist procedure	0	1	—
Takes focused medical history: • allergies/medications • respiratory problems • cardiac problems • high blood pressure • previous adverse reaction to anaesthesia • liver impairment	0	1	2
States intention to carry out physical examination, including Mallampati scoring	0	1	—
Explains procedure to patient	0	1	2
Obtains consent for sedation and procedure	0	1	—
Puts patient on full monitoring and oxygen	0	1	—
Checks that cannula is patent	0	1	—
Ensures that resuscitation equipment and drugs are available: • airway trolley • suction • naloxone • flumazenil • suitable resuscitation trolley with head tilt-down function	0	1	2
Chooses appropriate drugs: • midazolam • morphine	0	1	—
Carries out appropriate sedation and manipulation of the fracture	0	1	—
Ensures adequate postoperative recovery and gives adequate instructions: • driving • discharge with adult • follow-up for injury	0	1	2
Score from patient	/5		
Global score from examiner	/5		
Total score	/28		

It is possible to build on the sedation and safety theme and create a more complex OSCE scenario in which you are asked to review a patient who has been oversedated in the emergency department by one of your junior colleagues without proper supervision. The key to this scenario is not only to manage the pseudo-resuscitation scenario but also to look at the clinical governance issues related to the incident.

SCENARIO 3.5: OVERSEDATION

You are urgently called to see a 29-year-old woman by a staff nurse who is concerned about the management of this patient. She is being sedated by an F2 without supervision. You understand that an orthopaedic SpR asked the F2 to sedate the patient for the manipulation of a distal radial fracture. The F2 was asked by the SpR to give 10 mg of morphine and 10 mg of midazolam and await his arrival.

On arrival, the patient is not responding to voice, but responds to pain. Her oxygen saturation is 94% on air, BP 110/70 mmHg and pulse 70 bpm regular.

SUGGESTED APPROACH

This is almost a resuscitation OSCE, and could easily appear in Chapter 2.

Oversedation and consequent loss of verbal responsiveness equates with general anaesthesia in terms of the level of patient care required. You should start with resuscitation of the patient and ask for additional anaesthetic assistance if required. Ask your assistant to set up the airway trolley in preparation.

The priority should be the airway. You should perform a rapid assessment of the airway and check for the presence of an obstruction. If the airway is obstructed, be prepared to perform basic airway measures (chin lift/jaw thrust, as well as inserting an oropharyngeal airway). If the patient tolerates the airway, they may need to be artificially ventilated with a bag–valve mask. This patient is at particular risk of aspiration, since she may not have been fully starved for what was not an elective procedure.

It is important to find out exactly what has been given and when. In this case, the patient's reduced level of consciousness is due to a combination of morphine and midazolam, and you may need to administer reversal agents, which are discussed below. Ask for the patient's medical history to see if there are any medical reasons for the adverse event.

While you secure the airway, you should ask your colleague to listen to the chest and support the circulation with fluids if the patient is hypotensive.

If the patient does not respond to the reversal agents or her level of consciousness drops further despite administration of the reversal agents, you should suggest that she be intubated in order to protect the airway; ideally, this should be done by an anaesthetist. However, it is likely that your OSCE patient will recover after administration of naloxone.

Reversal agents

Flumazenil

Flumazenil is a competitive antagonist of the benzodiazepine class of drugs. The onset of action is within 1–2 minutes after intravenous administration, with peak effects within 10 minutes. The duration of action is dose-related, but it is typically shorter than that of longer-acting benzodiazepines. Repeat dosing may be required. The total recommended dose in adults is 1 mg, which will sustain reversal for up to 48 minutes. Flumazenil is generally given in increments of 0.2 mg, titrated to effect. One must exercise caution in patients receiving long-term benzodiazepine therapy, because seizures can occur.

Naloxone

Naloxone is a competitive opioid antagonist. The onset of action following intravenous administration is rapid, with effects appearing within 2–3 minutes. The duration of action is dose-related. The initial dose in adults is 0.4 mg intravenously. It can be repeated to a total dosage of 2 mg. This antagonist may have shorter duration of action compared with that of the longer-acting opioids. In that case, the patient may need multiple doses. If the patient is exhibiting signs of respiratory depression before the end of the procedure, one can give 0.1–0.4 mg for partial reversal. Virtually no side-effects occur when naloxone is given for procedural oversedation.

Conflict resolution and clinical governance

This scenario has great potential for a management-type OSCE in which there is not only a clinical governance issue where a junior is performing a potentially unsafe sedation on their own on the instructions of a speciality team – the examiners could also add a degree of conflict between the F2 and the nurse or the orthopaedic SpR, making it a highly sophisticated OSCE. After the patient has been stabilized, you should suggest that you talk to all those concerned to ascertain the facts. This is a serious clinical incident, and you should encourage the F2 to complete a clinical incident form.

You should also explain to the patient what happened, with full disclosure, and ensure that their injury is appropriately followed up.

You should avoid blaming the F2 or the orthopaedic SpR, but should suggest that the F2 be made aware of the departmental protocols on sedation and may need to undergo more sedation training under supervision. You should also suggest to the examiner that the departmental guidelines should be reviewed to ensure that future sedations in the emergency department are performed by an appropriate number of adequately trained staff. This could be extended to inform other specialities of the sedation protocols in the emergency department. Although a scenario of this complexity may be beyond the scope of the MCEM examination, there is no reason why it could not be turned into an FCEM OSCE.

Scoring Scenario 3.5: Oversedation

	Inadequate/ not done	Adequate	Good
Recognizes airway obstruction	0	1	—
Attempts simple airway manoeuvre	0	1	—
Gives supplemental oxygen	0	1	—
Applies appropriate monitoring	0	1	—
Ensures that suction is available	0	1	—
Ascertains appropriate history	0	1	—
Ascertains the skill level of all the team members	0	1	—
Utilizes simple airway adjunct	0	1	—
Gives effective ventilation with bag and mask	0	1	2
Utilizes all team members effectively	0	1	—
Requests antagonist agents	0	1	—
Asks for patient's relevant past medical history	0	1	—
Gives opioid antagonist appropriately	0	1	—
Gives benzodiazepine antagonist appropriately	0	1	—
Ensures appropriate fracture management	0	1	—
Provides appropriate support to F2	0	1	—
Provides appropriate follow-up plan for patient, including full disclosure	0	1	2
Recognizes major issues involved: patient safety, clinical governance, teaching and supervision	0	1	2
Global score from examiner	**/5**		
Total score	**/26**		

4

Wound Management

SAVVAS PAPPASAVVAS AND CHETAN R TRIVEDY

CORE TOPICS

- Closure of wounds
- Wound infections
- Special wounds (puncture wounds, animal bites and amputations)
- Tetanus immunization schedules

SCENARIO 4.1: DOG BITE

A 35-year-old man has presented to the emergency department in severe pain. He was attacked by a pit bull terrier 3 hours ago and has sustained multiple bites to his right forearm.

Carry out a history and examination of the wound and outline your management.

SUGGESTED APPROACH

Dog bite injuries are a common presentation to the emergency department and, although usually not life-threatening, they can result in significant morbidity, disfigurement and psychological trauma. The outcome is influenced by correct early management.

Start by clearing the airway and assessing the breathing and circulation.

Look for any life-threatening injuries.

Hypovolaemic shock is uncommon in isolated distal upper limb injuries unless there is a tear to a major vessel or an amputation injury. It should be managed actively by transfusing warm fluids/blood and instigating urgent surgical intervention to stop further bleeding.

Take a focused history of the events surrounding the injury

Mechanism and timing of injury

Factors that should be considered include:

- breed of dog
- rabies risk (low in the UK)
- site of injury

Timing of injury is also important, since an ischaemic injury beyond 6 hours may result in permanent nerve injury, as well as loss of function.

Patient factors

These include:

- medications and allergies
- vaccination status (tetanus)
- past medical history (immunocompromised state)
- hand dominance and occupation

Pain control should be one of the priorities, and the limb should be splinted and elevated while intravenous access is obtained. Analgesia should be prescribed in accordance with the degree of pain

Examination

Carry out a secondary survey, which involves a top-to-toe inspection looking for other bite injuries.

The limb should be completely exposed and a detailed musculoskeletal, neurological and vascular examination should be carried out. A detailed description of the assessment of the upper limb is given in Chapter 5.

Removal of the splint may result in further haemorrhage; this should be controlled by applying direct pressure.

Fractures of the long bones caused by a dog's powerful jaw muscles may present with crepitus deformity and tenderness on palpation, and these should be treated in the same way as compound fractures.

The site and the size of the wounds should be recorded and, if possible, photographs should be taken for documentation.

You should conduct a neurological assessment of the motor and sensory components of the median, ulnar and radial nerves. The presence of neurological deficit coexists with vascular injuries in up to 50% of cases. A two-point discrimination test may be positive, and there may be hypoaesthesia and weakness in the affected area.

A detailed vascular examination should be carried out, including an assessment of the pulses as well as measurement of the capillary refill time (CRT). A delay in the CRT greater than 3 seconds may be indicative of vascular compromise. A handheld Doppler ultrasound scanner may also be used to assess the blood supply.

You should be aware of compartment syndrome (CS) as a potential complication of any soft tissue injury to a limb. This may present as a tense soft tissue swelling within the boundaries of the compartment on either surface of the forearm.

Signs of compartment syndrome

These include:

- **Pain**: this is often disproportional to the injury, and the patient may complain of severe pain on passive and active movement of the affected limb.
- **Pallor**: the hand may be swollen, pale and cold, with the fingers held in a claw position – extended metacarpophalyngeal (MCP) joints and flexed proximal interphalyngeal (PIP) joints.
- **Absent pulse**: a loss of the pulses is a late sign for CS, and the pulses are initially present.
- **Perishing cold**: progressive ischaemia can result in cold peripheries and an increase in CRT.
- **Paralysis**: this is another late feature of CS, which occurs as a result of hypoxic nerve damage. It is usually reversible with time.

You should appreciate that CS is a surgical emergency and tissue necrosis may occur within 12 hours. Urgent surgical decompression should be arranged to prevent complications, which include ischaemic contractures and rhabdomyolysis.

Investigations

Urgent bloods should be sent: full blood count (FBC), urea and electrolytes (U&E), coagulation screen, creatine kinase (CK), as well as a group and save.

An X-ray of the affected limb should be taken to look for fractures as well as fragments of tooth.

Wound swabs should be taken (*Pasteurella multocida* is the most common organism isolated from infected wounds).

Management

High-flow oxygen should be provided if indicated. Intravenous fluids should be given if the patient is hypotensive or tachycardic.

The wound should be debrided with copious amounts of 0.9% saline and covered with an iodine-soaked gauze dressing. It should be explored under local anaesthetic to look for tendon damage and to remove devitalized tissue. However, if there are extensive wounds with underlying damage to the neurovascular structures, they should be explored under general anaesthetic.

A limb that has its neurovascular status compromised represents a time-critical surgical emergency that should prompt an urgent surgical referral.

Patients with CS should also be referred for an urgent decompression fasciotomy.

Primary closure should be avoided where possible, to minimize the risk of infection.

Broad-spectrum intravenous antibiotics should be given (co-amoxiclav).

Anti-tetanus immunization (passive or active) may be necessary, depending on the patient's tetanus status.

Tetanus-prone wounds

- Wounds sustained over 6 hours before intervention.
- Any wounds that have:
  - a significant degree of devitalized or necrotic tissue
  - bites or puncture wounds
  - features of contamination
  - signs of infection

Immunization schedule

The typical UK tetanus immunization timetable is:

1. Primary three vaccines administered at 2, 3 and 4 months of age
2. Fourth vaccination given 3 years after the primary course (preschool)
3. Fifth and final vaccination given between ages 13 and 18

The triple vaccine containing diphtheria/typhoid/tetanus (DTP) is preferred.

If the patient has received a full five-dose course of tetanus vaccine, or is up to date with their tetanus immunization schedule, no further doses of vaccine are required. However, if the risk of tetanus is high because the wound is heavily contaminated, human tetanus immunoglobulin (250 or 500 iu) should be given intramuscularly.

If the immunization schedule is not up to date or the status is unknown, a booster dose of tetanus vaccine should be given, and the patient should receive further doses so that they complete their course of vaccinations. In addition, immunoglobulin should be given for any injury defined as a tetanus-prone wound.

Additional points

Unless there are child protection issues, it is the responsibility of the patient to inform the police/RSPCA.

You should complete the station by arranging appropriate follow-up and advice regarding wound infection and CS.

Scoring Scenario 4.1: Dog bite

	Inadequate/ not done	Adequate	Good
Gels-in with alcohol gel	0	1	—
Appropriate introduction	0	1	—
Rapid assessment of ABC and appropriate management	0	1	—
Suggests measures to achieve pain relief: • splints and elevates limb • nitrous oxide • oral analgesia • IV morphine/paracetamol	0	1	2
Takes a focused history: • timing of injury • sites of injuries • breed of dog • past medical history • allergies • tetanus status • occupation/hand dominance	0	1	2
States intention to conduct a general inspection to exclude additional injuries	0	1	—
Exposes limb and examines wound: • Comments on neurovascular status • Deals appropriately with haemorrhaging • Assesses motor function • Photographs and swabs wound • Soaks or wraps wound with disinfectant/iodine	0	1	2
Suggests exploration under local anaesthetic or referral to plastic surgeons for further management	0	1	—
Suggests that primary closure should be delayed	0	1	—
Advises on tetanus vaccination	0	1	2
Suggests antibiotics	0	1	—
Arranges follow-up and gives wound-care advice	0	1	—
Gels-out with alcohol gel	0	1	—
Score from patient	/5		
Global score from examiner	/5		
Total score	/27		

SCENARIO 4.2: SUTURING A WOUND

You have been asked to review a 24-year-old man who has come to the emergency department with a 4 cm laceration on the right side of the forehead after being accidentally head-butted while playing football. He has been seen by the F2, who has excluded a head injury as well any fractures to the facial skeleton. You assess the patient and feel that the wound needs suturing.

Carry out an examination of the wound and close it on the model provided. Demonstrate your hand-washing techniques.

SUGGESTED APPROACH

Suturing is a core skill for any emergency department physician, and ideally this station should not pose a problem for the trainee. However, the prospect of suturing a piece of foam in less than 7 minutes while pretending that it is attached to a real patient is another matter. The key to this station is not just placing the sutures but also talking through the skill and demonstrating to the examiner that you know how to manage lacerations in the emergency department. In addition, do not forget that there will be marks for effective hand hygiene as well as your ability to assess the wound and administer local anaesthetic. It is essential that you talk through your skill and say what you are doing as you go along. Again do not forget that, although you are suturing a foam pad, you are meant to treat it as if it were part of a patient. There will also be marks for your communication skills and arranging follow-up for the patient.

As you enter the station and introduce yourself, demonstrate your hand-washing technique as described at the end of this chapter. You may not have to physically do it, but should at least state your intention to perform a thorough hand washing.

Offer analgesia as appropriate.

Although you have not been asked to take a medical history, you should ask a few questions that may have direct bearing on your management. You can do this while you are getting your equipment ready or washing your hands.

- Is the patient allergic to local anaesthetic or iodine?
- Do they have a history of poor wound healing/scarring (keloid)?
- Do they use steroids?
- Do they have a history of immunosuppression or diabetes?

Emergency department physicians can suture most facial lacerations under local anaesthetic. However as the aesthetic result is a major concern with these types of injuries, it is essential that you be aware of injuries that may need referral to a specialist such as a plastic or maxillofacial team. These include:

- injuries crossing the vermillion border of the lip
- any laceration involving the eyelid
- any facial laceration with marked tissue loss
- infected wounds
- patients who have a history of scarring or poor wound healing

Explain to the patient that you would like to examine the wound, and then close it under local anaesthetic. Verbal consent is usually sufficient, but you should document that informed consent was taken, as well as any warnings on side-effects or complications. These include:

Early

- pain
- bleeding
- swelling/bruising

Late

- scarring
- infection

Prepare your equipment, including:

- a sterile dressing pack
- non-dissolving 5/0 sutures
- suture pack
- sterile gloves
- sterile saline and syringes
- sterile drapes
- local anaesthetic (1% lidocaine)
- chlorhexidine- or iodine-based disinfectant

Set up your equipment after washing your hands. It is essential that you use an aseptic technique and ask for an assistant if required to drop equipment onto your sterile field.

After you have donned your sterile gloves, the area around the wound edges should be cleaned with disinfectant and draped, creating a sterile field.

Administer local anaesthetic. You should be aware of the maximum safe dose of lidocaine and should state that you would aspirate before you inject, to prevent intravascular injection. You should suggest using a regional nerve block such as a supra-orbital nerve block. This would not only minimize any tissue distortion, which may arise from directly infiltrating the wound, but also reduce the overall amount of local anaesthetic required.

Wait for approximately 5 minutes before testing the area to make sure that it is adequately anaesthetized. Once this achieved, you should proceed to clean out and suture the wound.

Debridement is crucial for successful closure, and, after removing any obvious foreign bodies, you should perform a thorough irrigation with copious amounts of 0.9% saline to flush the wound. This should be repeated until the wound is free from any debris.

Explore the wound, and remove any ragged margins or devitalized tissue before proceeding to close the wound.

Wound closure

It is likely that you will have to place two or three simple interrupted sutures on a model. You should practise your suturing skills, bearing in mind the following points:

- Hold the instruments correctly – although this may seem obvious, it is surprising how many of us lapse into bad habits as the years go by.
- Take adequate bites through the wound edge 5 mm from the margin.
- Do not hold or palm your needle (no-touch technique).
- Space your sutures evenly.
- Avoid trauma to the soft tissues by excessive handling.
- Evert the wound edges.
- Ensure that all your knots lie on the same side of the wound.
- If the wound is deep, suggest that you would close it in layers.
- Dispose of all sharps safely.

Follow-up

The wound can be dressed with a light non-adhesive dressing, although facial wounds are often left uncovered.

The patient should be given clear written instructions on wound care and should be advised to return to have the sutures removed in 5–7 days if they are on the face. The patient should be advised to use sunblock over the wound to minimize scarring.

Tetanus vaccination should be discussed, and administered if appropriate.

Wash your hands with alcohol gel as you leave the station.

Scoring Scenario 4.2: Suturing a wound

	Inadequate/ not done	Adequate	Good
Gels hands with alcohol gel with appropriate steps	0	1	—
Introduces self appropriately	0	1	—
Offers analgesia as required	0	1	—
Enquires about mechanism (excludes glass in the wound with an X-ray if necessary)	0	1	—
Takes a focused medical history – asks about: • allergies to local anaesthetics • diabetes/steroids/immunosupression • scarring (keloid)	0	1	2
Explains procedure and complications, and obtains consent: • pain/swelling • bleeding • infection • scarring	0	1	2
Prepares equipment (selects 5/0 non-absorbable sutures for the face)	0	1	2
Hand hygiene and sterile gloves	0	1	—
Anaesthetizes the area – aspirates, and is aware of maximum doses (3 mg kg^{-1} lidocaine without adrenaline, 7 mg kg^{-1} with adrenaline)	0	1	—
Indicates a 5 min wait for local anaesthetic to work	0	1	—
Explores the wound and carries out a through irrigation and debridement of the wound	0	1	—
Prepares a sterile field	0	1	—
Places sutures: 1. Holds instruments correctly 2. Does not handle needle with hands 3. Does not traumatize soft tissue 4. Takes equal bites with needle 5. Everts wound edges 6. Sutures are equally spaced 7. Knots lie to one side 8. Sutures are not too tight	0	1	2
Disposes of sharps	0	1	—

Continued

Scoring Scenario 4.2 *Continued*

	Inadequate/ not done	Adequate	Good
Gives appropriate wound-care advice: • suture removal in 5–7 days • use sun cream to minimize scarring	0	1	—
Gives appropriate head-injury advice	0	1	—
Discusses tetanus vaccination	0	1	—
Gels hands with alcohol gel	0	1	—
Score from patient	**/5**		
Global score from examiner	**/5**		
Total score	**/32**		

HAND HYGIENE

This is an important topic; it has been tested in the examination and is of much current interest. You should start by removing watches, bracelets and rings. Sleeves should be rolled up so that the arm is exposed to the elbows.

Hand washing is carried out using soap and water and can be divided into six distinct steps (Figure 4.1). Each step is made up of six repetitions and should not last more than 10 seconds. At the end of the hand-washing cycle, the hands should be washed and dried.

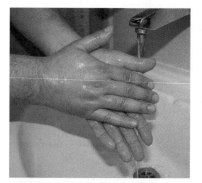
Step 1: Palm to palm

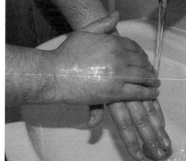
Step 2: Backs of hands

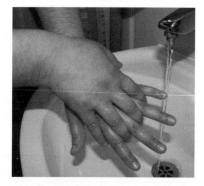
Step 3: Interdigital spaces

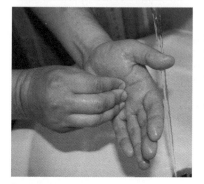
Step 4: Fingertips

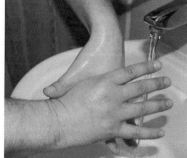
Step 5: Thumbs and wrists

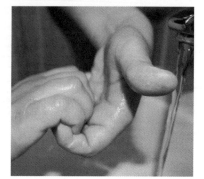
Step 6: Nails

Figure 4.1 Hand washing.

B) Breathing and ventilation
Look for:
SUGGESTED APPROACH
This is a common scenario, which you should have already encountered many times before you sit your OSCE. There are two elements in this OSCE: preparation and management.

5
Major Trauma
HARITH AL-RAWI

CORE TOPICS

- Major trauma
- Head injury
- Chest trauma
- Abdominal trauma
- Maxillofacial trauma

The management of major trauma is a major topic and is a near-certainty in the CEM OSCE. The key to the major trauma OSCE, regardless of the scenario, is a systematic and methodical approach to management. The advanced trauma life support (ATLS) method is the internationally accepted approach to major trauma. You should therefore ensure that if you are not ATLS-trained you at least read the *ATLS Student Course Manual* before your OSCE, since much of what is expected is contained in this manual.

To review the entire ATLS manual is beyond the scope of this chapter, the objectives of which are to provide guidance on how to:

- approach patients presenting with major trauma
- perform primary and secondary surveys
- take an 'AMPLE' history
- clear the C-spine and read a C-spine X-ray

SCENARIO 5.1: PRIMARY SURVEY (TENSION PNEUMOTHORAX)

You are informed of an urgent priority call. The ambulance crew has a 21-year-old man who was involved in a motor vehicle collision. He is an unrestrained driver who hit a tree and sustained chest injuries. His systolic blood pressure is 80 mmHg, pulse rate 120 bpm and GCS 10. The expected time of arrival is 5 minutes.

How would you prepare yourself in those 5 minutes and how would you manage this patient as the trauma team leader. You have an ATLS-trained nurse and an F2.

(D) Disability

This involves a focused assessment of the patient's neurological status. This is often difficult to assess in those who have a reduced level of consciousness or are intoxicated. However, it is essential to pick up a significant head injury.

- Calculate the Glasgow Coma Scale (GCS < 8 equates to loss of the gag reflex and is an indication for endotracheal intubation).
- Examine pupil size and reaction.
- Look for the presence of lateralizing signs.
- Do not forget to check the patient's blood sugar.
- Look for external signs of a head injury.
- Leakage of cerebrospinal fluid (CSF) from the ears/nose is also indicative of a severe head injury.
- Is there evidence of seizures?
- Is there abnormal limb posturing (as a consequence of intracerebral haemorrhage).
- Is the breathing pattern normal?

(E) Exposure and Environment control

The patient should be completely exposed in preparation for the detailed secondary survey. Following complete removal of the patient's clothes, both the front and back of the patient should be assessed after log rolling.

Make sure that the patient is covered adequately after exposure. Check their temperature.

Intervention in the primary survey

In the OSCE, it is highly likely that you will have to make one or more crucial interventions in order to stabilize the patient; this could be at any stage during your assessment in the primary survey. However, from reading the scenario, you should have a reasonable idea of what the problem might be. It is important that every time you make an intervention, you go back to the airway and restart your assessment. If you detect a pneumothorax, you should decompress it immediately and then arrange for a formal chest drain. You would be expected to know the relevant anatomical landmarks, explain the procedure to the patient and obtain the patient's verbal consent for it. The examiner will ask you to talk through the intervention; it is crucial that, once you have completed it, you ask to review the observations to see what impact the intervention has had on the patient. It is entirely possible that you may not get beyond assessing the breathing or circulation in the OSCE, particularly if you have a patient with a pneumothorax that needs to be treated. This should not put you off – the key is to keep going through your systematic assessment and treat any life-threatening injuries as you find them. Only once you are confident that the patient is stable do you move on to the secondary survey.

The examiners could choose a number of life-threatening conditions that require prompt intervention, and you should be familiar with diagnosing and managing the life-threatening conditions that can occur following a major motor vehicle collision (Table 5.1).

Imaging in major trauma

There will also be marks for arranging appropriate investigations. The trauma series consists of:

- lateral C-spine
- chest
- pelvis

The timing of the request for imaging is important, since it should not compromise the primary survey. Imaging should never delay life-saving treatment – more lives are saved by operations than by scans. A mode of imaging that you may consider specifically for this scenario is the focused assessment with sonography for trauma (FAST) scan, which is an effective tool for detecting free fluid in the abdomen. If you suspect that the patient has a head injury or that their C-spine cannot be clinically cleared, a CT scan of the head and/or neck should be organized. If the mechanism or the ECG is suggestive of myocardial injury, it may be prudent to organize a bedside echocardiogram.

Table 5.1 Potential life-threatening emergencies associated with a major motor vehicle collision

Potential critical event identified in the primary survey	Intervention required in OSCE
Airway	
Airway obstruction	Manage airway with adjuncts/ET tube/surgical airway
Significant C-spine injury	Demonstrate placement of collar and blocks
Breathing	
Tension pneumothorax	Immediate needle decompression, and arrange for a formal chest drain with an underwater seal
Haemothorax	Insert a chest drain
Haemopneumothorax	Insert a chest drain
Flail chest	Splint chest
Circulation	
Cardiac tamponade	Pericardiocentesis
Aortic dissection	Stabilize/CT and urgent vascular referral
Cardiac contusion	Bedside echocardiogram
Hypovolaemia from an abdominal injury (liver/spleen)	FAST scan/direct peritoneal lavage
Hypovolaemia from a bony injury (pelvis/femur)	Splint pelvis or traction-splint for the fractured femur
Disability	
Head injury	Manage head injury (see Scenario 2.4)
Reduced GCS and compromised airway	Maintain obstructed airway (see above)
Spinal injury	Demonstrate safe log roll technique/manage spinal shock
Seizures	Treat seizures as well as cause (see Scenario 2.1)
Exposure	
Hypothermia	Treat hypothermia

Scoring Scenario 5.1: Primary survey (tension pneumothorax)

	Inadequate/ not done	Adequate	Good
Appropriate introduction and handover	0	1	—
Puts out a trauma call, assembles the team and states that he/she will be team leader	0	1	2
Checks the availability of the equipment required; asks for patient to be put on oxygen and monitoring	0	1	—
Assesses the airway and makes appropriate use of airway adjuncts	0	1	—
Ensures that the C-spine is immobilized	0	1	—
Assesses 'B' and identifies the presence of a tension pneumothorax (auscultates appropriately)	0	1	—
Suggests immediate needle thoracocentesis; demonstrates landmarks accurately	0	1	2
Suggests formal underwater sealed chest drain: • Describes landmarks accurately • Explains procedure to patient • Administers local anaesthetic • Places drain in situ and connects appropriately to underwater seal • Secures drain appropriately	0	1	2
Rechecks observations following intervention	0	1	—
Assesses 'C': • Pulse • Central capillary refill • Blood pressure • ECG • External blood loss/abdomen/pelvis/femur	0	1	2
Gives warms fluids or O-negative blood if appropriate	0	1	—
Assesses 'D' accurately: • GCS • Pupils • Blood sugar • Abnormal breathing pattern	0	1	2
Assesses 'E' accurately: • Checks temperature • Exposes patient	0	1	—
Suggests appropriate imaging (trauma series): lateral C-spine/chest/pelvis	0	1	—
Effective team leader skill and use of team members	**/5**		
Global score from examiner	**/5**		
Total score	**/29**		

SCENARIO 5.2: SECONDARY SURVEY

You are called by your F2 to attend to the resuscitation area immediately, since he is unable to cope with a patient on his own. The paramedics have just brought in a 35-year-old woman who has jumped from her third-floor flat and sustained head injuries. The paramedics say that her pulse is 65 bpm, her blood pressure 124/84 mmHg and her GCS 10. Her C-spine has been secured with a collar and blocks.

How would you manage this patient and proceed to perform a secondary survey. There are the F2 and an ALS-trained nurse to help you.

SUGGESTED APPROACH

This represents a rather more complex type of scenario that would be suited to a double 14-minute OSCE scenario as is encountered in the FCEM examination. It requires you not only to review the primary survey performed by an F2 on their own (a management issue in its own right) but also to proceed to perform a secondary survey.

The initial preparation and assessment are the same as described for Scenario 5.1. However, when you assess 'D', you will find that this patient has a GCS of 6 with unequal pupils; on discovering this, you must suggest that this patient needs a definitive airway (patients with GCS < 8 need a definitive airway). At this stage, you should check to see if a trauma call has been put out and should request an anaesthetist. If the examiner wishes you to demonstrate your airway skills, you will be told that the anaesthetist is unavailable and you should proceed to secure the airway. As this OSCE is also about the secondary survey, the primary survey and intervention should be relatively straightforward, allowing you to complete the primary survey and move on to the secondary survey.

As you conclude your primary survey, you must suggest that this patient needs a full trauma series (which includes a lateral C-spine X-ray, a chest X-ray and a pelvic X-ray). In this particular scenario, a CT head is also required, and you should ensure that the patient is stable and safe for transfer to the CT scanner. For the purpose of the OSCE, you may have to arrange and oversee the transfer of the intubated patient for a CT scan.

The secondary survey does not begin until the primary survey has been completed. It is a complete head-to-toe evaluation of the trauma patient, i.e. a complete history and physical examination, including a reassessment of all vital signs.

In awake patients able to verbalize, you should take an 'AMPLE' history:

Allergies

Medications currently used

Past illnesses/Pregnancy

Last meal

Events/Environment related to the injury

In comatose patients, as much of this information as possible should be obtained from family, friends or ambulance crew.

In this case, any features suggesting that the patient has a psychiatric history are important. The possibility that the patient has taken a deliberate overdose is also important with regard to their management. If you suspect deliberate self-harm, paracetamol and salicylate levels should be checked in addition to the routine bloods.

The secondary survey

To avoid missing an injury, each region of the body is completely examined; a simple way of achieving this is to divide the body into:

- head and neck
- trunk
- pelvis
- limbs

Head and neck

The whole scalp, eyes (including visual acuity and fundoscopy), ears, nose, mouth, facial bones and neck are all thoroughly examined. Mention to the examiner that you would look for foreign bodies in any lacerations, as these can easily be overlooked.

Trunk

The chest, abdomen and back, including the spine, are all assessed thoroughly. You may be asked to perform a log roll in order to examine the back and/or clear the C-spine. You will have to ensure that you have the appropriate number of people to perform the log roll.

Pelvis

Carefully and gently assess the pelvis for any injury or deformity. If you suspect that the patient has an unstable pelvis, you should splint it temporarily. In an adult scenario, you should suggest that you would examine the genitalia as well as performing a digital rectal examination and a vaginal examination (with an appropriate chaperone present). Intimate examinations should not be performed on children – if they are absolutely essential, the child should be referred for a senior surgical opinion.

Limbs

Carry out a detailed limb examination, starting at the shoulder and ending at the toes. Examine each joint in detail and arrange X-rays as thought necessary. A detailed description of joint examinations is given in Chapter 6. If you find that the patient has an unstable ankle injury or a fractured femur, you may need to intervene and either reduce the fracture or splint the fractured femur following a femoral nerve block.

Depending on your progress in this OSCE, you may be shown a CT scan that reveals a right extradural haemorrhage. On diagnosing this, you must suggest contacting the neurosurgeons and getting the patient to theatre. Meanwhile, you should stabilize the patient and suggest that they have invasive monitoring and a urinary catheter (management of a patient with a major head injury is discussed in Scenario 2.4).

Management/debriefing

You should also suggest that a debriefing be held after the trauma call for all of the team. Some of the management issues – such as why the F2 was left alone with the trauma patient – can be discussed openly without assigning any blame. The management slant to this OSCE is more important in the FCEM examination, where the candidate has to play the role of an acting consultant.

Scoring Scenario 5.2: Secondary survey

	Inadequate/ not done	Adequate	Good
Appropriate introduction	0	1	—
Establishes the need to put out a trauma call, assembles the team and states that he/she will be team leader	0	1	—
Asks for airway trolley and states intention to check equipment	0	1	2
Assesses 'A' adequately, with C-spine immobilization	0	1	—
Asks for monitoring and high-flow oxygen	0	1	—
Assesses 'B' adequately	0	1	2
Assesses 'C' and the need for IV access and bloods	0	1	2
Assesses 'D' adequately; ascertains that the patient has a GCS of 6 and unequal pupils	0	1	2
Checks blood sugar	0	1	—
Indicates the need for a definitive airway and a CT	0	1	—
Assesses 'E' adequately	0	1	—
Takes an 'AMPLE' history and performs a secondary survey Ascertains that the patient is on antidepressants Must ask for bloods to be sent for paracetamol/salicylate level	0	1	2
Diagnoses right extradural bleed and contacts the neurosurgeons	0	1	2
Suggests management in emergency department: central line/arterial lines/urinary catheter/head-up position	0	1	2
Suggests debrief session and counsels/supports F2	0	1	—
Score from patient	/5		
Global score from examiner	/5		
Total score	/32		

SCENARIO 5.3: PAEDIATRIC TRAUMA

You are the emergency department registrar covering the paediatric emergency department. You are called to the resuscitation area because they have just heard that a 6-year-old boy has been hit by a bus and has sustained left-sided truncal injuries. He has a pulse rate of 140 bpm, a systolic blood pressure of 70 mmHg and a GCS of 11. The estimated time of arrival is 2 minutes.

Outline how you would prepare yourself and manage this child. You have an F2 and an advanced paediatric life support (APLS)-trained nurse to help you.

SUGGESTED APPROACH

You should be prepared for a paediatric scenario; in essence, this is very similar to an adult scenario, except that you have to know a few formulas in addition to your primary survey protocol.

This child has sustained major trauma and from the observations given is clearly haemodynamically unstable. As you start your OSCE, make sure that you introduce yourself to the parent/guardian accompanying the child and ascertain their relationship to the child. It is likely that they will be extremely anxious and may even interfere with your assessment. It is important that you remain calm and do not exclude them from the scenario. Explain what is going to happen and if possible ask the nurse to stay with them. This will boost your global score, and you would be unwise to ignore them.

You will need the first 2 minutes to make your calculations. A good way of remembering these is the mnemonic 'WET FLAG':

Weight = (age in years + 4) × 2 kg

Energy = 4 J kg^{-1}

T: endotracheal Tube diameter = (age in years/4) + 4 mm

Fluids = 10 mL kg^{-1} of crystalloid in trauma (10 mL kg^{-1} of packed red blood cells where needed)

Lorazepam 0.1 mL kg^{-1}

Adrenaline = 0.1 mL kg^{-1} of 1 in 10 000 adrenaline

Glucose = 5 mL kg^{-1} of 10% glucose

You can also state that you would use the Broselow tape to estimate the child's weight, and you can use this to calculate the doses of fluids, drugs and equipment that you need. Once you have completed your calculation, you will need to check that you have the appropriate equipment to manage this child; this will be displayed on a table or resuscitation trolley.

The next part of this OSCE involves managing the child. The first thing that you will need to do is to put out a paediatric trauma call and allocate roles to your team, stating that you will be the team leader.

The initial assessment is the same as that described in Scenarios 5.1 and 5.2, but this child has a 'C' problem and on this assessment is also noted to have a capillary refill time of 5 s, left upper quadrant tenderness and pain on palpating the pelvis. In this scenario, it is important to note that:

- After the second fluid bolus, blood will be needed.
- A surgeon must attend, since if there is no response to the third bolus, the child will need to go to theatre with a high suspicion of a splenic injury.

When asked about the blood, the most rapidly available is O-negative, which should be kept in the fridge in the resuscitation area. Type-specific blood takes 10–15 minutes to prepare, whereas a full cross-match would take 45–60 minutes. You will get bonus points for mentioning doing a FAST scan, but none for requesting a CT, since this child is unstable and may arrest in the scanner. In fact, the parents may push you to order a CT scan, and you should explain to them that this is potentially dangerous for the child.

Another important measure is to apply pelvic support, be it a Velcro belt or just wrapping a sheet around the pelvis to reduce pelvic volume and blood loss. You may not get the chance to assess 'D' or 'E' in this child, since 'C' is the main problem and must be addressed, with the definitive care being that the child ultimately needs to go to theatre for the surgeons to deal with the splenic injury and the orthopaedic surgeons to deal with the pelvic fracture.

You should also deal with the child's pain appropriately by giving morphine 100–200 µg kg^{-1} in a child over the age of 1 year. It is possible that the examiner will inform you that you are unable to get intravenous access; you should reply by telling the examiner that you will go for the intraosseous route.

Intraosseous (IO) access

This is a core skill, and is commonly tested in the OSCE. The marks can be divided into three areas for this skill:

- explaining the need for the procedure and getting consent from the parent(s)
- performing the skill after identifying the anatomical landmarks:
  - tibial approach (anterior surface of the tibia 2 cm below the tibial tuberosity)
  - femoral approach (anterolateral surface 3 cm above the lateral condyle)
- technique (outlined in Chapter 31)

Scoring Scenario 5.3: Paediatric trauma

	Inadequate/ not done	Adequate	Good
Appropriate introduction. Confirms identity of parents/guardians and engages them	0	1	—
Correct calculations and preparation: weight/energy/endotracheal tube/fluids/lorazepam/adrenaline/glucose ('WET FLAG')	0	1	2
Establishes the need to put out a trauma call, assembles the team and states that he/she will be team leader	0	1	—
Assesses 'A' adequately, with C-spine immobilization	0	1	—
Assesses 'B' adequately	0	1	—
Assesses 'C' and the need for IV access and bloods	0	1	2
Indicates two failed attempts at IV access and states intention to place IO needle Discusses with parents and informs verbal consent Describes landmarks and inserts IO needle	0	1	2
Makes rapid assessment of abdomen and pelvis and indicates that the child has possible splenic/pelvic injuries	0	1	2
Suggests a FAST scan to the examiner	0	1	—
Does not recommend a CT scan when asked by parent	0	1	—
States the need for blood after second bolus and calls for a surgeon	0	1	2
Stabilizes the pelvis by wrapping a sheet around it	0	1	—
Indicates that the child needs to go to theatre, since he is haemodynamically unstable	0	1	—
Score from parents	/5		
Global score from examiner	/5		
Total score	/28		

You should conclude the scenario by reviewing the important aspects of your objectives. Encourage questions and arrange for the next teaching session. Do not forget to thank your patient and answer any questions that they may have.

Scoring Scenario 5.4: C-spine injury

	Inadequate/ not done	Adequate	Good
Appropriate introduction to patient and student/F2	0	1	—
Gains patient's consent to examine C-spine and teach student/F2	0	1	—
Ensures that patient is comfortable and provides analgesia if required	0	1	—
Outlines objectives to student/F2 Clinical examination and log roll Discusses C-spine rules: either Canadian or NEXUS	0	1	2
Talks the student through assessing the C-spine and ascertains mechanism	0	1	2
Asks for assistance with log roll: • Requests 5 people in total • Assigns roles to team • Takes control of C-spine safely • Gives clear instructions and explanation to patient • Gives clear instructions to team about hand positioning and when to roll patient • Performs a safe and coordinated log roll • Examines C-spine after removing collar • Indicates that will perform digital rectal examination	0	1	2
Indicates that, after examination of the C-spine, imaging is indicated: lateral/AP/odontoid peg	0	1	—
Explains findings to patient and encourages questions	0	1	—
Summarizes objectives to student and sets out further learning objectives	0	1	2
Maintains patient's dignity	0	1	—
Score from patient	/5		
Score from student/F2	/5		
Global score from examiner	/5		
Total score	/29		

REFERENCES AND USEFUL RESOURCES

American College of Surgeons Committee on Trauma. *ATLS Student Course Manual*, 8th edn. Chicago: American College of Surgeons, 2008.

Hoffman JR, Mower WR, Wolfson AB et al. Validity of a set of clinical criteria to rule out injury to the cervical spine in patients with blunt trauma. *N Engl J Med* 2000; **343**: 94–9.

Stiell IG, Clement CM, McKnight RD et al. The Canadian C-spine rule versus the NEXUS low risk criteria in patients with trauma. *N Engl J Med* 2003; **349**: 2510–18.

Trauma Audit & Research Network website: www.tarn.ac.uk.

Trauma.org website: www.trauma.org.

6
Musculoskeletal Emergencies
EVAN COUGHLAN

CORE TOPICS

- Shoulder
- Elbow
- Wrist and hand
- Back
- Hip
- Knee
- Ankle

The diagnosis and management of musculoskeletal injuries in the emergency department is a core skill, and this is reflected in the CEM curriculum. All trainees should be competent in the examination of the joints listed above, as well as having a structured approach to the differential diagnosis and management of common musculoskeletal injuries.

It is also important to refresh yourself with the key anatomical landmarks of each joint.

The key to the musculoskeletal OSCE stations is to have a well-practised examination routine. All examinations begin with an appropriate introduction, confirmation of the patient's problem and a request to examine the site of injury. Consider other areas that may have been injured; it is appropriate to advise the examiner that you would like to exclude other associated possible injuries (e.g. head injury and cervical spine injury) if the mechanism is suggestive of these injuries, before moving on the appropriate area. Ask the patient if they require analgesia prior to examination.

Although the focus of the OSCE with respect to musculoskeletal injuries is on examination, it is appropriate to ask some focused questions, since these will often have an impact on your management. These include, as appropriate:

- mechanism of injury
- hand dominance
- occupation/hobbies
- smoking history
- tetanus prophylaxis
- history of previous problems in the specific area to be examined

If the area to be examined is a sensitive one, ask for a chaperone. Explain that you would wash your hands. Expose the area to be examined fully, while maintaining the patient's dignity.

We will now discuss the specific OSCEs.

EXAMINATION OF THE SHOULDER

SCENARIO 6.1: EXAMINATION OF THE SHOULDER

You are asked to see a 40-year-old man who was thrown off his bicycle and landed on his left shoulder 2 days ago. He is now complaining of pain in that shoulder.

Examine his shoulder and present your findings, including a differential diagnosis and management plan.

SUGGESTED APPROACH

Inspection

Look at the shoulder from the front, sides and behind. Assess for:

- asymmetry
- abnormal posturing of the upper limb
- scars
- bruising/haematoma
- sinus tracts
- loss of contour
- muscle wasting (deltoid, supraspinatus, infraspinatus)
- step deformities in the clavicle
- subluxation of the acromioclavicular joint

Palpation

Feel the skin overlying the shoulder joint for an increased temperature or crepitus. Proceed to palpate the following components of the shoulder joint for any tenderness:

- sternoclavicular joint (SCJ)
- clavicle
- acromioclavicular joint (ACJ)
- coracoid
- humeral head
- spine of the scapula

You should also palpate over the muscles that make up the rotator cuff for any tenderness:

- supraspinatus
- infraspinatus
- teres minor
- subscapularis

Specifically palpate the biceps tendon in the bicipital groove. Tenderness may be suggestive of tendonitis. A mass in the upper arm may represent rupture of the biceps tendon; this is associated with reduced flexion and supination of the forearm.

Movement

You should ask the patient to move the joint both passively and actively against resistance through a range of movements. Table 6.1 summarizes the main actions of the shoulder joint.

SCENARIO 6.4: CERVICAL SPINE INJURY

A 36-year-old man presents after a road traffic accident. He is complaining of neck pain and was collared at triage.

Examine his cervical spine and present your findings. There is an ATLS-trained F2 to assist you.

SCENARIO 6.5: EXAMINATION OF THE BACK

A 65-year-old woman presents with back pain and progressively decreased mobility.

Examine her spine in relation to her presentation and present your findings.

SUGGESTED APPROACH: CERVICAL SPINE

Inspection

Look out for the following:

- swelling
- deformity: kyphosis
- scars
- sinuses
- webbing of the neck: Klippel–Feil syndrome
- muscle spasms/shortening: torticollis
- thyroid enlargement
- lymphadenopathy
- erythema
- eye problems: uveitis, episcleritis, scleritis
- rheumatological abnormalities: evidence of arthropathies

Palpation

Palpate the neck for tenderness and swellings. Feel for uneven spacing between the spinous processes. Palpate the facet joints (one fingerbreadth lateral to the midline on either side). Palpate the paraspinal muscles.

Tenderness at the base of the neck is often associated with cervical spondylosis.

Feel for crepitus during flexion and extension, which is suggestive of cervical spondylosis.

Palpate any masses present, and examine for tenderness and temperature.

Palpate the supraclavicular fossa for a cervical rib and for lymphadenopathy. Asymmetry in the supraclavicular fossae may be caused by a Pancoast tumour.

Movement

Ranges of movement of the cervical spine are shown in Table 6.6. Always ask the patient if they develop any symptoms during their range of movement. Ask them to hold positions for a few seconds in extremes of range of movement and question whether they develop symptoms.

Table 6.6 Ranges of movement of the cervical spine

Movement	Normal range
Flexion	45°
Extension	45°
Lateral flexion	45°
Rotation	70–90°

Lhermitte's sign

On flexing the neck, the patient gets electric-shock-like sensations that run down the centre of the spine. There are multiple causes, among which multiple sclerosis is the most recognized.

Spurling's manoeuvre

Ask the patient to actively extend the neck and then laterally flex it and rotate the spine to both sides. Apply axial compression and ask about ipsilateral-side symptoms. This tests for foramina stenosis or nerve root irritation.

Neurological examination

Your examination should include a full peripheral neurological examination, with particular reference to the upper limb. Any abnormality may point to the level of cervical disturbance. Cervical myelopathy usually causes upper motor neuron signs, including a positive Hoffmann's sign (an inverted radial reflex and clonus). The sensory abnormalities tend to be tract-related and non-dermatomal.

Clearing the cervical spine

This involves deciding whether a trauma pati[ent] [...] [mult]icentre trials have looked at this question. From these stud[ies] [...] pine rules and the Canadian C-spine rules (see Table 5.2). Th[...] [cer]vical spine can be cleared clinically. Clearance of the cervical [...]

SUGGESTED APPROACH: LUMBOSACRAL

Inspection

Look for the following:

- swelling
- muscle spasm
- deformity: scoliosis, lordosis, kyphosis (m[...]
- scars
- sinuses
- erythema
- hair tuft, discolouration or dimpling at base of spine: spina bifida
- eye problems: uveitis, episcleritis, scleritis
- rheumatological abnormalities: evidence of arthropathies

Palpation

Palpate the spinous processes and the interspinous ligaments, looking for tenderness, prominences and widened interspinous distances. Feel the paraspinal muscles for tenderness and spasm. Check for increased temperature and tenderness in areas of swelling.

Examine the sacroiliac joints, looking for tenderness, erythema and swelling.

Movement

Ranges of movement of the thoracic and lumbar spine are shown in Table 6.7.

Table 6.7 Ranges of movement of the thoracic and lumbar spine

Movement	Expected range of movement	
	Thoracic	**Lumbar**
Flexion (Schober's test)	45°	60°
Extension	25°	35°
Lateral flexion	30°	
Rotation	40°	

Schober's test (modified)

This involves identifying the lumbosacral junction (at the level of the dimples of Venus). Horizontal lines are marked at this level and 10 cm above and 5 cm below. The end of a tape measure is held against the upper mark. The patient is asked to bend fully forward. The distance between the two lines is remeasured and 15 cm is subtracted from this new distance. The normal value obtained is 6–7 cm. A value less than 5 cm is indicative of spinal pathology.

Special tests

Straight leg raising (SLR)

Ask the patient to lift their leg off the bed and to stop when they develop pain. The normal angle of elevation at this point is approximately 60°. Check the site of the pain, it is not abnormal to have hamstring pain, but pain in the back (central disc protrusion), leg (lateral disc protrusion), or paraesthesia and pain down the back of the leg (root irritation) are highly suggestive of disc protrusion. While the patient is in this position, passive dorsiflexion of the foot often worsens pain and paraesthesia.

Bowstring test

While at SLR level, slightly flex the knee and apply firm pressure to the popliteal fossa. The test is positive if this causes paraesthesia and radiating pain; this is indicative of sciatic nerve root impingement.

Reverse Laségue test

With the patient in a prone position, flex the patient's knee. If this results in pain in a femoral distribution, it is suggestive of an upper lumbar disc lesion. Pain in the ipsilateral buttock or thigh is suggestive of a more distal disc problem.

Patrick's test

With the hip and knee flexed, the lateral malleolus is placed on the patella of the other leg. Pressing down on the knee causes pain in sacroiliac disease and osteoarthritis of the hip.

Completing the examination

It is important to follow up this examination by a lower limb neurological examination. Pay particular attention to flexion of the big toe, which will be reduced in cauda equina cord compression. Tell the examiner that you would like to perform an abdominal examination to assess for abdominal causes of back pain and to examine perianal sensation (S3–5) and rectal tone (both of which are abnormal in cauda equina lesions). You should also offer to examine the hip (see Scenario 6.6) and perform a vascular examination of the leg.

Spinal conditions

Common spinal conditions are listed in Table 6.8.

Table 6.8 Common spinal conditions

Condition	Features	Investigation in emergency department	Management
Cervical spine fracture and dislocation	• Neck pain dependent on site of fracture • Neck may feel unstable and patient may be actively supporting head	• Cervical spine X-ray (3 views) • CT spine to elucidate fracture • MRI spine to image cord and ligaments	• Collar immobilization until diagnosis made • Analgesia and collar with review in 2–3 weeks if stable fracture • Halo fixation if unstable
Whiplash injury	• Neck pain • Headache • Jaw pain	• Cervical spine X-ray (3 views) may be needed to rule out other pathology	• Analgesia • Return to activity • Physiotherapy
Cervical spondylosis	• Intermittent neck or shoulder pain, which may be associated with neurological symptoms	• Cervical spine X-ray is usually unhelpful • MRI is imaging modality of choice	• Analgesia and physiotherapy at onset • Surgery may be required for decompression
Spinal infections Osteomyelitis, subdural and epidural	• Back pain, which may or may not be associated with fever • Intravenous drug use or immunosuppression • Neurological abnormality may be present	• Full blood count, C-reactive protein, erythrocyte sedimentation rate, cultures • Plain films are usually normal for the initial 2–4 weeks in osteomyelitis • CT is better for osteomyelitis and MRI for spinal canal infections	• Antibiotics (6–8 weeks of therapy in osteomyelitis) • CT-guided biopsy in osteomyelitis • Surgical intervention may be required

Continued

Table 6.8 *Continued*

Condition	Features	Investigation in emergency department	Management
Spinal tumours Usually metastatic from breast (24%), gastrointestinal tract (9%), kidney (1%), lung (31%), prostate (8%), lymphoma (6%) and melanoma (4%)	• Back pain with neurology is usually associated with vertebral collapse • Pain at night with a history of carcinoma is an ominous sign • This may be followed by radicular pain and bladder and bowel dysfunction	• Plain films may show an abnormality, particularly loss of owl's eye on AP view (90%) • Osteosclerotic changes with prostate cancer and Hodgkin's lymphoma and occasionally with breast cancer and other lymphomas • MRI is modality of choice	• Steroids • Management of hypercalcaemia if present with bisphosphonates • Radiotherapy • Surgery if stabilization is required
Prolapsed intervertebral disc L5/S1 most common, followed by L4/L5 then L3/L4	• Back pain ± sciatic symptoms dependent on root involvement • Sensory abnormalities are dependent on level of lesion • Positive straight leg raising test	• MRI will show level of lesion and whether there is compression	*If no neurology:* • analgesia • physiotherapy • physical therapy *If neurological abnormalities:* • MRI spine • orthopaedic opinion
Cauda equina syndrome	• Urinary retention • Faecal incontinence • Decreased rectal tone • Sexual dysfunction • Saddle anaesthesia • Bilateral leg pain and weakness	• MRI spine	• Urgent surgical decompression
Lumbar compression fracture	• Back pain in the elderly • History of osteoporosis • Corticosteroid use	• Lumbar spine X-ray	• Compression fractures with <50% loss of height are usually stable injuries
Ankylosing spondylitis	• Back pain in 30s/40s that is worse in the morning and improves on exercise • May have alternating buttocks pain and iritis	• Pelvis X-ray will show fusion of sacroiliac joints	• Analgesia and referral for rheumatology opinion would be appropriate

Scoring Scenario 6.4: Cervical spine injury

	Inadequate/ not done	Adequate	Good
Appropriate introduction	0	1	—
History: • mechanism of injury (flexion, extension, rotation, compression) • protective forces (seatbelt, airbag) • ambulation • sites of pain • onset of pain • bladder or bowel symptoms • neurological abnormalities (weakness, pins and needles)	0	1	2
Uses assistant and appropriate places for in-line immobilization	0	1	2
Asks patient if they are in pain and offers analgesia	0	1	—
Palpation: • Checks for central midline tenderness • Comments on swelling, tenderness, widening of spinous processes • Palpates paraspinal muscles	0	1	2
Neurological: • Checks tone, power, coordination, reflexes and sensation in arms	0	1	2
Neurological: • Checks tone, power, coordination, reflexes and sensation in legs	0	1	2
Asks patient to rotate neck laterally	0	1	—
Appropriate use of Canadian or NEXUS C-spine rules	0	1	2
Clears C-spine without X-ray and explains why	0	1	—
Outlines management and follow-up	0	1	2
Score from patient	/5		
Global score from examiner	/5		
Total score	/28		

Scoring Scenario 6.5: Examination of the back

	Inadequate/ not done	Adequate	Good
Appropriate introduction	0	1	—
Asks about bladder and bowel symptoms	0	1	—
History (red flags): • age > 55 • progressive disability • history of malignancy • corticosteroid use • systemic symptoms • unexplained weight loss • intravenous drug abuse • immunosuppression • HIV • fevers	0	1	2
Inspection: • swelling • muscle spasm • deformity • scars • sinuses • erythema • hair tuft, discolouration or dimpling at base of spine • eye problems • rheumatological abnormalities	0	1	2
Asks patient if they are in pain and offers analgesia	0	1	—
Palpation: • Checks for central midline tenderness • Comments on swelling, tenderness, widening of spinous processes • Palpates paraspinal muscles	0	1	2
Movement: • Assesses movement of spine for flexion, extension, lateral flexion and rotation	0	1	2
Neurological: • Checks tone, power, coordination, reflexes and sensation in legs	0	1	2
Neurological: • straight leg raising • bowstring test • reverse Laségue test	0	1	2
Asks to perform abdominal and vascular examination	0	1	—
Asks to assess for saddle anaesthesia and rectal examination	0	1	—
Outlines management and follow-up	0	1	2
Score from patient	/5		
Global score from examiner	/5		
Total score	/29		

SCENARIO 6.6: EXAMINATION OF THE HIP

You are asked to see a 65-year-old man who has been having pain in his right hip for the last month. He has taken analgesia for this, but is having problems with his mobility.

Examine his hip and present your findings, including a differential diagnosis and management plan.

SUGGESTED APPROACH

To perform the hip examination properly, you will need a tape measure. The examination begins with the patient standing. Ask him to walk and take note of his gait:

- A **Trendelenburg gait** is one where weakened adductors allow the pelvis to tilt to the other side during walking.
- An **antalgic gait** occurs when the patient shortens the stance phase of movement on the painful side.

Other gait abnormalities include stiff leg gait and short leg gait.

Trendelenburg sign

Ask the patient to stand on one leg. Normally, the pelvis tilts upwards on the side with the leg lifted; if it tilts downwards this test is said to be positive. This is a sign of abductor weakness on the stance side (Figure 6.8). Causes include an L5 root lesion, proximal myopathy or congenital hip problems.

Inspection

Inspection of the hip is performed best while the patient is standing. Look for the following:

- muscle wasting
- rotational deformities
- plantarflexion of the foot
- spine: scoliosis, lordosis
- scars
- sinuses
- erythema
- ecchymoses
- swelling
- deformity

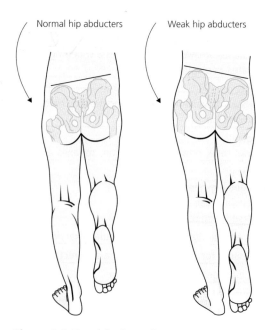

Normal hip abducters   Weak hip abducters

Figure 6.8 Trendelenburg sign.

Leg length

Assessment of leg length comes next, with the patient lying on the bed.

Apparent leg length

This should be measured first, as you do not need to reposition the patient before doing so. Measure the length from the xiphisternum to the medial malleolus on both sides.

True leg length

This should be measured from the anterior superior iliac spine (ASIS) of the pelvis to the medial malleolus and the sole of the foot on both sides. It is important that you position the patient properly to do this by straightening up the pelvis and placing the legs parallel to each other. If there is an abnormality then you must decide whether the problem is above or below the trochanter. Place your thumb on the ASIS and your index finger on the greater trochanter. If there is a shorter distance between thumb and finger on the affected side then the cause is above the trochanter. If not then ask the patient to flex their knees with their feet together and compare sides.

Be wary, since there may also be a discrepancy in the width of the foot – but you should have an idea of this if you also measure true length to the soles on each side.

Palpation

Palpate over the head of the femur and feel for crepitus during motion of the leg. Feel for tenderness over the lesser trochanter (iliopsoas strain), adductor longus tendon (adductor strain), ischial tuberosity (hamstring strain) and greater trochanter. Feel for increased temperature.

Movement

Ranges of movement of the hip are shown in Table 6.9.

Table 6.9 Ranges of movement of the hip

Movement	Expected range	Comment
Flexion	120°	The good hip is first flexed and held in position by the patient while the bad hip is flexed
Abduction	40°	Steady pelvis by holding the opposite ASIS and steadying the other with your forearm
Adduction	25°	Again steady the pelvis with your forearm
Internal rotation	45°	With knee flexed to 90°
External rotation	45°	With knee flexed to 90°
Extension	5–20°	With patient on their front and your hand on the pelvis. Loss is the first sign of a hip effusion
Internal rotation in extension	35°	Knees flexed to 90°
External rotation in extension	45°	With knees flexed to 90°

Special tests

Thomas's test

This test checks to see if the patient has a fixed flexion deformity. Ask the patient to lie flat, with your hand under the lower part of their back to remove any lumbar lordosis. With your hand in position, flex each leg fully in turn and see if the other leg remains lying flat on the bed. If it does not then this may indicate a fixed flexion deformity involving the iliopsoas muscle.

FABER (flexion, abduction, external rotation of the hip) test

The patient is asked to lie in the supine position. You should then flex the leg being tested and put the foot on the opposite knee. Proceed by pushing down on the superior aspect of the tested knee joint, lowering the leg into further abduction (Figure 6.9). The test is positive if there is pain at the hip or sacral joint, or if you cannot lower the leg to the same plane as the other leg.

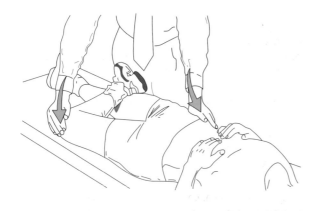

Figure 6.9 FABER test.

Completing the examination

You should inform the examiner that you would like to examine the patient's back, knee, and hernial orifices and the vascular supply to the leg. Do not forget to thank the patient and cover them up. Offer help in dressing if necessary.

Hip conditions

Common hip conditions are listed in Table 6.10.

Table 6.10 Common hip conditions

Condition	Features	Investigation in emergency department	Management
Hip fracture	• Pain in hip post trauma • Unable to weight-bear	• Pelvis and lateral hip views may show a fracture	• Analgesia • Femoral nerve block • Orthopaedic fixation
Perthes' disease	• Painful limp in 3- to 12-year-old child • M > F • Decreased range of movement	• Pelvis and lateral hip views	• Analgesia • Orthopaedic opinion
Slipped upper femoral epiphysis	• Children aged 10–16 years • There is often a history of minor trauma • Decreased abduction and internal rotation	• Pelvis, lateral hip and frog-leg views	• Analgesia • Orthopaedic opinion for reduction and fixation
Transient synovitis	• Hip pain and limp • May follow a viral illness	• X-rays are normal. White cell count (WCC), erythrocyte sedimentation rate (ESR) and C-reactive protein (CRP) are often mildly elevated • Ultrasound will show an effusion, which can be aspirated if clinically indicated	• Rest and analgesia • Reassessment in a few days if clinically well and bloods normal • Aspiration to exclude septic arthritis
Osteoarthritis of hip	• Pain, stiffness and loss of mobility • Loss of internal rotation is often the earliest sign	• X-ray will show changes suggestive of osteoarthritis	• Analgesia and physiotherapy • Total hip replacement may be required if symptoms are severe
Trochanteric bursitis	• Lateral hip pain radiating down lateral thigh • May be associated with snapping or clicking sensation • Tenderness and crepitus over greater trochanter	• X-rays may rule out other conditions	• Analgesia • Rest • Local anaesthetic injection
Septic arthritis	• Pain and severely reduced movement • More common in patients with rheumatoid arthritis, on immunosuppressants or steroids, and at extremes of ages	• X-ray may rule out other pathology • WCC, ESR and CRP are elevated • Joint aspiration for urgent microscopy and culture	• IV antibiotics • Analgesia • Joint washout

Scoring Scenario 6.6: Examination of the hip

	Inadequate/ not done	Adequate	Good
Appropriate introduction	0	1	—
Assessment of gait	0	1	—
Inspection: • muscle wasting • rotational deformities • plantarflexion of the foot • spine: scoliosis, lordosis • scars • sinuses • erythema • ecchymoses • swelling • deformity	0	1	2
Trendelenburg sign	0	1	—
Asks the patient if they are in pain and offers analgesia	0	1	—
Assesses apparent and true leg length	0	1	—
Palpation: checks for tenderness and temperature over hip joint and tenderness over: • adductor longus tendon • lesser trochanter • greater trochanter • ischial tuberosity	0	1	2
Movement: • flexion • extension • abduction • adduction • internal rotation (flexion and extension) • external rotation (flexion and extension)	0	1	2
Thomas's test	0	1	—
FABER test	0	1	—
Asks to perform back, knee and vascular examination	0	1	—
Outlines management and follow-up	0	1	2
Score from patient	/5		
Global score from examiner	/5		
Total score	/26		

SCENARIO 6.7: EXAMINATION OF THE KNEE

You are asked to see a 28-year-old man who sustained an injury to his right knee earlier today while out jogging. He is complaining of knee pain and swelling. He is finding it difficult to weight-bear.

Examine his knee and present your findings, including a differential diagnosis and management plan.

SUGGESTED APPROACH

Knee problems are common and can be quite complex. It is very important to have a good idea of the structure of the joint when performing this examination.

Inspection

Look for:

- swelling
- erythema
- ecchymosis
- scars
- sinuses
- rashes
- eye signs
- muscle wasting
- deformity
- evidence of rheumatoid arthritis

Palpation

Feel for tenderness and temperature over the joint. Palpate the joint line and feel for localized tenderness over the line suggestive of a meniscal tear. Palpate over the medial and lateral collateral ligaments, the patella, and the fibular head. Feel over the tibial tubercle to assess for tenderness. Feel for crepitus in the joint on movement.

The first evidence of an effusion may be loss of the knee dimple.

Patellar tap

Squeeze any excess fluid out of the suprapatellar pouch with one hand. Press quickly downwards with the fingers of the other hand. A click indicates a positive test.

Fluid displacement test

Squeeze any excess fluid out of the suprapatellar pouch with one hand. Stroke the lateral side of the joint and look for distension on the medial side suggestive of an effusion.

X-rays

The decision to X-ray or not can be made using the Ottawa knee rules: X-ray if any of the following apply:

- age 55 or over
- isolated tenderness of the patella
- tenderness over the head of the fibula
- inability to flex to 90°
- inability to weight-bear (at least 4 steps) both immediately and in the emergency department

Movement

Ranges of movement of the knee are shown in Table 6.11.

Table 6.11 Ranges of movement of the knee

Movement	Expected range
Flexion	135°
Extension	0°

Test the extensor apparatus by sitting the patient with their leg over the side of the bed. Ask the patient to straighten their leg while you support it with one hand. Feel for contraction of the quadriceps and look for active limb movement. This may be abnormal if there is a quadriceps rupture, a patellar fracture, rupture of the patellar ligament or avulsion of the tibial tubercle.

Special tests

Medial collateral stretch

With one hand on the thigh and the other on the lower leg, hold the upper hand stable and push the lower leg laterally. The test is positive if you feel the ligament give way.

Lateral collateral stretch

With one hand on the thigh and the other on the lower leg, hold the upper hand stable and push the lower leg medially. The test is positive if you feel the ligament give way.

Anterior drawer test

Flex the knee to 90° with the foot pointing straight forward. Grab the leg firmly with both hands while keeping the foot stable. Pull the leg towards you. The test is positive if the anterior cruciate ligament gives way.

Posterior drawer test

The same position is taken as described in the anterior drawer test. Pull the leg away from you. Again the test is positive if there is give.

McMurray's test

First flex the knee fully with your hand over the joint line to detect a click should one occur. Externally rotate the foot and abduct the lower leg; then extend the joint smoothly while maintaining abduction. A palpable click and associated pain suggests a medial meniscal tear. Reverse to test for a lateral meniscal tear.

Completing the examination

Finish the examination by telling the examiner that you would also like to examine the patient's hip and back. Present your findings in a logical fashion and give a differential diagnosis and management plan. Common knee conditions are listed in Table 6.12.

Table 6.12 Common knee conditions

Condition	Features	Investigation in emergency department	Management
Quadriceps rupture	• Inability to straight-leg raise • Tenderness and swelling along the course of the tendon	• Ultrasound of the quadriceps will confirm diagnosis	• Analgesia • Orthopaedic opinion in relation to surgical repair
Medial and lateral collateral ligaments	• Pain with medial or lateral ligament stretch • Peroneal nerve injuries can occur with lateral collateral ligament injuries	• Nil	• Analgesia • Physiotherapy • Orthopaedic follow-up if give is present • Follow-up and reassessment by GP in 2 weeks
Anterior and posterior cruciate injury O'Donoghue's triad: anterior cruciate injury, medial meniscal injury and/or medial collateral injury	• Sudden-onset haemarthrosis associated with injury • Positive drawer test	• X-ray may show Segond's fracture in some cases	• Analgesia • Physiotherapy • Orthopaedic follow-up or reassessment by GP after analgesia and elevation for 2 weeks
Septic arthritis	• Swelling and inability to move joint • Multiple sexual partners or recent infection	• Elevated white cell count, erythrocyte sedimentation rate and C-reactive protein • Blood cultures • Aspiration	• Analgesia • Aspiration • Antibiotics • Orthopaedic referral for joint washout
Meniscal tear	• General sports-related, associated with synovitis • May be associated with locking	• Nil	• Analgesia • Orthopaedic outpatients follow-up
Tibial plateau fracture	• Severe trauma • Haemarthrosis	• X-ray diagnosis	• Analgesia • Orthopaedic assessment for fixation

Continued

Table 6.12 *Continued*

Osteochondritis dissecans	• Male in 20s • Usually presents with knee pain	• X-ray diagnosis	• Rest • Analgesia • Orthopaedic outpatients follow-up, since may need foreign body removed

Bursitis	• Swelling and redness over a bursa:
	  ○ anterior patella for prepatellar bursitis
	  ○ over patellar ligament for infrapatellar bursitis
	  ○ in popliteal region for semimembranosus bursitis
		• Aspiration of the bursa may help to distinguish between septic and aseptic bursitis	• Conservative management with analgesia and rest
			• Steroid injections may help if aseptic
			• Oral antibiotics if felt to be septic bursitis

Osgood–Schlatter disease	• Generally 10–14 years old with pain over the tibial tuberosity that is worse on movement	• X-ray confirms diagnosis	• Analgesia • Rest until pain subsides, then physiotherapy • Rarely surgery is required

If the history is suggestive of a DVT, ask further about:

- pregnancy
- recent episode of immobility, including recent long-haul air travel
- previous DVT
- malignancy
- recent major surgery (especially pelvic or orthopaedic)
- thrombophilia
- smoking history
- drug history (oestrogen contraceptive pill)
- family history of DVT

A reasonable differential diagnosis at this stage includes DVT, cellulitis or trauma.

Examination

State to the examiner that you would like to go on to examine the patient. You would also like to have her baseline vital signs (if not given) and a blood glucose level.

Mild fever may be present.

The leg may be erythematous and swollen, with dilated superficial veins and calf discomfort on dorsiflexion of the foot (Homans' sign). Mention the test – but do not perform it, since there is a risk of dislodging thrombus to produce emboli. The thrombus may also be palpable as a fibrous cord in the popliteal fossa.

Confirm swelling by measuring the limb circumference in both legs 15 cm above and 10 cm below the tibial tuberosity. In all cases, abdominal and rectal examinations must be performed to exclude an abdominal cause or venous obstruction, such as an ovarian mass.

You should perform a formal examination of the venous system and examine for venous ulcers, varicose veins and venous eczema.

Trendelenburg test (tourniquet test)

This can be performed to test the competency of the venous system:

- The patient is asked to lie flat and the leg is elevated to empty the venous system.
- A tourniquet or two fingers is placed to occlude the saphenous opening, which lies 5 cm below and medial to the femoral pulse.
- While the saphenous opening is occluded, the patient is asked to stand up. If the valve is competent, you will observe a slow filling of the veins from below the tourniquet. If the valve is incompetent, you will see a sudden filling of the veins from above the tourniquet when you remove it.
- This procedure should be repeated at different levels.

Completing the examination

Examine the abdominal system, looking particularly for masses that may impair venous drainage, causing venous stasis, or that may indicate an underlying abdominal malignancy.

Management of DVT in the emergency department

Investigations

D-dimers have a high predictive value for DVT and can be useful in combination with a clinical assessment scoring system such as the Wells score (Table 7.1). If there is a low clinical probability of DVT and a negative D-dimer result, no further investigation is required. A positive D-dimer result should be followed by ultrasonography.

Table 7.1 Wells score for a pre-test clinical probability scoring for a DVT

Clinical features	Points
Active cancer (treatment within last 6 months or palliative)	1
Paralysis, paresis or recent plaster immobilization of leg	1
Major surgery or recently bedridden for >3 days in last 4 weeks	1
Local tenderness along distribution of deep venous system	1
Entire leg swollen	1
Calf swelling >3 cm compared with asymptomatic leg	1
Pitting oedema	1
Collateral superficial veins (non-varicose)	1
Alternative diagnosis as likely or more likely than that of DVT	−2

Venous compression ultrasonography of the leg veins is quick and non-invasive, with sensitivity and specificity of over 90%. It can simultaneously assess the extent of proximal progression of the thrombus, in particular extension into pelvic vessels.

Consider baseline full blood count, urea and electrolytes, ECG, chest X-ray, urinalysis, and pulse oximetry on all patients.

Look for an underlying cause if appropriate, with a coagulation screen and a procoagulant screen, and screen for specific malignancies.

Wells score and guidelines for DVT management

- **≥3 points: high pre-test probability.** Treat as suspected DVT and perform compression ultrasound scan.

- **1–2 points: intermediate pre-test probability.** Treat as suspected DVT and perform compression ultrasound scan.

- **0 points: low pre-test probability.** Perform D-dimer test. If the test is positive then treat as suspected DVT and perform compression ultrasound scan. If it is negative then DVT is reliably excluded.

Treatment for positive DVT

Low-molecular-weight heparin (LMWH) (e.g. enoxaparin 1.5 mg kg^{-1}/24 h) is superior to unfractionated heparin. Start warfarin at the same time, and stop heparin once the INR is 2–3. Consider the use of local anticoagulation services or the patient's GP for ongoing care.

Scoring Scenario 7.2: DVT – history and examination

	Inadequate/ not done	Adequate	Good
Appropriate introduction and asks about analgesia	0	1	—
Enquires about the risk factors for a DVT: • procoagulant states (acquired and congenital) (gives 3 examples) • venous stasis (gives 3 examples) • previous history of DVT/PE • family history of DVT/PE	0	1	2
Takes focused medical, drug and social history	0	1	2
Obtains patient's consent for vascular examination and exposes the patient appropriately, preserving their dignity and with chaperone if appropriate	0	1	—
Examines leg, looking for: • erythema/cellulitis • swelling • pitting oedema • scars indicating previous surgery • stigmata of peripheral vascular disease Looks for varicose veins (venous eczema) Palpates peripheral pulses Assesses skin temperature Palpates for tenderness along venous system	0	1	2
Mentions Homans' sign, but does not perform test	0	1	—
Mentions Trendelenburg test to assess venous competency (does not have to perform it)	0	1	—
Measures leg circumference appropriately at two sites	0	1	—
Suggests examination of the abdomen for masses	0	1	—
Calculates Wells pre-test probability (PPT) for DVT (examiner to provide criteria) and stratifies patient as high/intermediate/low-risk for a DVT	0	1	2
Outlines management according to Wells score (requests ultrasound scan and treats for DVT if intermediate- or high-risk; only asks for D-dimers if low-risk PPT)	0	1	2
Arranges appropriate follow-up	0	1	—
Score from patient	/5		
Global score from examiner	/5		
Total score	/27		

8
Abdominal Emergencies
CHETAN R TRIVEDY AND ANDREW PARFITT

CORE TOPICS

- Differential diagnosis of acute abdominal pain
- Examination of the abdominal system
- The management of upper and lower gastrointestinal bleeds
- Infective gastroenteritis

SCENARIO 8.1: ABDOMINAL PAIN

A 44-year-old woman presents to the emergency department with an 8-hour history of acute epigastric pain and vomiting; she is in marked discomfort. She has a history of drinking 15 units of alcohol a day.

Her initial observations at triage are:

Temperature 38.2 °C
Pulse 118 bpm
BP 98/66 mmHg
Blood glucose 9.4 mmol L^{-1}
Oxygen saturation 94% on air
Urine dipstick negative; urine β-hCG negative

Take a focused history and at the end of your assessment offer a differential diagnosis and management plan.

SUGGESTED APPROACH

Even after just reading the instructions for the scenario, you should be alerted that this patient is unwell, since she is pyrexial, tachycardic and hypotensive. You should be considering significant underlying pathology and ascertain the location of the patient in the department. You should suggest that the patient is unwell and should be transferred to the resuscitation area.

After introducing yourself appropriately, you should begin by characterizing the nature of the patient's pain:

- site
- severity (scale of 1–10)
- character (e.g. colicky, constant)

Box 8.1 Glasgow Prognostic Score for acute pancreatitis

- Age > 55 years
- WBC > 15×10^9 L^{-1}
- Urea > 16 mmol L^{-1}
- Glucose > 10 mmol L^{-1}
- Po_2 < 60 mmHg
- Albumin < 32 g L^{-1}
- Calcium < 2 mmol L^{-1}
- LDH > 600 units L^{-1}
- AST/ALT > 100 units L^{-1}

WBC, white blood cell count; LDH, lactate dehydrogenase; AST, aspartate aminotransferase; ALT, alanine aminotransferase

Box 8.2 Ranson's criteria for acute pancreatitis

Present on admission
- Age > 55 years
- WBC > 15×10^9 L^{-1}
- Glucose > 11 mmol L^{-1}
- LDH >350 units L^{-1}
- AST > 250 units L^{-1}

Developing during first 48 hours
- Haematocrit fall 10%
- Urea rise 1.8 mmol L^{-1}
- Serum calcium < 2 mmol L^{-1}
- Arterial Po_2 < 60 mmHg
- Base deficit > 4 mmol L^{-1}
- Fluid sequestration > 6 L

The Glasgow Prognostic Score provides a useful immediate guide of severity. A score of 3 or more indicates severe pancreatitis. The *UK Guidelines for the Management of Acute Pancreatitis*, produced by the British Society of Gastroenterology (BSG), recommend that these patients should be managed in HDU/ITU.

These guidelines, published in *Gut* 2005; **54** (Suppl III): iii1–9, are available at: www.bsg.org.uk/clinical/general/guidelines.html.

Differential diagnosis

Although a discussion of each cause of the acute abdomen is outside the scope of this book, it is recommended that you be familiar with the common differential diagnosis of an acute abdomen specified in the syllabus and listed below. It is essential that you be knowledgeable in the discriminatory clinical features and investigations of each of these conditions in order to be able to make a working diagnosis and institute appropriate treatment in the emergency department.

Hepatobiliary disorders

- Pancreatitis
- Biliary colic
- Cholecystitis

Upper gastrointestinal tract disorders

- Small bowel obstruction
- Peptic ulcer

Vascular disorders

- Mesenteric ischaemia
- Abdominal aortic aneurysm

Lower gastrointestinal disorders

- Diverticulitis
- Appendicitis
- Infective gastroenteritis
- Incarcerated inguinal hernia

Renal disorders

- Renal colic
- Pyelonephritis

Gynaecological disorders

- Ectopic pregnancy
- Ovarian cyst/torsion
- Fibroids
- Endometriosis
- Pelvic inflammatory disease

Scoring Scenario 8.1: Abdominal pain

	Inadequate/ not done	Adequate	Good
Appropriate introduction	0	1	—
Addresses the fact that the patient is in pain and offers pain relief	0	1	—
Takes a focused abdominal history: • site of pain • radiation • severity • character • relieving/exacerbating factors	0	1	2
Enquires about: • vomiting • diarrhoea • melaena • haematemesis	0	1	2
Enquires about changes in bowel habits/weight loss	0	1	—
Takes a focused medical history: • serious illnesses • medications • allergies • operations • asks about alcohol intake	0	1	2
Takes a focused gynaecological history: • vaginal bleed/discharge • dysmenorrhoea • dyspareunia • menorrhagia	0	1	—
Makes a working differential diagnosis from the history	0	1	2
Asks for appropriate investigations	0	1	2
Constructs an appropriate treatment plan	0	1	—
Arranges appropriate follow-up	0	1	—
Conducts examination in a fluent and logical manner	0	1	—
Score from patient	/5		
Global score from examiner	/5		
Total score	/27		

Completing the examination

You should thank the patient and offer to assist them with getting dressed.

Scoring Scenario 8.2: Abdominal examination

	Inadequate/ not done	Adequate	Good
Appropriate introduction	0	1	—
Addresses the fact that the patient is in pain and offers pain relief	0	1	—
Adequately exposes and positions the patient	0	1	—
Carries out a general inspection from the end of the bed, looking for: • scars • abdominal distension • jaundice • masses (transplanted kidney)	0	1	2
Examines the hands	0	1	—
Examines the eyes	0	1	—
Examines the mouth	0	1	—
Palpates the neck for lymphadenopathy/masses	0	1	—
Conducts a superficial and deep palpation of all four quadrants : • Palpates the liver • Palpates the spleen • Ballots the kidneys • Feels for an abdominal aortic aneurysm	0	1	2
Percusses over liver and spleen	0	1	—
Auscultates for bowel sounds and bruits	0	1	—
States intention to conduct an examination of the hernial orifices and testes	0	1	—
States intention to conduct a digital rectal examination and urinalysis	0	1	—
Carries out examination in a fluent manner	0	1	—
Offers a differential diagnosis	0	1	2
Suggests appropriate investigations	0	1	2
Score from patient		/5	
Global score from examiner		/5	
Total score		/30	

SCENARIO 8.3: UPPER GI BLEED

You are asked to review a 65-year-old man who has presented with a 2-hour history of vomiting blood. He has a history of atrial fibrillation and was recently started on oral amoxicillin and non-steroidal anti-inflammatory drugs (NSAIDs) for a dental infection.

His initial observations at triage were:

Temperature 36.9 °C
Pulse 110 bpm, irregular
BP 110/80 mmHg
Oxygen saturation 97% on air
GCS 15

Take a focused history and make a management plan. You are not expected to examine the patient.

SUGGESTED APPROACH

Gastrointestinal (GI) bleeds are a common presentation to the emergency department. It is important that all emergency department trainees be familiar with the differential diagnosis and management of GI bleeding. This is summarized in the national clinical guideline *Management of Acute Upper and Lower Gastrointestinal Bleeding*, produced by the Scottish Intercollegiate Guidelines Network (SIGN) and adopted by the BSG.

This guideline is available at: www.sign.ac.uk/guidelines.

History and immediate management

The initial observations suggest that this patient is haemodynamically stable. OSCE scenarios, which require you take a history, will invariably involve a stable patient. However, the tachycardia is worrying, despite his normal blood pressure. It would be prudent to tell the examiner from the outset that you would move the patient to an area where he can be monitored and that you would obtain a repeat set of observations, since those carried out at triage may have changed.

The immediate management would to secure two large-bore cannulae for intravenous access and obtain a venous gas to check haemoglobin and electrolytes. Send blood samples, including a coagulation screen and a group and save. The patient should be cross-matched if still actively bleeding or if there is low haemoglobin on the initial blood gas. Fluid resuscitation should be carried out as required.

The key to this scenario is to first ensure that you have stabilized the patient and then take a focused history so that you can make a definitive management plan. The important features in this patient's history are as follows:

- It is important to ascertain if the blood is fresh or whether it has been partially digested ('coffee grounds'), since this will localize the site of the upper GI bleed, which may differentiate between a variceal bleed and a duodenal ulcer.
- The passage of melaena, which usually presents as black, offensive tarry stools, also supports the diagnosis of an upper GI bleed. Although a patient may vomit small amounts of blood, they may suffer massive blood and fluid loss through melaena.

Scoring Scenario 8.3: Upper GI bleed

	Inadequate/ not done	Adequate	Good
Appropriate introduction	0	1	—
Identifies that the patient is shocked and institutes immediate treatment if unstable: • Asks for repeat observations and arranges appropriate monitoring (postural drop) • Secures bilateral large-bore IV access • Requests bloods, including a cross-match, coagulation screen, liver function tests, and urea and electrolytes • Institutes fluid resuscitation and oxygen	0	1	2
Takes a focused past medical history: • previous illnesses • previous operations • medications (anticoagulants/steroids) • allergies • family history of bowel disorders • shortness of breath/faints/dizziness/lethargy	0	1	2
Enquires about : • colour of blood: fresh/'coffee ground' vomiting • presence of melaena • abdominal pain • use of NSAIDs/corticosteroids • anticoagulants (patient on warfarin for atrial fibrillation) • history of peptic ulcer disease • use of alcohol • other medications (interaction of warfarin with amoxicillin)	0	1	2
Suggests appropriate investigations: • erect chest X-ray to exclude a perforation • urgent endoscopy	0	1	—
Offers a differential diagnosis: • bleed secondary to increase in INR • variceal bleed • peptic ulcer • upper GI malignancy	0	1	2
Offers management plan: • fluid/blood resuscitation • intravenous proton pump inhibitors • reversal of warfarin (vitamin K/FFP) • urgent gastroenterology opinion • upper GI endoscopy • HDU/ITU involvement	0	1	2
Correctly calculates and interprets Clinical Rockall Score	0	1	—
Score from patient	**/5**		
Global score from examiner	**/5**		
Total score	**/23**		

SCENARIO 8.4: LOWER GI BLEED

You are asked to see a 70-year-old man who has presented with a 2-week history of passing blood per rectum. He appears pale and his initial observations are:

Temperature 36.8 °C
Pulse 110 bpm, regular
BP 90/60 mmHg
Oxygen saturation 96% on air
GCS 15

Take a focused history, and give a management plan, including the investigations that you would request.

SUGGESTED APPROACH

This patient is tachycardic and also hypotensive, suggesting that he is unwell. The fact that he has been bleeding for at least 2 weeks and is pale suggests that he may require a transfusion.

As this OSCE asks you take a focused history and outline your management, your strategy should be to tell the examiner what immediate measures you would undertake to stabilize the patient. You should then proceed to take the history and follow up with your definitive management plan for this patient in the emergency department.

The immediate management of a lower GI bleed is the same as for an upper GI bleed (Scenario 8.3), and the patient should be resuscitated as necessary with fluids or crash O negative blood. Urgent bloods should be sent, and an arterial or venous gas should be used to assess the baseline haemoglobin. Often, direct examination of the anus and rectum will identify an obvious cause, such as bleeding haemorrhoids or an anal fissure. However, bleeding from the more proximal lower GI tract may be difficult to diagnose, and the patient may require endoscopic examination or imaging to find the source.

In addition to a standard medical history, enquiring about previous illnesses, operations, medications and allergies, you should ask focused questions to characterize the bleed with regard to when it started and any factors that make it better or worse. Ask about recent intake of foods such as beetroot that can give the impression of blood in the stool. Ask about symptoms such as shortness of breath and dizziness or evidence of postural hypotension, since these will indicate significant blood loss.

You should ask the following:

- What colour is the blood (bright red or dark red) and is the bleeding associated with bowel opening? Lower GI bleeds usually present with fresh red blood, and it is important to quantify the volume of blood passed and whether it was mixed in with stool or whether the stool was covered with blood.
- Is there any abdominal pain? Is there is any change in bowel habit? Diarrhoea is a more sinister sign than constipation.
- Has there been any weight loss?
- Is any mucus passed with the stool?
- Is the patient taking any medications such as anticoagulants that can potentiate a lower GI bleed?
- Is there a past history of inflammatory bowel disease (IBD): Crohn's disease, ulcerative colitis or diverticulitis? Features of IBD include mouth ulcers, glossitis, rashes (erythema nodosum) and perianal tags.
- Has there been local trauma or anal intercourse? In children, you may have to consider a non-accidental injury.
- Are there any associated features such as fever or vomiting that in the presence of bloody diarrhoea would support an infective cause?

Note that a painless lower GI bleed accompanied with weight loss and a change in bowel habit in an elderly patient is highly suggestive of an underlying malignancy.

Investigation and management

Blood tests should be as for an upper GI bleed (see Scenario 8.3). In addition, blood and stool cultures should be requested if you suspect an infective cause.

In addition to the routine observations, ask for a lying and standing blood pressure and a urine specimen.

Plain abdominal X-rays should not be routinely requested for every lower GI bleed unless you suspect a toxic megacolon or a malignant stricture causing a bowel obstruction.

Colonoscopy or flexible sigmoidoscopy is the investigation of choice, but is rarely indicated in the emergency setting.

Other investigations include:

- mesenteric angiography
- double-contrast barium enema
- red blood cell labelling scintography
- helical CT

The main goal of management in the emergency department is to resuscitate and stabilize the patient. Patients who are haemodynamically stable and have a normal haemoglobin can be discharged home and be followed up for an outpatient colonoscopy. Where the cause is external (e.g. haemorrhoids or an anal fissure), the patient should be managed conservatively and have follow-up with their GP in the first instance. Patients with an acute flare-up of ulcerative colitis should be managed with a combination of anti-inflammatories and steroids and referred to the gastroenterology team.

Scoring Scenario 8.4: Lower GI bleed

	Inadequate/ not done	Adequate	Good
Appropriate introduction	0	1	—
Identifies that the patient is shocked and institutes immediate treatment: • Asks for repeat observations and arranges appropriate monitoring (postural drop) • Secures bilateral large-bore IV access • Requests bloods, including a group and save and cross-match, coagulation screen, liver function tests, and urea and electrolytes • Institutes fluid resuscitation and oxygen • Requests blood transfusion	0	1	2
Takes a focused past medical history: • previous illnesses • previous operations • medications (anticoagulants/steroids) • allergies • family history of bowel disorders • shortness of breath/faints/dizziness/lethargy	0	1	2

Continued

Scoring Scenario 8.4 *Continued*

	Inadequate/ not done	Adequate	Good
Enquires about: • colour of blood (fresh/melaena) • change in bowel habit • weight loss • associated abdominal pain • features to suggest an infective aetiology (fever/diarrhoea/travel) • history of inflammatory bowel disease (diverticulitis/ulcerative colitis/Crohn's disease) • use of anticoagulants • local trauma	0	1	2
Suggests appropriate investigations: • plain abdominal X-ray • double-contrast barium enema • flexible sigmoidocopy/colonoscopy	0	1	—
Offers a differential diagnosis: • diverticulitis • inflammatory bowel disease • benign anorectal disease • malignancy • coagulopathy • angiodysplasia	0	1	2
Offers management plan: • fluid/blood resuscitation • correction of any coagulopathy • urgent colonoscopy • use of anti-inflammatories/steroids in ulcerative colitis	0	1	2
Arranges appropriate referral and/or follow-up	0	1	—
Score from patient	**/5**		
Global score from examiner	**/5**		
Total score	**/23**		

SCENARIO 8.5: GASTROENTERITIS

You are asked to see a 20-year-old female medical student who has had a 2-day history of diarrhoea.

Her initial observations are:

Temperature 37.8 °C
Pulse 100 bpm
BP 118/84 mmHg
Oxygen saturation 96% on air

Take a focused history and outline your investigations and management plan.

SUGGESTED APPROACH

This scenario represents a common presentation to the emergency department, and you should have a sound knowledge of the differential diagnosis and management of acute gastroenteritis. A key feature in the scenario is that the patient is a medical student, which is likely to have a significant impact on the management. The bulk of the marks will be for taking a history, but there will also be marks for suggesting a differential diagnosis and suggesting a management plan. As this patient is infective, you should inform the examiner that you would like to put on gloves and an apron before you proceed.

The history should include the following:

- Determine the onset of symptoms and establish what the patient perceives as diarrhoea. How often is the patient opening their bowels? (By definition, diarrhoea is the passage of more than three watery stools a day.)
- Is there an association with abdominal pain (possibly indicating appendicitis or inflammatory bowel disease)?
- Are there any exacerbating or relieving factors?
- Is there associated nausea or vomiting?
- Is there associated fever or rash?
- Determine the dietary history in the preceding 24 hours.
- Is blood, mucus or pus present in the stool?
- Obtain a description of stool consistency and colour (black tarry stools suggests an upper GI bleed). Fatty offensive stools that do not flush easily (steatorrhoea) may suggest a small bowel or pancreatic disorder resulting in malabsorption.
- Are there any features of inflammatory bowel disease (IBD), such as mouth ulcers, weight loss, anaemia or perianal tags?
- Has there been any previous bowel surgery?
- Ask about any recent travel (student elective in this scenario).
- Are there any occupational factors? (In this scenario, ask if the student has been working on a ward where there been an outbreak of any diarrhoeal illnesses.)
- Ask about drug history and if there has been any recent use of antibiotics or any laxative use or abuse. Has the patient used antimotility drugs, which may prolong the symptoms?
- Is there a history of:
  - hepatitis/jaundice?
  - diabetes?
  - a thyroid disorder?
- Is there a history or features of irritable bowel syndrome (IBS)?
- Is there any history of constipation (overflow diarrhoea)?
- Is there a history or any features of immunosuppression (HIV or immunosuppressive drugs)?

Differential diagnosis

Diarrhoea in a young otherwise healthy medical student presenting with a fever is likely to be infective in origin (Table 8.2). A detailed travel history is important here, especially if she has recently been on her elective. It is also important to find out if there has been an outbreak of diarrhoea on any of the wards she has been working on (*Clostridium difficile* or norovirus). Other causes in the differential diagnosis include:

- IBD
- IBS
- malabsorption sydrome or coeliac disease
- laxative abuse

Table 8.2 Incubation times for common infective causes of diarrhoea

Organism	Incubation time	Comments[a]
Vibrio cholerae	2 h–5 days	P
Staphylococcus aureus	1–6 h	
Bacillus cereus	1–6 h	
Salmonella	6–48 h	Bloody diarrhoea, P
Norovirus	12–48 h	H
Escherichia coli	24–48 h	P
VTEC 0157[b]	24–48 h	P
Campylobacter	24–72 h	Most common bacterial cause, P
Cryptosporidium	2–5 days	P
Shigella	24–72 h	P
Rotavirus	1–7 days	Most common viral cause
Giardia lamblia	1–25 days	P
Clostridium difficile	1 day–6 weeks	H
Hepatitis A	2–6 weeks	P
Entamoeba histolytica	Days–months	P

[a]P, refer to public health laboratories; H, hospital-acquired infection.
[b]Verocytotoxin-producing *E. coli* 0157.

Investigations and management

No investigations are usually necessary in those who present with a short history of diarrhoea, are haemodynamically stable and are otherwise well. If the patient is acutely unwell or presents with bloody diarrhoea, marked dehydration or a high fever, the following tests can be ordered:

- full blood count
- urea and electrolytes (look for electrolyte disturbances)
- liver function tests (giardiasis and other parasitic infections)
- C-reactive protein (CRP) (if you suspect IBD)
- coagulation screen (if you suspect hepatic involvement)
- blood culture (if the patient is pyrexial or is systemically unwell)
- urine dipstick
- stool analysis for microscopy and culture (*C. difficile* antigen test)
- venous/arterial blood gas to look at lactate and the severity of the acid–base disturbance (if the patient is acutely unwell)

A plain abdominal X-ray is not indicated unless you suspect that the patient has a toxic megacolon.

Those working with food, in a school or with patients should have stool cultures sent to have the pathogen identified.

Management for the majority of cases is supportive with oral hydration therapy, where 200–400 mL can be taken after each loose bowel motion. It is important that you advise on strict hand hygiene instructions. Those working with food, in a school or in a clinical setting should refrain from attending work for 48 hours after the diarrhoea has stopped. Furthermore, it is important that the medical student in this scenario be informed that if the stool culture is positive for the following pathogens, she may need clearance to work (in the form of negative stool specimens):

- *Entamoeba histolytica*
- VTEC 0157
- *Shigella dysenteriae*

Severe dehydration should be managed with intravenous fluids, and antibiotic treatment should be reserved for serious bacterial infections with positive stool cultures after consultation with the infectious diseases team. Antidiarrhoeal medications are rarely necessary except when the patient may be travelling.

A useful resource for the management of gastroenteritis can be found at: http://cks.library.nhs.uk/gastroenteritis.

Scoring Scenario 8.5: Gastroenteritis

	Inadequate/ not done	Adequate	Good
Appropriate introduction	0	1	—
Puts on protective apron and washes hands before entering cubicle	0	1	—
Enquires about: • onset of symptoms • number of bowel motions a day • associated vomiting/nausea • profession (placement on a surgical ward) • travel (student elective) • presence of blood, mucus or pus in the diarrhoea • recent use of antibiotics/other medications • features/history of IBD • features/history of IBS • relevant medical history (diabetes, thyroid disorders)	0	1	2
Suggests appropriate investigations: stool culture, since patient is based on a surgical ward. Blood tests and imaging are not necessary	0	1	—
Offers a differential diagnosis: • infective gastroenteritis • IBD • IBS • antibiotic-related	0	1	2
Offers management plan: • Oral rehydration therapy • Stops antibiotics • Advises patient to refrain from work for 48 hours after diarrhoea has stopped • Stool cultures • Reinforces hand hygiene • Does not recommend antidiarrhoeal medications	0	1	2
Arranges appropriate follow-up with occupational health before patient returns to clinical work (may need negative stool cultures)	0	1	—
Washes hands and disposes of apron before leaving cubicle	0	1	—
Score from patient	/5		
Global score from examiner	/5		
Total score	/21		

9

Genitourinary Emergencies

FRANCESCA GARNHAM

CORE TOPICS

- Acute urinary retention
- Acute scrotal pain
- Priapism
- Ureteric colic/renal calculi
- Phimosis
- Paraphimosis
- Fracture of the penis
- Haematuria
- Fournier's gangrene
- Prostatitis
- Skills: urethral catheterization, suprapubic catheterization

---

SCENARIO 9.1: TESTICULAR TORSION

A young man presents with a history of scrotal pain. Take a relevant history from the patient and demonstrate your examination on the model. Outline your investigations and management.

SUGGESTED APPROACH

A history of acute testicular pain in an otherwise fit and healthy young adult is highly suspicious of testicular torsion, and this should be at the top of your differential diagnosis. You should start by ensuring that the patient is given appropriate analgesia.

History

Ask when the pain started: a short history of sudden onset is more characteristic of testicular torsion.

Enquire about the following:

- nature of the pain (dull or sharp, continuous or colicky)
- exacerbating or relieving factors
- site of the pain (unilateral or bilateral)
- referred pain to abdomen, back or flank
- urinary symptoms (dysuria or haematuria)
- nausea or vomiting
- abdominal pain
- fever
- penile discharge
- previous history of sexually transmitted disease (STD)
- previous history of orchitis, epididymitis or mumps
- any risk factors for torsion:
  - congenital abnormality
  - undescended testicle
  - vigorous sexual activity
  - trauma
  - exercise
  - active cremasteric reflex in cold weather
- any other medical problems
- medications and allergies

Examination

After ensuring the patient's privacy and the presence of a chaperone, the patient should be exposed so that the scrotum and hernial orifices are exposed.

Look for scrotal swelling and for any discoloration of the scrotum (erythema or dusky appearance).

Is the scrotum hot to touch?

Gently palpate each of the testes in turn. Comment on the size, shape, consistency and lie of the testes. In torsion, the testicle may be high-riding and have a horizontal lie.

Check for any masses and their size and consistency (soft or hard, smooth or irregular). Is there a mass separate from the body of the testicle, for example an inguinal hernia or hydrocele (which feels like a bag of worms)?

Palpate the epididymis. Is it thickened? Is it tender on palpation?

Check for any testicular tenderness. Lift the scrotum to see if this alleviates the tenderness (Prehn's sign). This test is positive in epididymo-orchitis, but negative (no pain relief on elevation of the scrotum) in testicular torsion.

Does the scrotum transilluminate (hydrocele)?

Examine the hernial orifices for any masses or lumps.

Examine the penis. Look for any discharge, ulcers, erythema or vesicles.

You should complete the examination by examining the abdomen.

Investigations

Ultrasound is a helpful adjunct in the diagnosis of torsion, but if there is a high clinical suspicion it is not sufficiently sensitive to rule out torsion. Radionuclide scans and colour Doppler ultrasound can also be helpful in identifying arterial blood flow and other testicular disorders.

Note that a full blood count may be performed, but is not discriminatory, since up to 60% of patients with testicular torsion have an elevated white cell count. Other blood tests include urea and electrolytes, C-reactive protein, a coagulation screen, and a group and save.

Where you suspect epididymo-orchitis, you should perform a urine dip (for pyuria), urine microscopy (including Gram stain and presence of threads), culture and sensitivities, a urethral swab, and a urine nucleic acid amplification test (for *Neisseria gonorrhoeae* and *Chlamydia*).

If an STD is present then the patient should be screened for other STDs.

Differential diagnosis

Testicular torsion

Testicular torsion has two peaks, at 1 and 14 years of age. It is uncommon in men over 35. Patients often present with sudden-onset pain in the left iliac fossa. Fifty percent have had previous episodes of intermittent torsion. In addition, 20–30% have nausea and vomiting and/or abdominal pain, 16% are pyrexial, and 4% have urinary frequency.

It is essential that you convey that testicular torsion is a **SURGICAL EMERGENCY** and that the prognosis is time-critical. Most cases are salvageable with detorsion within 6 hours, 20% with detorsion within 12 hours and 0% after that. You should arrange an urgent referral to the surgical team on call for further management.

Manual detorsion is described as a temporary measure: the respective testis should be rotated outwards along its vertical axis in units of 90° as if opening a book (clockwise on the right side and anticlockwise on the left). Even if this procedure is successful, an urgent surgical referral is mandatory.

Torsion of the testicular appendix

In torsion of the testicular appendix, on examination, at the upper pole of the testis, there may be focal discoloration ('blue dot' sign) and a palpable hard, pea-sized mass.

Epididymitis ± orchitis

Epididymitis, with or without orchitis, is the most common cause of acute scrotal pain in adolescents worldwide. Organisms are usually spread from the prostatic urethra or the seminal vesicles or are blood-borne (less commonly).

Predisposing factors include:

- STDs (e.g. *Chlamydia trachomatis* and *N. gonorrhoeae*) – especially in those aged under 35
- urinary tract infections – especially in those aged over 35
- urinary tract anatomical abnormalities
- urethral instrumentation

Note that Gram-negative enteric organisms may also be transmitted through anal intercourse.

Non-infective epididymitis is also recognized with drugs (e.g. amiodarone) and Behçet's disease.

Onset may be more gradual than is seen with torsion and the patient may have associated systemic signs (fever, tachycardia, etc). There is tenderness in the epididymis and/or the testis. Prehn's sign is positive (pain is relieved on elevating the scrotum). There may be urethral discharge or erythema of the overlying scrotum.

Complications include chronic epididymitis, testicular atrophy, infarction, abscess formation, and reduced fertility or infertility (from fibrotic obstruction of the epididymal tubes).

Management involves analgesia (non-steroidal anti-inflammatory drugs may be particularly helpful), scrotal support and bed rest.

Contact partners for investigation and advise avoidance of sexual intercourse until treatment has been completed.

Antibiotics should be provided before results of investigations are available; they should be determined by the likely organism from the history using national and local guidelines.

Strangulated hernia

With a strangulated hernia, there is a firm, tender irreducible swelling, possibly with a previous history of a lump. There may be signs of obstruction and/or sepsis. Precipitating factors include:

- raised intra-abdominal pressure due to straining while defecating, urinating or lifting heavy weights or when coughing (note any history of chronic obstructive pulmonary disease)
- ascites
- ventriculoperitoneal shunt and peritoneal dialysis
- family history of hernias
- obesity

Trauma

It is usually obvious from the history that trauma has occurred, although the patient may require encouragement to reveal assault or trauma secondary to sexual activities.

Tumours

Usually a tumour will appear as a painless lump or swelling, but approximately 10% of men present with acute pain and 20–30% experience an ache. Half of testicular tumours are seminomas (found in older patients), with the remainder comprising teratomas, mixed tumours and others (more commonly found in younger patients).

Testicular malignancies account for 1% of cancers in men in the UK, with a peak incidence in the age range 25–35 years.

Risk factors include developmental abnormality (e.g. dysgenesis or maldescent), previous cancer in the opposite side, HIV/AIDS, torsion, Klinefelter's syndrome and a family history of testicular cancer.

The prognosis is generally good: the 5-year survival rate for seminomas is nearly 90%.

More than half of solid swellings in the body of the testis are due to cancer.

Scoring Scenario 9.1: Testicular torsion

	Inadequate/ not done	Adequate	Good
Appropriate introduction	0	1	—
Ensures privacy and chaperone	0	1	—
Offers analgesia	0	1	—
Ascertains time of onset of pain	0	1	—
Characterizes pain: • site • radiation • severity • character	0	1	2

Continued

Scoring Scenario 9.1 *Continued*

	Inadequate/ not done	Adequate	Good
Asks about: • dysuria • haematuria • nausea/vomiting • abdominal pain • penile discharge	0	1	2
Elicits risk factors for torsion: • vigorous sexual activity • undescended testis • congenital abnormality • trauma • exercise	0	1	2
Suggests taking a sexual history	0	1	—
Washes hands	0	1	—
Exposes genitalia and inguinal region	0	1	—
Inspects for: • swelling • discoloration	0	1	—
Palpates the testes, commenting on: • size and shape • consistency • lie of the testes • pain • palpates spermatic cord • any masses	0	1	2
Transilluminates scrotum for a hydrocele	0	1	—
States intention to examine for hernias	0	1	—
Recognizes that testicular torsion is a surgical emergency and makes an urgent referral	0	1	—
Demonstrates manual detorsion with appropriate analgesia (nitrous oxide)	0	1	2
Arranges investigations: • Doppler ultrasound • bloods • midstream urine	0	1	—
Score from patient	/5		
Global score from examiner	/5		
Total score	/32		

Acute angle closure glaucoma

Acute angle closure glaucoma should be considered in a patient over the age of 50 with a painful red eye. The attack comes on quite quickly, characteristically in the evening, when the pupil becomes semi-dilated. There is pain in one eye, which is severe and accompanied by vomiting. There is impaired vision, and haloes appear around light sources owing to oedema of the cornea. There may have been similar attacks in the past that were relieved by going to sleep (the pupil constricts during sleep, thereby relieving the attack). The patient may be systemically unwell, with severe headache, nausea and vomiting.

Acute angle closure glaucoma must not be missed, or the eye may be damaged permanently. The eye is inflamed and tender. The cornea is hazy and the pupil is semi-dilated and fixed. Vision is impaired according to the state of the cornea. On gentle palpation, the affected eye feels harder than the other eye. The anterior chamber appears shallower than usual, with the iris being close to the cornea.

Management includes urgent referral to ophthalmology. Intravenous acetazolamide 500 mg should be given and pilocarpine 4% instilled in the eye to constrict the pupil. Initially, the pressure must be decreased medically and a hole then made in the iris with a laser (iridotomy) or surgically (iridectomy) to restore normal aqueous flow. The other eye should be treated prophylactically. If treatment is delayed, adhesions may form between the iris and the cornea or the trabecular meshwork may be irreversibly damaged, necessitating a surgical drainage procedure.

Scoring Scenario 10.1: Acute red eye

	Inadequate/ not done	Adequate	Good
Appropriate introduction and offers analgesia	0	1	—
Conducts a focused ophthalmological history: • onset/duration of symptoms • associated visual impairment/loss • floaters/haloes • nausea/vomiting • discharge/watery eye • photophobia • associated pain • previous ophthalmological problems • history of trauma/foreign bodies • use of contact lenses/glasses • focused medical history (diabetes, high blood pressure, rheumatological disorders, medications)	0	1	2
Makes external assessment of eyes: • Looks for periorbital swelling • Looks for proptosis/exophthalmos • Looks for discharge/lacrimation • Looks for redness/subconjunctival haemorrhage/corneal injection • Examines pupil size/shape/response to light/afferent defect • Inspects inner surfaces of eyelids carefully for foreign bodies • Assesses eye movement (restriction/pain)	0	1	2
Checks visual acuity with a Snellen chart (suggests use of pinhole camera)	0	1	—
Checks for peripheral visual field defects	0	1	—
Suggests dilating pupils prior to fundoscopy	0	1	—
Performs fundoscopy appropriately and checks red reflex	0	1	—
Suggests a slit-lamp examination with fluorescein staining to look for ulcers/abrasions	0	1	—
States intention to test colour vision with an Ishihara chart	0	1	—
Ask for blood pressure and urine dipstick	0	1	—
Offers differential diagnosis: • conjunctivitis (bacterial/viral) • iritis • episcleritis • glaucoma (older patient)	0	1	2
Arranges follow-up and gives appropriate advice (viral conjunctivitis is highly contagious)	0	1	—
Score from patient	/5		
Global score from examiner	/5		
Total score	/25		

SCENARIO 10.2: ACUTE LOSS OF VISION

A 70-year-old woman attends the emergency department with a complaint of sudden visual loss in the left eye this morning. Take a focused history and perform an appropriate examination of the visual system. Give the possible causes and outline a management plan.

SUGGESTED APPROACH

Sudden visual loss requires rapid assessment and treatment. It is important to determine the onset and duration of the visual loss and whether there has been any progression or recovery.

Introduce yourself appropriately. Confirm the patient's name. The patient may understandably be upset, and accurate diagnosis will often depend on your ability to reassure them in order to obtain an accurate and swift history and examination.

It is essential to establish that this is truly a sudden loss of vision and not simply a longstanding loss that has gone unnoticed.

Identification should be made of any associated features, such as visual symptoms or pain, that preceded visual loss. Obtain clarification of general medical history, such as diabetes or hypertension.

Examination

Examine the eye as described in Scenario 10.1.

Differential diagnosis and management

The causes of sudden onset of visual loss are numerous (Box 10.1). They can be classified anatomically from the anterior to the posterior axis of the eye.

Box 10.1 Causes of sudden visual loss

Painful	**Painless**
• Angle closure glaucoma	*Fleeting*
• Retrobulbar optic neuritis	• Embolic arterial occlusion
• Giant cell arteritis	• Migraine
• Orbital cellulitis	• Raised intracranial pressure
• Uveitis	• Prodromal in giant cell arteritis
• Endophthalmitis	*Prolonged*
• Corneal ulcer/keratitis	• Ischaemic optic neuropathy
	• Retinal artery occlusion
	• Retinal vein occlusion
	• Vitreous haemorrhage
	• Retinal detachment
	• Age-related macular degeneration
	• Other macular disease
	• Orbital disease affecting the optic nerve
	• Intracranial disease affecting the visual pathway

Corneal ulcer/keratitis

The development of a corneal ulcer or keratitis may lead to rapid visual loss – usually, but not always, with severe pain.

Anterior uveitis

Anterior uveitis may cause some blurring of vision when inflammatory cells adherent to the back of the cornea (keratitic precipitates) lie on the visual axis.

Posterior uveitis

With posterior uveitis, visual loss may be caused by vitritis (inflammation of the vitreous). This may be associated with local retinitis or choroiditis, with further visual loss due to retinal damage. The eye may be painful and photophobic.

Acute angle closure glaucoma

Sudden onset of corneal oedema and clouding in acute angle closure glaucoma causes blurred vision, severe pain and redness of the eye. A history of attacks of blurred vision and eye pain or headache that then subsided is given by the patient. These prodromal attacks may be precipitated in the dark, by pupil dilatation.

Proliferative diabetic retinopathy

A common cause of sudden, painless visual loss is a bleed into the vitreous, which may result from the rupture of abnormal capillary vessels growing from the surface of the retina in proliferative diabetic retinopathy.

Wet age-related macular degeneration

Wet age-related macular degeneration can cause a sudden loss of vision. Central vision is lost, but peripheral vision is retained. Central serous retinopathy or a macular hole may cause a sudden central visual loss.

Retinal detachment

Retinal detachment (Figure 10.1) may be preceded by floaters, due to a small vitreous bleed or to a vitreous detachment and condensation of the vitreous gel. Vitreous detachment also puts traction on the retina, giving symptoms of flashing lights. Patients may report premonitory flashing lights or a 'snowstorm', before developing cloudy vision. Retinal detachment occurs commonly in people with myopia or diabetes, in elderly people and following trauma. The affected retina is dark and opalescent, but may be difficult to visualize. Urgent referral to ophthalmology is needed for surgery and reattachment.

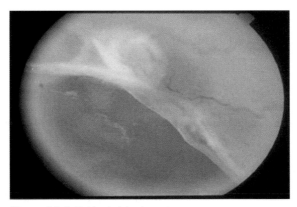

Figure 10.1 Retinal detachment.

Venous or arterial occlusion

Sudden painless loss of vision involving the whole visual field may result from total occlusion of the central retinal vein or retinal artery. A partial loss of vision is caused by a branch occlusion. Direct pupil reaction is sluggish or absent in the affected eye, but the pupil reacts to consensual stimulation (afferent pupillary defect). The retina is pale, with a swollen pale optic disc and 'cherry-red macula' (the retina is thinnest here and the underlying choroidal circulation is normal) (Figure 10.2). The retinal blood vessels are attenuated and irregular ('cattle-trucking' in arteries).

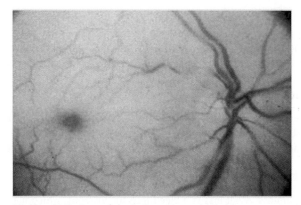

Figure 10.2 Central retinal artery occlusion.

Put out an urgent call for the ophthalmologist. Meanwhile, start treatment by digitally massaging the globe for 5 seconds every 10 seconds to decrease intraocular pressure and dislodge the embolus. Sublingual glyceryl trinitrate (GTN) and intravenous acetazolamide 500 mg (which decrease intraocular pressure) can be started.

Central retinal vein occlusion is a more frequent cause of sudden painless visual loss than arterial occlusion. Old age, chronic glaucoma, arteriosclerosis, hypertension and polycythaemia are the main predisposing factors. There is markedly reduced visual acuity and often an afferent pupillary defect. Ophthalmoscopy shows a 'stormy sunset' appearance (hyperaemia with engorged veins and adjacent flame-shaped haemorrhages) (Figure 10.3). The disc is obscured by haemorrhages and oedema. Cotton-wool spots may be visible. There is no specific treatment, but underlying causes may be treatable and so provide protection for the other eye.

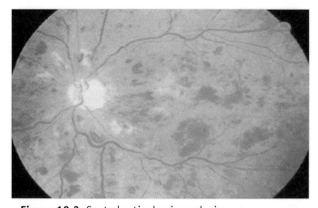

Figure 10.3 Central retinal vein occlusion.

Amaurosis fugax

A transient loss of vision, lasting minutes and said to be like 'a shutter coming quickly across the vision', is known as amaurosis fugax. This is caused by a platelet embolus passing through the retinal circulation. This is usually classified as a form of transient ischaemic attack (TIA) and should be investigated and managed accordingly.

Migraine

Occasionally, visual loss is attributable to a migraine attack causing vasospasm of the retinal vessels.

Anterior ischaemic optic neuropathy

Anterior ischaemic optic neuropathy (AION) results from a sudden decrease in blood supply to the optic nerve head. It presents with loss of vision. It may be caused by giant cell arteritis, with associated symptoms of pain in the temple, jaw claudication, shoulder pain and tiredness. There is profound loss of vision in the affected eye. AION is also seen in patients with vascular disease, and with ageing, diabetes or hypertension. The risk is increased in those with small, crowded optic discs. The loss of field is painless. Symptoms often occur in the morning, perhaps because of decreases in blood pressure and optic nerve head perfusion pressure during sleep. The visual loss affects the upper or lower visual field.

Giant cell (temporal) arteritis

In giant cell arteritis, inflammation of the posterior ciliary arteries results in rapid and profound visual loss. Usually this presents in people over 50 years of age (with a female predominance) and is associated with polymyalgia rheumatica. Visual loss is preceded by headache, jaw claudication and muscular pains. The temporal arteries are tender to palpation. The ischaemic disc is pale, waxy and elevated and has splinter haemorrhages. On suspicion, give intravenous hydrocortisone 200 mg or oral prednisolone 60 mg and check the erythrocyte sedimentation rate (ESR) (typically this is much greater than 40 mm h^{-1}, but can be normal) before referral to the acute medical team.

Pathology images

With this type of OSCE, you may be asked to take a history from a healthy patient/actor, perform your fundocopy on a model and describe your findings to the examiner. Alternatively, you may be shown an image of retinal pathology to comment on. You should be able to identify the following:

- hypertensive retinopathy
- diabetic retinopathy
- retinal detachment (Figure 10.1)
- retinal artery occlusion (Figure 10.2)
- retinal vein occlusion (Figure 10.3)

Scoring Scenario 10.2: Acute loss of vision

	Inadequate/ not done	Adequate	Good
Appropriate introduction and offers analgesia	0	1	—
Conducts a focused ophthalmological history: • onset/duration of symptoms • associated visual impairment/loss • floaters/haloes • characteristics of visual field loss (partial/total) • discharge/watery eye • photophobia • whether marked pain is associated with visual loss and whether there is jaw claudication/scalp tenderness • previous ophthalmological problems • history of trauma • use of contact lenses/glasses • focused medical history (diabetes/high blood pressure/rheumatological disorders/medications) • history of migraines	0	1	2
Makes external assessment of eyes: • Looks for periorbital swelling • Looks for proptosis/exophthalmos • Looks for discharge/lacrimation • Looks for redness/subconjunctival haemorrhage/injection • Examines pupil size/shape/response to light • Inspects inner surfaces of eyelids carefully for ulceration • Assesses eye movement (restriction/pain)			
Checks visual acuity with a Snellen chart (suggests use of pinhole camera)			
Checks for peripheral visual field defects	0	1	—
Does not recommend dilating pupils, since this may exacerbate glaucoma	0	1	—
Performs fundoscopy appropriately and checks the red reflex	0	1	—
Suggests a slit-lamp examination with fluorescein staining to look for ulcers/abrasions	0	1	—
States intention to test colour vision with an Ishihara chart	0	1	—
Ask for blood pressure and urine dipstick	0	1	—
Offers differential diagnosis: • temporal arteritis • glaucoma • optic neuritis • uveitis	0	1	2

If dx glaucoma

do not dilate pupil = 1 exac. glaucoma

Continued

Scoring Scenario 10.2 *Continued*

	Inadequate/ not done	Adequate	Good
Orders blood tests, including ESR	0	1	—
Makes urgent referral to ophthalmology and suggests commencing patient on steroids	0	1	—
Addresses patient's concerns about coping with disabled husband	0	1	—
Score from patient		/5	
Global score from examiner		/5	
Total score		/27	

SCENARIO 10.3: TRAUMATIC EYE INJURY

A 20-year-old man has been involved in a fight, during which he sustained injuries to the left eye. You are asked to assess the patient and manage as appropriate.

SUGGESTED APPROACH

Introduce yourself appropriately. Early on in your assessment, you should double-check the mechanism of injury, and any other injuries that may have occurred. Note that if the patient is inebriated or has a reduced level of consciousness, it may be necessary to proceed with advanced trauma life support (ATLS) guidelines and carry out a primary survey to exclude life-threatening emergencies.

Assess exactly how the injury occurred. Blunt trauma from objects may result in severe damage to the globe, particularly when there is high-velocity impact (e.g. a squash ball injury). Penetrating trauma can also damage ocular structures, and it is important to examine the globe carefully for an entry point and also for foreign bodies.

In all cases, it is vital that visual acuity be recorded in both the injured and the uninjured eye. Where a penetrating injury is suspected, pressure to the globe should be avoided and it may only be possible to measure vision approximately in the injured eye. The skin around the orbit and eyelids should be examined carefully for a penetrating wound.

Damage to the orbit itself (a blow-out fracture) should be suspected if there is:

- paraesthesia below the orbital rim, suggesting infraorbital nerve damage
- air emphysema in the region of the maxillary sinus
- restriction of eye movement due to entrapment of the rectus muscles resulting in ophthalmoplegia

The eye may subsequently become recessed into the orbit (enophthalmos).

A laceration involving the medial canthus may result in damage to the lacrimal canaliculi, causing epiphora (excessive tear production) if untreated.

The eyelids should be everted to exclude a subtarsal foreign body. Proceed to examine the conjunctiva and sclera after administering local anaesthetic eye drops and performing a slit-lamp examination using fluorescein dye.

Examine the fundus with a direct ophthalmoscope, looking for damage to the optic disc as well as retinal haemorrhage. Absence of the red reflex may indicate a vitreous haemorrhage. The pupil may also show a fixed dilatation as a result of blunt trauma (traumatic mydriasis).

The optic disc may be pale from a traumatic optic neuropathy caused by avulsion of the blood vessels supplying the optic nerve.

Blunt trauma may cause haemorrhage into the anterior chamber, where blood collects, with a fluid level becoming visible (hyphaema). This is caused by rupture of blood vessels in the root of the iris; alternatively, the iris may be torn away from its insertion into the ciliary body (iris dialysis to produce a D-shaped pupil).

Dislocation of the lens may be suggested by a fluttering of the iris diaphragm on eye movement (iridodonesis). The lens clarity should be assessed with the slit lamp and against the red reflex after pupil dilatation. Cataracts can develop abruptly following direct penetrating trauma to the eye. Blunt trauma also causes a transient posterior subcapsular cataract within hours of injury.

Management of traumatic eye injuries

If there is any doubt as to the diagnosis, referral should be made to the on-call ophthalmology team.

Lacerations to the skin and lids

Lacerations to the skin and lids require careful suturing, especially if the lid margin is involved. This may necessitate referral to a plastic surgeon.

Corneal abrasions

Abrasions of the cornea are very painful, but normally heal rapidly. Treatment is with antibiotic ointment, with or without an eye pad. Dilatation of the pupil with cyclopentolate 1% can help to relieve the pain caused by spasm of the ciliary muscle.

Corneal foreign bodies

Foreign bodies in the cornea should be removed with a needle under topical anaesthesia. A rust ring may remain, but can be removed with a small rotating burr. Subtarsal objects can often be swept away from the everted lid with a cotton-wool bud. Treatment is then as for an abrasion. A CT scan may also be indicated if an intraocular foreign body is suspected, and imaging should be discussed with the ophthalmologist on call.

Hyphaema

Hyphaema (Figure 10.4) usually settles with rest, but a re-bleed may occur in the first 5–6 days after injury. Children usually require admission to hospital for a period of observation, whereas adults can be treated at home, provided that they rest. Steroid eye drops are given for a short time, with dilatation of the pupil. Steroids reduce the risk of re-bleeds. The commonest complication is raised ocular pressure.

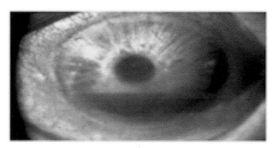

Figure 10.4 Hyphaema.

Chemical injury

In chemical injury, the most important aspect of treatment is immediate irrigation of the eye with copious quantities of clean water at the time of the accident. The nature of the chemical is ascertained by history and measuring tear pH with litmus paper.

Blow-out fracture

If a blow-out fracture is suspected, a CT scan will delineate the bony and soft tissue injury. If this is not possible, plain facial X-rays are performed. Treatment may be delayed until the periorbital swelling has settled, and the patient should be referred for a maxillofacial opinion.

Scoring Scenario 10.3: Traumatic eye injury

	Inadequate/ not done	Adequate	Good
Appropriate introduction and offers analgesia	0	1	—
Ascertains mechanism of injury	0	1	—
Suggests performing a rapid primary survey to exclude life-threatening injuries	0	1	—
Provides adequate analgesia	0	1	—
Conducts a focused ophthalmological history: • associated visual impairment/loss • diplopia • characteristics of visual field loss (partial/total) • photophobia • previous ophthalmological problems • use of contact lenses/glasses (trauma may result in corneal abrasions) • takes a focused medical history	0	1	2
Makes external assessment of eyes: • Looks for periorbital swelling • Looks for proptosis/exophthalmos • Looks for bony tenderness/step deformity of orbital rim/zygoma • Looks for subconjunctival haemorrhage • Looks for hyphaema • Examines pupil size/shape/response to light/afferent defect • Inspects inner surfaces of eyelids carefully for foreign bodies/ulceration • Assesses eye movement (restriction/pain may suggest blow-out fracture)	0	1	2
Checks visual acuity with a Snellen chart (suggests use of pinhole camera)	0	1	—
Checks for peripheral visual field defects	0	1	—
Performs fundoscopy appropriately and checks the red reflex	0	1	—
Suggests a slit-lamp examination with fluorescein staining to look for ulcers/abrasions	0	1	—
States intention to test colour vision with an Ishihara chart	0	1	—
Checks tetanus status if there is a contaminated wound	0	1	—
Arranges appropriate imaging (facial views to exclude blow-out fracture) Recognizes signs on a plain film	0	1	—
Makes referral to maxillofacial surgeon Gives head injury advice prior to discharge	0	1	—
Score from patient	/5		
Global score from examiner	/5		
Total score	/26		

11
Ear, Nose and Throat Conditions
SHUMONTHA DEV

CORE TOPICS

- History, examination and investigation of patients presenting with ear, nose and throat (ENT) problems, ensuring appropriate treatment and referral.
- Painful ear: otitis media, otitis externa, cholesteatoma, perforated tympanic membrane, mastoiditis
- Epistaxis
- Sore throat: epiglottitis, Ludwig's angina, tonsillitis, pre-tonsillar abscess
- Retropharyngeal abscess
- Foreign bodies
- Other problems: causes of vertigo, salivary gland problems, sinusitis, facial pain, VII nerve palsy, laceration to ear, post-tonsillectomy bleed
- Traumatic ear conditions in children
- Earache or discharge in children

SCENARIO 11.1: ACUTE OTITIS MEDIA

A 6-year-old boy is brought by his parents to the emergency department with pain in his right ear. You are asked to take a full history from the parents and to examine the ear on the model provided. You are also asked to provide a differential diagnosis and outline your management plan.

SUGGESTED APPROACH

Introduce yourself to the child and his parents appropriately. Explain that you need to ask some questions and examine the child before determining how best to proceed. Offer analgesia if appropriate.

The key to this type of station is to have a good rapport with the child as well as the parents, and it is worth spending a few seconds interacting with the child so that the examination does not come across as a frightening procedure. Explain to the parents and the child what you are going to do; this will vary according to the age of the child. It is important to have a calm and reassuring approach to your examination, since there will be marks from the parents on how you come across. If the child is not cooperating, do not be forceful or persistent.

The history should elicit the duration, site, nature, characteristics and radiation of the pain. Ask about fever, deafness, irritability, any discharge and its nature. Note any previous episodes and how they have been managed (e.g. antibiotic treatment or grommet insertion). You should also ask about activities such as swimming and whether the parents use cotton buds to clean the ears. You should also ask about aller... ...inations and other ENT conditions such as tonsillitis ...

It is often a ... ... lay with it while you explain what you are ... ...much smoother.

Examination ... ...h the parent's arms embracing th ... ...on yourself to one side and ensure that y ... ...ears (post-auricular and endaural scar...

In adults, the ... ...raighten the bend. In infants, pull t ... ...sential that you talk to the child and reas ... ...chniques. You should look at the good ea ... ...ikely to be painful.

Insert the larg... ... in turn. Identify the pars tensa, the ... ...that points to the toes (Fig... 11.1) ... e. In addition, look for a per...

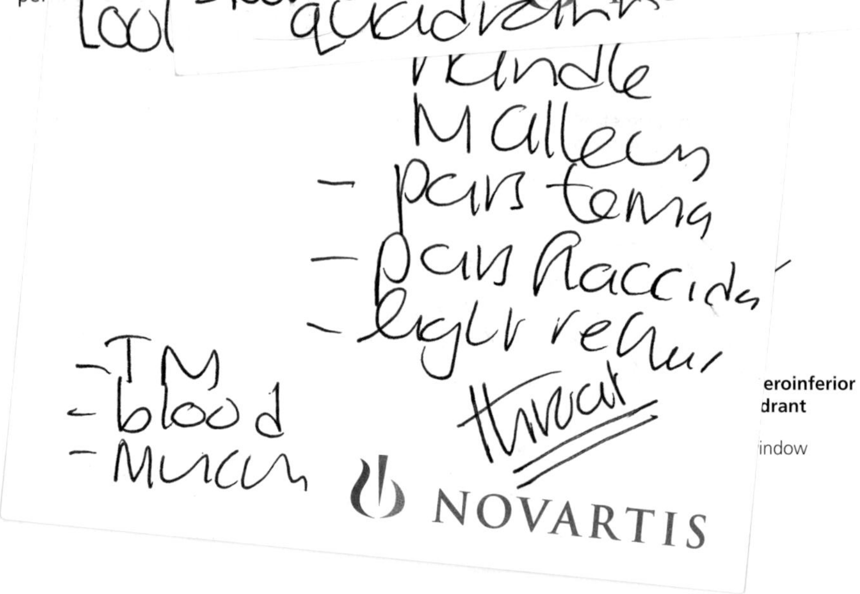

Handwritten notes:

Otoscope
- familiar
- objectives
- check equip
- dim, child o mum
- position,
- child - down & back
- adult - up & back.
- look @ all @
  accidents
- handle
  Mallens
- pars tens
- pars flaccida
- light refl.
Throat

- TM
- blood
- Mucus

NOVARTIS

NOVARTIS

...eroinferior
...drant

...indow

Figure 11.1 Normal tympanic membrane.

Continue your ENT examination by examining the mastoid region for swelling and tenderness. You should get into the habit of examining the oral cavity as a routine part of your assessment. The throat may appear inflamed in the presence of an upper respiratory tract infection (URTI). Poor dentition is a common cause of earache, and you should have a cursory look at the teeth. If the child is cooperative and not distressed, you should continue to examine the regional lymph nodes for lymphadenopathy.

State that you would like to complete the examination with free-field voice testing and tuning-fork tests, although this can be challenging in a 6-year-old!

Differential diagnoses

There are many causes of ear pain. The cause is non-otological in 50% of cases. Pain is referred from other sources, for example from infections of the pharynx and from dental abscesses.

Otitis externa

In otitis externa, there is discharge and tragal tenderness due to acute inflammation of the skin of the meatus from moisture, trauma, high humidity, absence of wax, a narrow ear canal or hearing aids. *Pseudomonas* is often the organism involved, and the condition is often seen in swimmers. Aural toilet is the mainstay of treatment.

Furunculosis of the external ear

In furunculosis of the external ear, hair follicle infection in the outer third of the ear causes severe pain. Examination shows a localized inflamed swelling. Treatment is with analgesia and antibiotics.

Acute otitis media

Acute otitis media is most common in the 3–6-year age group and may follow a URTI. *Streptococcus pneumoniae* and *Haemophilus influenzae* are the most common pathogens. Treatment is with oral analgesia and antibiotics (e.g. amoxicillin or erythromycin), although their efficacy is debated. If symptoms have persisted for several days, it is reasonable to start antibiotics. If there is perforation, ENT follow-up is arranged and swimming should be avoided.

Acute mastoiditis

Acute mastoiditis is now uncommon, but it must be considered in view of the risk of intracranial infection. It is an unusual complication of acute otitis media. There is pain, redness, swelling, bogginess or tenderness over the mastoid process. This needs urgent ENT referral for admission and antibiotics.

Cholesteatoma

Cholesteatoma is an erosive condition that affects the middle ear and mastoid and can result in life-threatening intracranial infection. The resultant discharge is offensive, and severe cases result in conductive hearing loss with vertigo and facial nerve palsy. There is granulation tissue and possible perforation of the tympanic membrane, with visible white debris. The patient needs referral to ENT for further management.

Traumatic tympanic membrane rupture

The tympanic membrane may be ruptured as a result of direct penetrating injury, blunt injury or basal skull fracture. The rupture is painful and is associated with decreased hearing. Perforation is visible on examination. Most cases heal with conservative measures, including analgesia and oral antibiotics. ENT follow-up is needed.

Barotrauma

In barotrauma, there is pain and hearing loss, with fluid behind the tympanic membrane from sudden changes in atmospheric pressure when the eustachian tube is blocked. Usually, this resolves spontaneously with analgesia.

Scoring Scenario 11.1: Acute otitis media

	Inadequate/ not done	Adequate	Good
Appropriate introduction	0	1	—
Develops rapport with parent and child	0	1	—
Offers analgesia	0	1	—
Focused history about complaint: • onset and duration of symptoms • characteristics of pain • radiation • dicharge (pus/blood) • fever • deafness • features of URTI • swimming/cotton-bud use • childhood vaccinations • previous ENT complaints • allergies • medications	0	1	2
Explains procedure to child and parent appropriately according to age of child	0	1	—
Engages child using distraction/play therapy	0	1	—
Positions child appropriately on parent's lap	0	1	—
States intention to look at good ear first	0	1	—
Holds the otoscope and ear correctly, maintaining finger guard	0	1	—
Uses otoscope to examine the ear on the model appropriately	0	1	—
Correctly describes findings	0	1	2
Maintains rapport with child throughout the examination	0	1	—
States intention to examine: • throat • lymph nodes • teeth	0	1	2
Offers differential diagnosis: • acute otitis media • otitis externa • traumatic perforation	0	1	2
Outlines management plan to parents and child	0	1	—
Encourages questions	0	1	—
Arranges appropriate follow-up and advice on swimming/use of cotton buds/antibiotics	0	1	—
Score from parents	**/5**		
Global score from examiner	**/5**		
Total score	**/31**		

SCENARIO 11.2: ACUTE EPISTAXIS

A 60-year-old man presents to the emergency department with epistaxis. As the emergency department registrar, you are asked to take a focused history and describe the possible management options available (demonstrate on the manikin as appropriate).

His observations are:

Temperature 36.5 °C
Pulse 92 bpm, irregular
BP 164/102 mmHg

SUGGESTED APPROACH

As always, approach the patient by introducing yourself and explaining the task that you are about to undertake. Confirm the patient's name and obtain his consent to proceed.

Management begins quickly with the principles of basic first aid. The patient should be sitting up with their head tilted downwards to prevent blood trickling backwards. A firm pressure is applied on the cartilaginous nose using finger and thumb for 10–15 minutes (Trotter's method).

You should assess for shock and resuscitate as needed, and place two large-bore intravenous cannulae. Bloods should also be sent to check the haemoglobin level and the INR if the patient is on warfarin. A postural drop in blood pressure can also indicate significant blood loss.

A focused history should try and establish the likely cause. Remember that epistaxis is the most common ENT emergency and is potentially fatal. Ask about minor trauma such as nose picking, isolated nose injury, history of hypertension and coagulation disorders, and use of non-steroidal anti-inflammatory drugs (NSAIDs) and anticoagulants. Septal perforation and, rarely, neoplasms can be a cause. Other rare causes to consider include hepatic coagulopathy, leukaemia, malaria, typhoid and Osler–Weber–Rendu syndrome (hereditary haemorrhagic telangiectasia).

Most epistaxis is from blood vessels on the nasal septum. The bleeding is from Little's area, where there is convergence of the anterior and posterior ethmoidal arteries, the septal branches of the sphenopalatine arteries, the superior labial arteries, and the greater palatine artery. From middle age onwards, the bleeding sites move posteriorly.

Then examine the nose. Direct visualization is the key to treatment. Anterior bleeds are easily seen with rhinoscopy and are generally simpler to treat. Always check the oropharynx, since bleeding may still be identifiable along the posterior wall. You should use a Thudicum speculum and preferably a head light to inspect the nasal mucosa for a bleeding point. Alternatively, you can raise the nasal tip with your thumb to visualize the source of the bleed.

Management of anterior epistaxis

Remove any clots gently with suction.

Insert a cotton-wool pledget (e.g. a Merocel tampon) soaked in lidocaine with adrenaline into the nostril, along the floor of the nose, and leave for 5 minutes.

Anterior bleeding that is clearly visible can be cauterized with silver nitrate sticks. This is done with application of firm pressure to and around the bleeding site for 10 seconds. Ensure that both sides of the septum are not cauterized and avoid excessive cautery. If cautery is successful, the patient can be discharged with advice to avoid sniffing, picking or blowing the nose.

If bleeding persists, a nasal pack consisting of 1.25 cm-wide ribbon gauze soaked in oily paste (e.g. bismuth iodoform paraffin paste) can be inserted. Nasal packs that have the effect of tamponading the bleed are commercially available.

These patients will need admission under the ENT team for observation to ensure that airway obstruction does not occur.

Management of major or posterior epistaxis

In major epistaxis, the bleeding site is likely to be posterior, and bleeding can be rapid, causing hypovolaemic shock. Therefore, resuscitate as appropriate.

In this situation, access is difficult and the bleeding is not localizable by anterior rhinoscopy. The gold standard treatment for posterior epistaxis is with endoscopy and bipolar cautery under the ENT team.

If the bleeding site cannot be found, a 16G or 18G Foley catheter can be passed through the nostril into the nasopharynx, inflated with 10 mL sterile water and then pulled forward until it lodges to close off the posterior choanae. Refer to the ENT team for further management.

Packing is left for 48 hours, and therefore the patient should be admitted and monitored. Infections and hypoxia are well-known complications, but infarcts, strokes and death have also been reported.

Persistent posterior epistaxis can be treated by examination under anaesthesia and endoscopic ligation of the maxillary/sphenopalatine artery around the sphenopalatine foramen.

Any coagulopathy should be corrected appropriately. A raised INR can be reversed either by omitting the next dose of warfarin or, if there is active bleeding, by giving vitamin K or fresh frozen plasma (FFP). Patients who have frequent episodes of epistaxis secondary to high blood pressure should have a review of the medical management of their blood pressure.

Scoring Scenario 11.2: Acute epistaxis

	Inadequate/ not done	Adequate	Good
Appropriate introduction	0	1	—
Performs first aid to arrest bleeding, assesses ABC and treats shock appropriately	0	1	—
Secures IV access and checks bloods (FBC/INR/group and save)	0	1	—
Focused history about complaint: • onset and duration of symptoms • characteristics of bleed • bright/dark blood • history of epistaxis • blood plus pus suggests infection/malignancy • history of high blood pressure • history of bleeding disorders/liver impairment • trauma • medications (aspirin/warfarin/antihypertensives)	0	1	2
Examines nasal mucosa appropriately using Thudicum speculum	0	1	2
Suggests removal of clots with suction/nose blowing	0	1	—
Identifies bleed in Little's area	0	1	—
States intention to cauterize chemically with silver nitrate if a bleeding point is identified	0	1	—
Suggests packing an anterior bleed with nasal packs (needs admission post packing)	0	1	—
Suggests use of Foley catheter for posterior bleeds	0	1	—
Suggests correction of any coagulopathy if appropriate: • vitamin K to reverse INR • specific clotting factors • FFP • platelet transfusion	0	1	2
Makes urgent ENT referral	0	1	—
Suggests treating hypertension	0	1	—
Score from patient	/5		
Global score from examiner	/5		
Total score	/26		

12

Maxillofacial Emergencies

CHETAN R TRIVEDY

CORE TOPICS

Maxillofacial trauma

- Nasal fractures
- Le Fort classification of maxillary fractures
- Mandibular fractures
- Zygomatic fractures
- Temporomandibular joint dislocation
- Tongue lacerations
- Soft tissue injuries

Dental emergencies

- Dental anatomy
- Dental abscesses
- Avulsed permanent teeth
- Post-extraction complications
- Dental nerve blocks

Maxillofacial and dental injuries are common presentations seen in the emergency department. Although the majority of emergency department trainees receive no formal training on how to manage these types of emergencies, this area is included in the CEM curriculum and hence can be tested in the examinations. The detailed management of specific dental/maxillofacial injuries is beyond the remit of this book, and you are advised to contact your local maxillofacial unit for local guidelines.

SCENARIO 12.1: MAXILLOFACIAL INJURY

As the registrar on duty, you are asked to review a 45-year-old man who has been assaulted with a baseball bat. Carry out an examination of his maxillofacial system and outline your management plan. You are not expected to take a history.

SUGGESTED APPROACH

You may be faced with a simulated patient, and have approximately 7 minutes to conduct a thorough examination of the maxillofacial system. As with all emergencies, it is essential that the primary survey be reviewed, and this should form the starting point of your examination. The airway/C-spine control, breathing, circulation and GCS should be assessed and managed appropriately before you conduct a detailed survey of the facial skeleton.

It is essential that you introduce yourself to the patient and explain the procedure that you are about to undertake. Some of the examination may be uncomfortable for the patient, and it is useful to provide analgesia as appropriate before you examine them.

Examine the scalp for any lacerations. You should also feel for the presence of any swellings or irregularities. A soft 'boggy' haematoma may be indicative of a skull fracture and should be investigated with appropriate imaging.

Palpate the supraorbital ridges for any bony tenderness or step deformities. Crepitus or surgical emphysema in this area suggests a fracture involving the nasoethmoidal complex or the roof of the orbit. You should proceed to examine for any sensory loss in the distribution of the supraorbital nerve.

A detailed ophthalmological examination is an essential part of the assessment. You should start by looking for any signs of asymmetry and widening of the intracanthal distance. Each eyelid should be everted and examined for abrasions, foreign bodies and lacerations.

A formal test of visual acuity should be carried out as part of the assessment. This should be followed by checking the pupillary and accommodation reflexes and examining for visual field defects. Cranial nerves II, III, IV and VI should be assessed; the presence of ophthalmoplegia may represent a traumatic injury either to the brain or to the nerves as they pass through the orbit. Entrapment or snagging of the rectus muscles in orbital floor fractures may also result in diplopia.

The globe should be inspected for trauma or penetrating injuries; if these are suspected, you should proceed to conduct a slit-lamp examination after administering local anaesthetic eye drops and fluorescein dye. All penetrating injuries to the globe should be referred to an ophthalmologist for specialist management.

The nasal complex should be examined carefully, looking for any obvious asymmetry, swelling, epistaxis, rhinorrhea and the presence of a cerebrospinal fluid leak. The nasal cavities should be examined with a good light source and nasal prongs for septal haematomas.

The ears should be examined with an otoscope, looking for any disruption to the tympanic membrane and the presence of blood in the middle ear. These may be due to a fracture of the base of the skull and may warrant further imaging. You should also look for bruising behind the ears, which is referred to as Battle's sign, which results from blood accumulating beneath the skin around the tip of the mastoid process. Although this is also often quoted as another sign suggestive of a fracture of the base of the skull, it is a relatively late sign, since it takes time for the blood to accumulate and so may not appear for several days following the injury.

The zygomaticomaxillary complex should be inspected, looking for any asymmetry or flattening of the zygomatic arch. This should be followed by gently palpating the infraorbital rim for a step deformity. This is often difficult to demonstrate when there is swelling of the overlying periorbital tissues.

Check for the presence of paraesthesia in the cheek, signifying potential trauma to the infraorbital nerve as it leaves the infraorbital foramen. Ask the patient if they have any numbness in the cheek, anterior teeth or upper lip. A displaced fracture involving the zygomatic arch may also interfere with the coronoid process of the mandible, resulting in a restriction in normal mouth opening.

Fractures of the midface have classically been referred to as Le Fort fractures:

- **Le Fort I:** The fracture extends in a plane parallel to the upper teeth, passing horizontally above the roots of the upper teeth. The patient may complain of an inability to bite their teeth together or that they have loose teeth. When the anterior teeth are grasped with thumb and forefinger, the palatal arch can be felt to move.

- **Le Fort II:** This is also referred to as a pyramidal fracture. It extends from the nasal bridge through to the frontal process of the maxilla and the infraorbital margin. It also extends laterally, involving the zygomatic arch and the pterygoids.

- **Le Fort III:** This is the most severe of the midface fractures. It is a craniofacial fracture in a plane that separates the maxilla from the base of the skull. The fracture usually extends posteriorly from the bridge of the nose through the orbit, ethmoid and sphenoid bones.

The temporomandibular joint (TMJ) should be examined using an extra- and intraoral approach. The joint should be palpated by placing your hands in front of the ears while you ask the patient to open and close their mouth.

An inability to open the mouth (trismus) suggests trauma to the TMJ or to the condylar head of the mandible or a displaced fracture of the zygomatic arch. Also look for any deviation in the excursion of the mandible during opening and closing. Feel for any clicks and crepitus during mouth opening. You should be aware that pain from the TMJ can be referred to several places, including the ear, eye, head, mandible and neck. Tenderness over the masseter and lateral pterygoids may also indicate a traumatic injury to the TMJ. Masseteric spasm can be elicited by placing a gloved finger between the upper posterior molars and the cheek. The patient is then asked to clench their teeth together. If this elicits pain, it may signify joint pathology.

A thorough inspection of the oral cavity should be carried out, paying special attention to any soft tissue trauma and traumatic injuries to the dentition. The emergency physician should have a basic understanding of adult and paediatric dental anatomy. The eruption dates of permanent and deciduous teeth are shown in Table 12.1.

Table 12.1 Eruption dates of permanent and deciduous teeth

Permanent maxillary teeth		Eruption dates	Deciduous maxillary teeth		Eruption dates
1	Central incisor	7–8 years	A	Central incisor	8–12 months
2	Lateral incisor	8–9 years	B	Lateral incisor	9–13 months
3	Canine	11–12 years	C	Canine	16–22 months
4	First premolar	10–11 years	D	First molar	13–19 months
5	Second premolar	10–12 years	E	Second molar	25–33 months
6	First molar	6–7 years			
7	Second molar	12–13 years			
8	Third molar	17–21 years			
Permanent mandibular teeth		Eruption dates	Deciduous mandibular teeth		Eruption dates
1	Central incisor	6–7 years	A	Central incisor	6–10 months
2	Lateral incisor	8–9 years	B	Lateral incisor	10–16 months
3	Canine	11–12 years	C	Canine	17–23 months
4	First premolar	10–11 years	D	First molar	14–18 months
5	Second premolar	10–12 years	E	Second molar	23–31 months
6	First molar	6–7 years			
7	Second molar	12–13 years			
8	Third molar	17–21 years			

Examination of occlusion (bite) is a crucial part of the assessment, since a change in the patient's bite may suggest a shift in the tooth-bearing part of the maxilla or mandible. This sign is quite subtle, and most patients will complain that their teeth do not meet the way they used to. Look for a new cross-bite, premature contacts or a step deformity in the occlusion. The teeth should also be examined for any cracks or shearing injuries.

The soft tissues of the oral cavity should be examined carefully under direct lighting, paying particular attention to the presence of any lacerations or tears over the opening of the major salivary glands in the floor of the mouth (submandibular and sublingual glands) and in the cheek adjacent to the upper first molar (parotid gland). If these are missed, they often heal with scarring, resulting in salivary gland obstruction.

Look for any bruising or laceration around the chin. In the presence of limited mouth opening and a painful bite, this is suggestive of a 'guardsman's fracture' – so-called because of the mechanism of injury. Any direct impact on the symphysis menti will result in a fracture of the mandible at three sites: the midline and one or both condylar heads. The resulting triad presents as a patient who has a limited opening, with bruising or laceration on the chin and tenderness around the lower anterior teeth.

You should complete the examination by making a visual inspection of the patient's neck, looking for any bruising, puncture marks or tenderness over the thyroid cartilage and trachea, which may be indicative of trauma to the airways.

The management and the appropriate imaging in the emergency department are summarized in Table 12.2.

Table 12.2 Imaging and management of common facial fractures

Injury	Imaging	Management
Isolated undisplaced zygomatic fracture	• Occipitomental 15° and 30° views	• Soft diet • No nose blowing • Analgesia • Maxillofacial outpatients review • Head injury advice sheet • Tetanus cover if appropriate
Complex fractures involving the floor of the orbit	• Occipitomental 15° and 30° views. CT of facial skeleton, with 3D reconstruction	• Ophthalmology review • Urgent maxillofacial review • Tetanus cover if appropriate • Admit under specialist team with neurological observations
Nasal complex injury	• No imaging in the emergency department	• Nasal tampons to treat epistaxis • Analgesia • Tetanus cover if appropriate • Head injury advice sheet • Avoid nose blowing • Discharge with ENT follow-up unless you detect a septal haematoma
Injury to base of skull	• CT head	• Neurosurgical referral • Admit under specialist team • Neurological observations • Antibiotics • Tetanus cover if appropriate
Le Fort fractures	• CT face	• These are serious midface injuries and there is a risk of airway compromise • Senior anaesthetic opinion • Urgent maxillofacial opinion • Admission in preparation for surgery • Tetanus cover if appropriate
Undisplaced mandibular fracture	• An orthopantomogram (OPG) is the X-ray of choice for all mandibular fractures. • If an OPG is not available, posteroanterior (PA) mandible and lateral oblique views are useful	• Soft diet • Antibiotics if there is an open fracture • Analgesia • Outpatient follow-up with maxillofacial surgeons • Head injury advice sheet • Oral hygiene instructions • Tetanus cover if appropriate
Displaced mandibular fracture	• OPG • PA mandible • Lateral oblique view • CT face for comminuted fractures	• Secure airway if there is a bilateral mandibular fracture • Urgent referral to maxillofacial team for reduction and plating • Soft diet and antibiotics • Tetanus cover if appropriate
TMJ injury	• OPG • PA mandible/lateral oblique • No indication for TMJ views	• Soft diet • Maxillofacial OPD review • Analgesia

Scoring Scenario 12.1: Maxillofacial injury

	Inadequate/ not done	Adequate	Good
Appropriate introduction	0	1	—
Asks about pain; offers analgesia and obtains verbal consent	0	1	—
States intention to wash hands and glove-up	0	1	—
Examines scalp	0	1	—
Examines orbital margins	0	1	—
Rapid assessment of visual acuity: • asks about visual acuity • asks about diplopia	0	1	2
Examines nasal complex for stability and septal haematoma	0	1	—
Examines the TMJ and looks for Battle's sign	0	1	—
States intention to conduct an internal examination of the ear	0	1	—
Ascertains whether there is any: • trismus • change in occlusion • maxillary/mandibular bony tenderness • maxillary/mandibular deformity • sensory loss over the face	0	1	2
Examines the oral cavity for soft tissue trauma or evidence of dental trauma	0	1	—
Makes a working diagnosis from the clinical signs	0	1	—
Asks for appropriate imaging	0	1	—
Constructs an appropriate treatment plan	0	1	—
Arranges appropriate follow-up	0	1	—
Conducts examination in a fluent and logical manner	0	1	—
Score from patient	/5		
Global score from examiner	/5		
Total score	/28		

13
Obstetrics and Gynaecology
FRANCESCA GARNHAM

CORE TOPICS

Gynaecology

- Ectopic pregnancy
- Endometriosis
- Complications of ovarian/corpus luteum cysts
- Pelvic inflammatory disease (PID) – diagnostic criteria
- Ovarian torsion
- Fibroids and their complications
- Dysmenorrhoea
- Menorrhagia
- Postmenopausal vaginal bleeding
- Cervicitis
- Vaginal prolapse
- Bartholin's abscess
- Emergency contraception
- Sexual assault – forensic evidence, follow-up (i.e. STD screening)
- Skills: pelvic and speculum examination, including relevant swabs

Obstetrics

- Normal anatomical and physiological changes in pregnancy
- Inevitable abortion
- Missed abortion
- Threatened abortion
- Ectopic pregnancy
- Abruptio placentae
- Placenta praevia
- Radiology in pregnancy
- Anti-D
- HELLP
- Eclampsia
- Management of disseminated intravascular coagulation
- Trauma in pregnancy
- Emergency delivery and management of common complications
- Skills: management of haemorrhagic shock (including uterine displacement), use of Pinard stethoscope/Doppler ultrasound, resuscitation of newborn

Scoring Scenario 13.4: Emergency contraception

	Inadequate/ not done	Adequate	Good
Appropriate introduction	0	1	—
Ascertains who is accompanying the patient	0	1	—
Offers a chaperone if the patient is alone	0	1	—
Explains that questions may be personal	0	1	—
Reassures patient about confidentiality	0	1	—
Ascertains history around sexual intercourse: • Consensual? • Influencing factors (drugs or alcohol)? • Age of partner? • Casual or long-term relationship? • Establishes that penetrative vaginal intercourse took place • Was protection used? • Time since intercourse?	0	1	2
Takes a menstrual history: • last menstrual period • usual form of contraception • previous pregnancies, ectopic pregnancies, miscarriages or terminations	0	1	2
Takes a focused sexual history	0	1	2
Ascertains whether the patient is competent to consent to treatment (Gillick competency, Fraser guidelines)	0	1	2
Excludes contraindications to emergency oral contraceptive pill (EOCP): • porphyria (absolute) • liver disease • inflammatory bowel disease • >120 h since unprotected vaginal intercourse	0	1	—
Explains rationale and how to take EOCP	0	1	—
Explains side-effects (vomiting, breast tenderness, irregular periods)	0	1	—
Discusses use of IUCD if >120 h (mentions side-effects such as PID)	0	1	—
Arranges follow-up with GP/family planning clinic/sexual health clinic	0	1	—
Addresses any child protection issues and liaises with paediatrics/ social services	0	1	—
Suggests resources that may provide support	0	1	—
Is non-judgemental and has good rapport with patient	0	1	—
Score from patient	/5		
Global score from examiner	/5		
Total score	/31		

14
Respiratory Emergencies
BETH CHRISTIAN AND CHETAN R TRIVEDY

CORE TOPICS

Asthma

- Pathophysiology of asthma
- Medical management and magnesium

Spontaneous pneumothorax

- Primary and secondary causes
- Management

Pulmonary embolism

- Causes and risk factors
- Differential diagnosis
- Severity stratification, investigation and treatment

Chronic obstructive pulmonary disease

- NICE guidelines for management of acute exacerbations of COPD
- Medical therapy: oxygen and drug therapy
- Management of type II (hypercapnic) respiratory failure
- Principles of non-invasive ventilation

Pneumonia

- Community-acquired pneumonia
- Recognition of severity of pneumonia

Respiratory failure

- Identification of causes of respiratory failure and knowledge of appropriate investigations
- Indications for ventilation:
  - Medical therapy
  - Non-invasive ventilation
  - Invasive ventilation

Other topics

- Aspiration pneumonia
- Acute lung injury
- Pleural effusion
- Foreign-body inhalation

- Haemoptysis
- Presentation of tuberculosis, neoplasia and lung abscess

Respiratory emergencies make up a key component of the CEM syllabus and this topic is examined across the board in all parts of the CEM examinations. It is essential that you be familiar with the latest British Thoracic Society (BTS) guidelines on the topics listed above (see the list at the end of this chapter).

SCENARIO 14.1: SEVERE ASTHMA

You are asked to attend a priority call in the resuscitation area. The patient is a 33-year-old man with difficulty in breathing.

His initial observations are:

GCS 11
RR 12 breaths min^{-1}
Oxygen saturation 92% on 15 L of O_2
HR 120 bpm
BP 90/65 mmHg

The expected time of arrival is 2 minutes. Prepare your team, consisting of a senior emergency department nurse and an F2. Take the handover from the ambulance crew and outline your management of this priority call.

This is a three-part OSCE that essentially tests your ability to organize your team for a priority call, take an effective handover from a fellow health care professional, and identify and treat a potentially life-threatening respiratory emergency.

SUGGESTED APPROACH

Preparation for the priority call

The key to approaching this OSCE is to be able to appreciate how unwell this patient is and that a patient who has a saturation of 92% on 100% oxygen and a respiratory rate of 12 breaths min^{-1} is not far from respiratory arrest. With this in mind, you should use your 2 minutes before the patient arrives to prepare your team and equipment and get any other help that you may require.

Preparation

In the time that you have before the patient arrives, find out who you have in your team and what their background is. Given the gravity of the initial observations, it is likely that this patient may need intubating, so it is worth bleeping the on-call anaesthetist to attend.

Check the oxygen, bag–valve mask and suction equipment. Ask the emergency department nurse to check and lay out the airway trolley and warn them in advance that they may need to prepare the drugs for a rapid sequence induction (RSI).

For all priority calls, as the team leader you should allocate roles for your team so that each member knows clearly what their role is.

In this scenario, since the airway and breathing are compromised, it may be advisable for you as the team leader to deal with the airway and breathing until anaesthetic assistance arrives. You could ask the nurse to put on the monitoring and get the drugs ready, which would leave the F2 to assess the circulation and secure intravenous access.

Taking handover

'Mr Smith is a 33-year-old asthmatic who has had flu-like symptoms for three days. He is unable to speak and has a quiet chest. The ambulance crew state that he has deteriorated en route to hospital. The history given to them by the patient on scene was that he had been using his puffers for the last two days without effect. He has had two previous admissions to hospital, including once where he was put to sleep. He has received 5 milligrams of salbutamol and 500 micrograms of ipratropium bromide via a nebulizer'

Taking a handover from other health care professionals is an important test of communication and assimilating key information that will allow you to treat the life-threatening emergency. Listen to the handover while one member of your team scribes down the important points and the other puts the patient on oxygen and organizes the monitoring.

Do not interrupt or talk over the ambulance crew while they are handing over. Remember to thank the crew for their help.

Initial management

This patient has severe life-threatening asthma, as evidenced by his oxygen saturation of 92%, silent chest, reduced conscious state and reduced respiratory effort.

Immediate medical management should include the following:

- high-flow oxygen according to the BTS guidelines on oxygen delivery (see below)
- salbutamol 5 mg immediately via back-to-back oxygen-driven nebulizers (note that intravenous salbutamol should only be used if inhaled therapy cannot be administered)
- steroids: intravenous hydrocortisone 100 mg immediately
- ipratropium bromide 500 µg 4–6-hourly with salbutamol
- magnesium sulphate: a single dose of 1.2–2 g intravenously over 20 minutes should be given to patients with severe asthma not responding to initial treatment
- intravenous fluids (note that potassium replacement may be required following salbutamol and steroid treatment)

Ask for an arterial blood gas and a portable chest X-ray, Arrange for old hospital notes if available.

If possible, get a history from the patient. Depending on the severity, this may not be possible.

Arrange for anaesthetic/ITU cover to intubate and ventilate the patient.

Explain the treatment to the patient and reassure them.

BTS guidelines on oygen delivery

You should be aware of the 2008 BTS guidelines on emeregency oxygen:

- All patients who are critically ill or peri-arrest should receive high-flow oxygen via a reservoir mask at 15 L min^{-1}.
- Patients who are stable should receive oxygen to achieve an oxygen saturation of 94–98%, or 88–92% in patients with chronic obstructive pulmonary disease (COPD).
- You should also make sure that the oxygen is appropriately prescribed on the chart and you should ask the nurses to adjust the oxygen given according to the levels.

Ventilation issues in severe asthma

Patients with severe life-threatening asthma may require invasive ventilation when they become exhausted and are unable to adequately maintain oxygenation and ventilation. This patient shows evidence of exhaustion, with his reduced conscious state and reduced respiratory effort. The main issues are as follows.

In RSI, care should be used in choosing the anaesthetic and paralyzing agents. The key is to avoid drugs that have the potential to induce histamine release and therefore exacerbate bronchospasm, namely

- morphine
- propofol
- atracurium

Agents that facilitate bronchodilation are preferred:

- ketamine, which is a potent bronchodilator and cardiovascular-stable agent
- inhalational anaesthetic, i.e. halothane
- pancuronium
- adrenaline

Ventilation parameters should be as follows:

- prolonged I:E ratio, i.e. 1:3
- low respiratory rate to allow for the prolonged expiratory time
- normal to low tidal volumes according to peak inspiratory pressures
- a pressure-limited mode of ventilation if available

Once a patient has been intubated, their $PaCO_2$ becomes of less importance and there should be no rush to correct it. The limiting factor is the patient's pH, since once this has become less than 7.10, they are more susceptible to cardiovascular instability.

Sudden falls in blood pressure should alert the clinician to potential barotrauma or venous return obstruction secondary to hyperinflation. Tension pneumothorax must be excluded and the patient removed from the ventilator to allow chest decompression to occur.

The patient in this scenario clearly warrants an ITU admission in line with the BTS guidelines (Table 14.1), and you should also inform the ITU registrar on call.

Table 14.1 Initial assessment of acute asthma and criteria for ITU admission according to BTS guidelines

Moderate exacerbation	Acute severe	Life-threatening	Near-fatal
• Worsening of symptoms • PEFR > 50–75% of best or predicted • No features of acute severe asthma	**Any one of:** • PEFR 33–50% of best or predicted • RR ≥ 25 breaths min^{-1} • Inability to complete sentence in one breath • Heart rate > 110 bpm	**Any one of:** • PEFR < 33% • SpO_2 < 92% • Normal $PaCO_2$ (4–6 kPa) • Silent chest • Cyanosis • Feeble respiratory effort • Bradycardia • Hypotension • Exhaustion • Confusion • Coma	• Raised $PaCO_2$ • Requiring mechanical ventilation
Criteria for admission to ITU • Any patient with life-threatening asthma or acute severe asthma who is not responding to therapy, as evidenced by worsening PEFR, increasing $PaCO_2$, increasing acidosis, exhaustion or confusion • Any patient who requires invasive ventilation			

PEFR, peak expiratory flow rate; RR, respiratory rate, SpO_2, peripheral oxygen saturation measured by pulse oximetry; $PaCO_2$, partial pressure of carbon dioxide in arterial blood.

Scoring Scenario 14.1: Severe asthma

	Inadequate/ not done	Adequate	Good
Prepares for the priority call: 1. Delegates roles 2. Checks airway trolley 3. Checks oxygen, bag–valve mask and suction 4. Asks for anaesthetic cover	0	1	2
Takes appropriate handover from ambulance crew: • Does not interrupt/talk over ambulance crew • Scribes points on board	0	1	—
Appropriate introduction	0	1	—
Performs a rapid assessment of ABCDE: A: Patent B: Silent chest, poor air entry C: Tachycardic and increased capillary refill D: GCS 11 E: Apyrexial	0	1	2
Appreciates that patient has life-threatening asthma and highlights features without prompting: • saturation of 92% on high-flow oxygen • reduced GCS • silent chest • reduced respiratory effort	0	1	2
Institutes immediate management: • high-flow oxygen according to BTS guidelines, prescribes oxygen • monitoring • salbutamol and ipratropium nebulizers • IV hydrocortisone • IV fluids • considers IV magnesium • ABG • portable chest X-ray • ECG • suggests placement of central line	0	1	2
Prepares for an RSI: 1. Asks for medications 2. Prepares equipment 3. ITU referral	0	1	2
Score from patient	**/5**		
Global score from examiner	**/5**		
Total score	**/22**		

SCENARIO 14.2: PNEUMOTHORAX

You are asked to see a 27-year-old man who has presented to the emergency department complaining of left-sided pleuritic chest pain and breathlessness.

His initial observations are:

Temperature 36.8 °C
Oxygen saturation 98% on air
RR 12 breaths min^{-1}
BP 110/76 mmHg
Pulse 90 bpm

Take an appropriate history and outline your investigations and management plan.

SUGGESTED APPROACH

The approach to this station is to take a focused history from a patient who is breathless and has pleuritic chest pain. You should start the examination by informing the examiner that you would repeat the observations and that if there were any deterioration you would act appropriately by moving the patient to an appropriate area and managing them accordingly. As the patient is stable, it would be prudent to continue with the history.

History

Features in the respiratory history to elicit include:
- history of onset of symptoms: acute versus chronic
- character of pain (sharp or dull); worse on inspiration
- radiation of pain
- exacerbating and relieving factors
- shortness of breath on exertion or at rest
- preceding coryzal symptoms
- any history of stress/anxiety or palpitations
- presence of productive or non-productive cough (colour of sputum)
- any recent travel, flights, immobilization or surgery
- family history of clotting disorders
- history of deep vein thrombosis
- social history: occupation/smoking/alcohol
- haemoptysis, weight loss, fever, night sweats or lymphadenopathy
- risk factors for immunosuppression: HIV/tuberculosis/*Pneumocystis* pneumonia
- history of previous chest trauma or fractured ribs
- previous history of pneumothorax
- history of asthma or chronic obstructive pulmonary disease (COPD)
- regular medications; oral contraceptive pill if female
- allergies/pets

Management

On concluding your history, you should outline your management plan:
- Oxygen should be given according to the BTS guidelines on oxygen therapy.
- Measure oxygen saturations.
- Provide intravenous access.
- An ECG may demonstrate changes of pulmonary embolism (PE).

- Examine the patient and look for reduced breath sounds (pneumothorax), consolidation or a wheeze.
- A chest X-ray will demonstrate a pneumothorax or areas of consolidation.
- If you suspect a PE and you have low pre-test probability, you can send for D-dimers (see Scenario 14.3).

Differential diagnosis

The differential diagnosis for a young apyrexial patient with pleuritic chest pain and breathlessness is:

- pneumothorax
- pulmonary embolism
- pneumonia

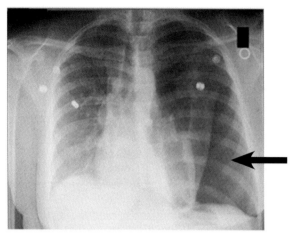

Figure 14.1 Chest X-ray of the patient in Scenario 14.2.

The chest X-ray of this patient (Figure 14.1) clearly demonstrates a left-sided pneumothorax.

BTS guidelines on the management of pneumothoraces

You should be familiar with the BTS guidelines on the management of pneumothoraces.

Clinical history and examination may suggest the presence of a pneumothorax, but they do not reliably correlate with the size of a pneumothorax. The BTS guidelines divide pneumothoraces into 'small' and 'large' depending upon the presence of a visible rim of <2 cm or >2 cm between the lung margin and the chest wall. A plain chest X-ray typically underestimates the size of a pneumothorax. As a rough estimate, a pneumothorax of 1 cm on a posteroanterior X-ray is equal to 27% and 2 cm is equal to 49%. Pneumothoraces can also be classified as primary or secondary: primary pneumothoraces are spontaneous with no underlying pathology, while secondary pneumothoraces are associated with underlying disease.

Treatment options

For small closed pneumothoraces, the treatment of choice is observation.

Patients with small (<2 cm) pneumothoraces not associated with breathlessness should be considered for discharge with early outpatient review. They must be provided with clear instructions to return if they become breathless.

If a patient is to be admitted overnight for observation, high-flow oxygen (10 L min^{-1}) should be administered unless contraindicated (i.e. in COPD). The rate of resolution/reabsorption of spontaneous pneumothoraces is 1.25–1.8% every 24 hours. A 15% pneumothorax would be expected to take 8–12 days to resolve fully. Oxygen administration increases the rate of reabsorption fourfold.

Breathless patients should not be left without intervention, regardless of the size of the pneumothorax. Simple aspiration is recommended as first-line treatment for all primary pneumothoraces requiring intervention. Successful re-expansion of the lung is less likely after simple aspiration of a secondary pneumothorax compared with a primary pneumothorax. Large secondary pneumothoraces (>2 cm), especially in patients over 50 years of age, should be considered at high risk for failure following simple aspiration, and chest drain insertion is therefore recommended.

Catheter aspiration of pneumothorax (CASP) will permit repeated aspirations without detriment to the patient in the event that the first aspiration fails to re-inflate the lung.

If, after two attempts, simple aspiration or CASP fails to re-inflate the lung of a symptomatic patient, an intercostal chest drain is required. You should be aware of the 2008 BTS guidance on the insertion of chest drains.

Chest drains are associated with a high complication rate of 18%. Fifteen percent of these complications are related to failure to resolve the pneumothorax. Incorrect tube placement, damage to major organs, infection (i.e. empyema) and surgical emphysema have all been reported.

The size of the intercostal drain is not thought to influence the effectiveness of pneumothorax resolution. A small (10–14F) chest drain should be used initially and should only be replaced by a large-calibre drain if a persistent air leak is present.

Chest drain suction should only be applied after 48 hours for persistent air leaks or failure of a pneumothorax to re-expand.

Scoring Scenario 14.2: Pneumothorax

	Inadequate/ not done	Adequate	Good
Appropriate introduction	0	1	—
Confirms observations	0	1	—
Asks about: • onset of symptoms • exacerbating factors • pleuritic chest pain • haemoptysis • history of spontaneous pneumothorax • previous history of chest trauma • history of asthma • other medical problems • medications • allergies • bleeding disorders • hobbies such as diving that might be affected by diagnosis of pneumothorax	0	1	2
Offers to conduct a full respiratory examination	0	1	—
Management: • oxygen according to BTS guidelines • chest X-ray • IV access • blood tests after reviewing chest X-ray	0	1	2
Offers differential diagnosis: • pneumothorax • pulmonary embolism • chest infection	0	1	—
Confirms pneumothorax on chest X-ray: >2 cm (large)	0	1	—
Correctly applies BTS guidelines on management	0	1	—
Advises that patient will no longer be able to dive	0	1	—
Score from patient	/5		
Global score from examiner	/5		
Total score	/21		

SCENARIO 14.3: DIAGNOSIS OF PULMONARY EMBOLISM

A 37-year-old woman presents to the emergency department complaining of right-sided pleuritic chest pain. She is breathless and appears very anxious. She has a swollen and tender left calf.

Her vital signs are:
Oxygen saturation 97% on room air
RR 16 breaths min^{-1}
Heart rate 105 bpm
BP 130/60 mmHg
She is afebrile

She is seen by the F2, who suspects that she may have a pulmonary embolism (PE). The F2 has requested a D-dimer test, which is negative, and a chest X-ray, which is normal. The F2 wishes to discharge the patient, but would like you to review the case. Take a focused history from the patient and explain to the F2 your rationale for the interpretation of the D-dimer results.

This OSCE tests not only your knowledge of the Wells pre-test probability score for using D-dimers to exclude a PE, but also your ability to take a focused respiratory history relevant to making a diagnosis of PE.

SUGGESTED APPROACH

A focused respiratory history should be taken (see Scenario 14.2), and you should ensure that you have asked about the risk factors for a PE. This information will allow you to formulate a Wells score for this patient.

Risk factors for PE

- recent (last 4 weeks) abdominal, pelvic or lower limb orthopaedic surgery
- recent immobilization
- splinting of lower limb in a cast
- previous history of deep vein thrombosis (DVT)/PE
- malignancy
- factor V Leiden, protein C, protein S , antithrombin deficiency
- family history of DVT/PE
- recent long-haul flight or long drive (e.g. long-distance lorry drivers)
- pregnancy or recent childbirth
- pelvic mass
- intravenous drug use
- recent femoral line
- medications: oral contraceptive pill/tamoxifen
- recent chemotherapy
- autoimmune disorders such as systemic lupus erythematosus (SLE)

The second part of this OSCE tests your understanding of the Wells score (Table 14.2). You should ask the FY2 what they know about the Wells score and pre-test probability (PTP). Depending on the risk factors that you confirm from the history, you should calculate the Wells score.

Table 14.2 Wells score for pre-test probability (PTP) of PE

Features	Score (points)
Clinical signs or symptoms of DVT (minimum of leg swelling and palpation of the deep leg veins)	3
Alternative diagnosis less likely than PE	3
Heart rate > 100 bpm	1.5
Immobilization or surgery in previous 4 weeks	1.5
Previous DVT or PE	1.5
Haemoptysis	1
Malignancy (at treatment, treated in the last 6 months or palliative)	1
Total score	
Score < 2 points = low PTP (1.6% chance of a PE) Score 2–6 points = moderate PTP (16.2% chance of PE) Score > 6 points = high PTP (37.5% chance of a PE)	

Assessing a patient's pre-test probability

It is crucial to make an assessment of a patient's risk of having a PE before embarking on any investigations. A PE may be reliably excluded in a 'low-risk' patient who has a negative D-dimer, but not if the risk is moderate or high.

From the information given, this patient would have a Wells score of 7.5 (she has a swollen, tender calf and tachycardia and an alternative diagnosis is less likely than a PE). Hence she has a high PTP and therefore cannot be discharged on the basis of her D-dimer result.

A low PTP with a negative D-dimer result can safely exclude a PE. The management of suspected PE with intermediate and high PTP is outlined in the algorithm shown in Figure 14.2. Those patients who have a low PTP should be started on prophylactic low-molecular-weight heparin (LMWH) only if the D-dimer test is positive. Those with an intermediate or high PTP should be commenced on LMWH while waiting for further investigations. Patients who have an intermediate or high PTP and who are unstable should be commenced on intravenous heparin, with a bolus of 10 000 units followed by an infusion or LMWH.

Investigations

Chest X-ray

The chest X-ray is often non-diagnostic, and is used more as a screen to exclude other pathology such as pneumonia or pneumothorax. There may be features that demonstrate hyperinflation, oligaemia in the upper zones and 'pruning' of hilar vessels, which may be suggestive of a proximal thrombus. If the chest X-ray is abnormal and further imaging is required, a ventilation/perfusion ($\dot{V}/\dot{Q}$) scan would of limited value, since it is difficult to interpret if there is pre-existing lung pathology. In these circumstances, it is better to request a computed tomography pulmonary angiogram (CTPA).

ECG interpretation

The ECG is a poor diagnostic test in diagnosing PE, but the following features may strengthen the support for a diagnosis of PE. The 12-lead ECG may show sinus tachycardia. Deep S waves in lead I suggesting a right bundle

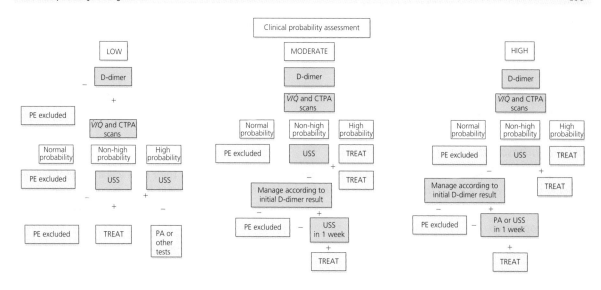

Figure 14.2 Decision algorithm for management of pulmonary embolism. $\dot{V}/\dot{Q}$, ventilation/perfusion; CTPA, computed tomography pulmonary angiography; USS, bilateral leg vein ultrasound scan; PA, pulmonary angiography.

branch block (RBBB), Q waves in lead III and T-wave inversion in lead III (S1Q3T3) are classical features of 'acute cor pulmonale' or 'right heart strain', but are not seen consistently. Poor R-wave progression across anterior–lateral leads and P-pulmonale suggestive of pulmonary hypertension also support a diagnosis of PE. These features are demonstrated in the ECG shown in Figure 14.3.

Imaging

$\dot{V}/\dot{Q}$ scans

As noted above, a $\dot{V}/\dot{Q}$ scan should not be performed unless the chest X-ray is normal. Also, there should be no significant cardiopulmonary disease. In low-PTP cases, a $\dot{V}/\dot{Q}$ scan should be performed only if the D-dimer test is positive. Moderate- to high-risk patients should have a $\dot{V}/\dot{Q}$ scan regardless of their D-dimer result.

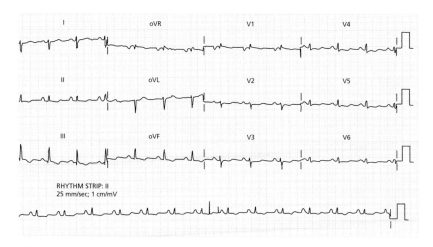

Figure 14.3 ECG showing features suggestive of pulmonary embolism.

Note that a negative $\dot{V}/\dot{Q}$ scan in a low- or moderate-risk patient reliably excludes PE, but does not do so for high-risk patients

CTPA

This is the recommended modality for non-massive PE. Patients with a good-quality negative CTPA will not require further investigation or treatment.

Bilateral ultrasound scan of the leg veins

This is recommended when the $\dot{V}/\dot{Q}$ scan is equivocal regardless of the PTP or when the PTP is low and the $\dot{V}/\dot{Q}$ scan is highly suggestive of a PE. If the ultrasound scan confirms a thrombus then treatment for PE is commenced.

Echocardiography

This is diagnostic in massive PE, but allows a firm diagnosis in only a minority of other PEs.

Classification of the severity of PE

PEs may be classified as follows:

- **massive PE**: haemodynamic instability and hypoxaemia
- **submassive PE**: tachycardia and mild hypoxaemia
- **minor PE**: normal oxygenation and cardiovascular state

Management
Supportive treatment

This comprises oxygen and intravenous fluids, plus inotropes if cardiovascular compromise is present.

Thrombolysis and embolectomy

Thrombolysis is recommended for massive PEs. Invasive approaches (i.e. thrombus fragmentation or inferior vena cava filter insertion) should be considered when available. Thrombolysis is not recommended for non-massive PEs.

Anticoagulation

Anticoagulation with LMWH is recommended for patients prior to imaging if the PTP is intermediate or high. Oral warfarin should only be commenced after diagnosis has been confirmed.

Action in the present case

You should explain to the F2 that the patient is not safe to be discharged and should be started on LWMH and have a chest X-ray. If this is normal, she should have an urgent $\dot{V}/\dot{Q}$ scan:

- If the $\dot{V}/\dot{Q}$ scan is normal, a PE can be excluded and the patient discharged, since the D-dimer test was negative.
- If the $\dot{V}/\dot{Q}$ scan is intermediate, the patient should have an ultrasound scan of her leg veins:
  ○ If the ultrasound scan is normal and the D-dimer test is negative, a PE can be excluded.
  ○ If the ultrasound scan is negative but the D-dimer test is positive, the scan should be repeated in a week; if this second scan is negative, a PE can be excluded.
- If the result of the $\dot{V}/\dot{Q}$ scan is high, the patient should be treated for a PE.

You should ensure that the F2 understands the role of the Wells score and PTP when interpreting D-dimer assays. You should recommend that they look up the 2006 BTS statement on D-dimers in suspected PE.

Scoring Scenario 14.3: Diagnosis of pulmonary embolisms

	Inadequate/ not done	Adequate	Good
Appropriate introduction	0	1	—
Ascertains the risk factors and features for a PE from the history: • onset of symptoms • difficulty in breathing/haemoptysis • history of thrombophilia • calf swelling/tenderness • recent immobilization • long-haul flights • previous history of DVT • oral contraceptive pill • recent diagnosis or treatment for malignancy	0	1	2
Asks the F2 about their understanding of the Wells PTP. Lists criteria: • malignancy • tachycardia • previous history of DVT • a diagnosis less likely than a PE • immobilization • haemoptysis • signs of a DVT	0	1	2
Calculates the PTP as being moderate	0	1	—
Suggests that a negative D-dimer test cannot rule out a PE unless the PTP is low and that further investigations should be carried out	0	1	2
Asks for a 12-lead ECG and knows about changes expected in a PE (S1 Q3 T3)	0	1	—
Suggests an urgent $\dot{V}/\dot{Q}$ scan based on the normal CXR	0	1	—
Treats with LMWH until the $\dot{V}/\dot{Q}$ scan is available	0	1	—
Explains management plan and need for admission to patient	0	1	2
Score from patient	**/5**		
Global score from examiner	**/5**		
Total	**/23**		

Scoring Scenario 14.5 *Continued*

	Inadequate/ not done	Adequate	Good
Examine the face and eyes for: • Horner's syndrome • nasal patency • central cyanosis • swollen tonsils	0	1	2
Examines the JVP	0	1	—
Palpates the trachea for midline shift	0	1	—
Examines the cervical lymph nodes	0	1	—
Checks for chest expansion	0	1	—
Percusses across: • front of chest • axillae • back of chest	0	1	—
Listens for vocal fremitus	0	1	—
Auscultates across: • front of chest, including apices • back of chest • axillae	0	1	2
Concludes examination by asking to check peak flow and sputum pot	0	1	—
Conducts examination in a fluent and logical manner	0	1	—
Score from patient		/5	
Global score from examiner		/5	
Total score		/34	

SCENARIO 14.6: ASTHMA IN PREGNANCY

You are asked to review a 28-year-old asthmatic patient who has been feeling wheezy for the last 48 hours. She is speaking full sentences.

Her observations are:

RR 16 breaths min^{-1}
Oxygen saturation 98% on air
Pulse 90 bpm
BP 120/78 mmHg
PEFR 78% of expected

She is 18 weeks pregnant and is concerned about the side-effects of her inhalers on the baby. Take a history, addressing her concerns, and check her inhaler technique.

This station requires you take an appropriate history, explore and address the patient's concerns, and be able to demonstrate to the patient how to use her inhalers. You should be familiar with the BTS guidelines on the management of asthma in pregnancy.

SUGGESTED APPROACH

After the appropriate introductions, you should take a focused respiratory history:

- onset of symptoms
- exacerbating factors: worse at night and during cold weather, stress-induced
- how long she has been an asthmatic
- previous hospital attendances
- previous admissions to ITU/HDU
- when the diagnosis of asthma was made
- who is following up her asthma
- pregnancy history
- compliance with inhalers
- compliance with peak flow
- social history: smoking, pets, housing, occupation and stress
- allergies
- other medications and allergies

According to the 2009 update of the BTS guidelines on asthma in pregnancy, asthma improves in one-third of women, deteriorates in one-third and remains the same in one-third. There is no evidence that β_2 agonists such as salbutamol are harmful during pregnancy. The guidelines suggest that $Pa0_2$ should be kept at greater than 94–98% in order to prevent fetal and maternal hypoxia. The patient should be reassured that it is important that she be compliant with her inhalers, since a severe asthma attack can have serious consequences. Many patients are concerned about the effects of inhaled steroids on the developing fetus, but there is no data indicating that inhaled steroids cause any congenital abnormalities. Oral steroids have been shown to increase the risk of eclampsia and hypertension, and a few studies have suggested a relationship between oral steroids and cleft palate. However, these latter links have not been proved, and the current recommendation is that the small risk of taking oral steroids during pregnancy is greatly outweighed by their benefit during a severe asthma attack.

You should take the opportunity to go through the patient's inhalers with her and ensure that she is using them correctly. You should explain how and when to use the 'reliever' and 'preventor' and the difference between the two.

Ask the patient to demonstrate her inhaler technique using a dummy inhaler. Check that she is following the instructions correctly:

- Remove the cap and shake the canister gently before use.
- Hold upright.
- Breath out.
- Make a good seal around the mouthpiece and breath in gently.
- While breathing in, press down on the canister.
- Hold the breath for 10 seconds after inhaling.
- Wait 30 seconds and repeat the process if required.
- Rinse the mouth after using inhaled steroids.

As the patient's PEFR is over 75% and she is speaking full sentences, she can be discharged home, with a follow-up appointment with her GP or midwife. It is crucial that you stress the importance of compliance with her medications.

Scoring Scenario 14.6: Asthma in pregnancy

	Inadequate/ not done	Adequate	Good
Appropriate introduction	0	1	—
Checks that the patient is stable	0	1	—
Takes a focused history: • onset of symptoms • previous admissions • medications • compliance • social history: smoking • allergies • pregnancy history • triggers: cold, infection or pets	0	1	2
Makes a diagnosis of mild asthma according to the BTS classification	0	1	—
Elicits patient's understanding of the term asthma. Explains asthma	0	1	—
Elicits concerns: • impact of inhalers on pregnancy • when to use inhalers	0	1	—
Advises that there is little evidence to support that her inhalers will harm the baby	0	1	—
Offers guidance on the difference between steroid and β_2-agonist inhalers	0	1	—
Demonstrates and checks inhaler technique	0	1	—
Demonstrates and checks the peak flow	0	1	—
Reassures the patient	0	1	—
Arranges appropriate follow-up	0	1	—
Encourages questions	0	1	—
Explains importance of compliance, without: • being judgemental • being confrontational • using technical jargon	0	1	2
Makes an agreed treatment plan	0	1	—
Score from patient	**/5**		
Global score from examiner	**/5**		
Total score	**/27**		

BRITISH THORACIC SOCIETY (BTS) GUIDELINES

All of these guidelines are available (under 'Clinical Information') from the BTS website: www.brit-thoracic.org.uk.

Asthma

BTS/ Scottish Intercollegiate Guidelines Network (SIGN). *British Guideline on the Management of Asthma: A National Clinical Guideline.* BTS/SIGN, May 2008 (revised June 2009).

Oxygen therapy

O'Driscoll BR, Howard LS, Davison AG; BTS Emergency Oxygen Guideline Development Group. Guideline for emergency oxygen use in adult patients. *Thorax* 2008; **63**(Suppl VI): vi1–vi73 (appendices are available at the BTS website).

Pneumothorax

Henry M, Arnold T, Harvey J; BTS Pleural Disease Group. BTS guidelines for the management of spontaneous pneumothorax. *Thorax* 2003; **58**(Suppl II): ii39–ii52.

Chest drain insertion

Chest Drain Insertion – Improving Patient Safety: A Symposium on Chest Drain Insertion Held at the BTS Winter Meeting, 3 December 2008. The presentations given at this meeting are available at the BTS website.

Pulmonary embolism

BTS Standards of Care Committee Pulmonary Embolism Guideline Development Group. British Thoracic Society guidelines for the management of suspected acute pulmonary embolism. *Thorax* 2003; **58**: 470–84.

D-dimer in Suspected Pulmonary Embolism (PE): A Statement from the BTS Standards of Care Committee. This statement is available at the BTS website.

Chronic obstructive pulmonary disease

National Institute for Health and Clinical Excellence. *Chronic Obstructive Pulmonary Disease. National Clinical Guideline on Management of Chronic Obstructive Pulmonary Disease in Adults in Primary and Secondary Care* (NICE Clinical Guideline 12). London: NICE, February 2004 (available at: http://guidance.nice.org.uk/CG12). The full version of the guideline is published in *Thorax* 2004; **59**(Suppl 1): i1–i232 (available at: http://thorax.bmj.com/content/vol59/suppl_1).

Non-invasive ventilation

Royal College of Physicians (RCP)/BTS/Intensive Care Society (ICS). *Non-Invasive Ventilation in Chronic Obstructive Pulmonary Disorder: Management of Acute Type 2 Respiratory Failure.* Concise Guidance to Good Practice Series No. 11. London: RCP, October 2008.

BTS/RCP/ICS. *The Use of Non-Invasive Ventilation in the Management of Patients with Chronic Obstructive Pulmonary Disease Admitted to Hospital with Acute Type II Respiratory Failure (With Particular Reference to Bilevel Positive Pressure Ventilation).* October 2008.

BTS Standards of Care Committee. Non-invasive ventilation in acute respiratory failure. *Thorax* 2002; **57**: 192–211.

15
Cardiological Emergencies
JOBAN S SEHMI, CHETAN R TRIVEDY AND ANDREW PARFITT

CORE TOPICS

- Focused history taking, examination and investigation of patients with cardiac symptoms in the emergency department
- Acute coronary syndromes
- Cardiac syncope
- Heart failure
- Cardiac arrhythmias

SCENARIO 15.1: CHEST PAIN – HISTORY AND MANAGEMENT

In the resuscitation department, you are asked to see a 38-year-old year man who presented to the emergency department with central chest pain. He is on oxygen and the ambulance crew have given him 300 mg of aspirin and 5 mg of morphine.

His observations are:

BP 160/90 mmHg
Pulse 110 bpm
Oxygen saturation 98% on high-flow oxygen
Blood glucose 6.4 mmol L^{-1}
GCS 13
ECG: see Figure 15.1

Take an appropriate history and outline your management. There is an ALS-trained nurse to help you.

SUGGESTED APPROACH

From the history given, there is a strong possibility that this patient is having an ischaemic cardiac event. The key to this station is to make a rapid assessment, institute emergency treatment and refer to the on-call cardiology team if required. The history of central chest pain with tachycardia and reduced GCS in a young patient with no cardiac risk factors should lead you to suspect that the patient may be under the influence of recreational drugs, with cocaine-induced ischaemia being high on the list of differentials. In addition to obtaining a focused history, it is important that you outline your initial management and delegate appropriate tasks to your assistant.

Cocaine has both acute and chronic effects on the myocardium. Acute effects include:

- coronary artery vasospasm
- thrombus formation
- increased oxygen demand by the myocardial tissue

Chronic effects include:

- atherosclerosis
- left ventricular hypertrophy

Management of cocaine-induced ACS/MI

The management of a cocaine-induced ACS/MI is essentially the same as for a non-cocaine cause, with few notable exceptions:

- Beta-blockers are contraindicated, since they exacerbate the vasospasm.
- Intravenous benzodiazepines are recommended to manage the tachycardia. It is not uncommon for large doses to be required to control symptoms.
- GTN is useful to treat vasospasm.
- Calcium-channel blockers can be used as second-line treatment if the pain is not responsive to benzodiazepine and GTN therapy.
- Phentolamine may be used a third-line agent, since it reduces vascular resistance in the coronary arteries.
- Primary angioplasty is the preferred intervention in the case of an acute MI.

Differential diagnosis

The differential diagnosis and management of a patient with chest pain is a core skill for every emergency physician. The OSCE scenario can be easily modified to include a variety of cardiac pathologies. A detailed discussion of all of the cardiac causes of chest pain is outside the scope of this book, but you should ensure that you can differentiate between common differential diagnoses based on the clinical history and ECG changes.

Atypical presentations

Atypical chest pain in the absence of risk factors does not usually merit a 12-hour troponin investigation to exclude myocardial injury. However, it is essential to look for other causes of the chest pain in these patients.

If there are symptoms that are atypical, you should attempt to identify whether there are any typical precipitants such as effort or emotion and you should also consider relieving factors such as rest, nitrates and oxygen.

The presence of risk factors, in particular diabetes mellitus, should lead to a low threshold to investigate for an ischaemic event. Since these patients may present without chest pain (silent infarct), they should have a troponin test to rule out an acute cardiac event as well as a treadmill test to screen for underlying coronary artery disease.

Acute coronary syndromes

'Acute coronary syndrome' is an umbrella tern that covers a spectrum of clinical conditions ranging from unstable angina to non-Q-wave MI and Q-wave MI.

A diagnosis of an ACS requires two out of the following three:

- chest pain
- ECG changes
- elevated cardiac enzymes

Table 15.1 Anatomical significance of ischaemic ECG findings in myocardial infarction

Area affected	Leads showing ST elevation	Leads showing reciprocal changes	Occluded artery
Septal	V1, V2	None	LAD
Anterior	V3, V4	None	LAD
Anteroseptal	V1–V4	None	LAD
Anterolateral	V3–V6, I, aVL	II, III, aVF	LAD, circumflex or obtuse marginal
Anteroseptal with lateral extension	V1–V6, I, aVL	II, III, aVF	Left main coronary artery
Inferior	II, III, aVF	I, aVL	RCA or circumflex
Lateral	I, aVL, V5, V6	II, III, aVF	Circumflex or obtuse marginal
Posterior	V7–V9	V1–V4	Posterior descending branch of RCA or circumflex
Right ventricular	II, III, aVF, V1, V4R	I, aVL	RCA

LAD, left anterior descending; RCA, right coronary artery.

The leading symptom that initiates the diagnostic and therapeutic cascade is chest pain, but the classification is based on the ECG. The two categories are:

1. Patients with typical acute chest pain and persistent (>20 minutes) ST elevation.
2. Patients with acute chest pain but without persistent ST elevation.

1. Patients with typical acute chest pain and persistent (>20 minutes) ST elevation

This reflects acute total occlusion of a coronary artery. The relationship between the occluded arteries and typical ECG findings is shown in Table 15.1.

The therapeutic objective is to achieve rapid, complete and sustained reperfusion by primary angioplasty or thrombolytic therapy, as guided by local facilities. The use of primary angioplasty will vary according to local policies; patients who have presented with a significant delay after onset of chest pain or those who have ECG changes and are pain-free should be discussed with the on-call cardiologist.

Indications for thrombolysis

'Door-to-needle time' represents the time permitted for the administration of thrombolytic therapy from the moment the patient enters the emergency department. Effective clinical practice demands that this be no greater than 20 minutes.

The indications for thrombolysis or referral for primary angioplasty include chest pain that began 12 hours ago or less, with specific ECG criteria:

- new-onset left bundle branch block (LBBB)
- 2 mm ST elevation in two contiguous chest leads
- 1 mm ST elevation in two contiguous limb leads

The Thrombolysis in Myocardial Infarction (TIMI) score is a useful tool that can be applied simply to risk-stratify a patient presenting with an NSTEMI:

- age ≥ 65 years
- three risk factors for coronary disease
- established coronary artery disease (stenosis > 50%)
- two angina events in the past 24 hours
- elevated cardiac markers
- ST depression ≥ 0.5 mm
- aspirin within the last 7 days

A score of 0 predicts a 4% probability of death and future cardiac events, and a score of 6/7 indicates a 40% probability of future mortality and cardiac morbidity.

Aortic dissection

Aortic dissection is an important differential diagnosis to exclude in patients presenting with chest pain.

Classically, the pain is described as severe, sudden and tearing in nature, which typically radiates through to the interscapular area.

A full cardiovascular examination is mandatory, and may reveal an early diastolic murmur, renal bruits, and a significant difference in blood pressure following measurement in both arms. Note that only 3–4% of dissections actually exhibit a significant difference in arm blood pressure measurements (>20 mmHg), making this sign of reduced practical use outside the OSCE!

- **Type A dissections** involve the ascending arch of the aorta, and can cause chest pain radiating to the face.
- **Type B dissections** do not involve the ascending thoracic aorta, and typically present with back pain.

Risk factors include:

- hypertension, which is present in 85% of patients
- bicuspid aortic valve
- any stage following insertion of an aortic cannula in a bypass procedure

The ECG may be normal, although global ischaemia maybe a feature as a result of a low-cardiac-output state. Infarcts may be seen, and the presence of strange lead combinations (e.g. inferior and anterior) should increase clinical suspicion. Other ECG patterns that may be observed include heart block and voltage criteria for left ventricular hypertrophy.

Connective tissue disorders, particularly Marfan's syndrome, are recognized causes of aortic dissection.

Type A dissections usually require urgent surgical intervention, although the associated mortality is high.

All cases require medical therapy, involving intensive monitoring of renal function and urine output, invasive haemodynamic monitoring, ideally in a critical care setting.

Labetalol is a useful agent that acts to decrease systolic blood pressure and reduce the heart rate. Nitroprusside is an appropriate second-line agent.

Other causes of chest pain

Other presentations to exclude in a patient presenting to the emergency department with chest pain in the absence of ischaemic heart disease include:

- pulmonary embolism
- aortic stenosis
- coronary artery spasm
- oesophageal spasm

Scoring Scenario 15.1: Chest pain – history and management

	Inadequate/ not done	Adequate	Good
Introduction	0	1	—
Institutes immediate management: • high-flow oxygen • full cardiac monitoring • 12-lead ECG • IV access • appropriate bloods/blood gas • chest X-ray	0	1	2
Takes focused cardiac history: • accurate time of onset of pain • radiation • severity • exacerbating/relieving factors • use of cocaine in last 24 hours • family history of ischaemic heart disease • diabetes • smoking • high cholesterol • South Asian origin	0	1	2
Identifies additional symptoms to support a diagnosis of ACS: • nausea/vomiting • sweating • palpitations • tachycardia • dizziness	0	1	2
Takes brief recent medical history, including drug history and allergies	0	1	2
Social history	0	1	—
Identifies changes on ECG to make diagnosis of MI (nurse to hand ECG early in OSCE only if requested). Mentions territories involved	0	1	—
Makes diagnosis of cocaine-induced MI and outlines immediate management: • aspirin (300 mg) • clopidogrel (300 mg) • IV morphine • metoclopramide (10 mg) • IV benzodiazepines (10–40 mg titrated dose) • GTN infusion • suggests that beta-blockers are contraindicated • urgent referral to cardiology for percutaneous coronary intervention (examiner will tell candidate that this is not available)	0	1	2
Correctly identifies clinical indication for thrombolysis	0	1	—

Continued

Scoring Scenario 15.1 *Continued*

	Inadequate/ not done	Adequate	Good
Asks patient about potential contraindications for thrombolysis	0	1	2
Suggests serial ECG monitoring	0	1	—
Arranges urgent cardiology referral	0	1	—
Score from patient	/5		
Global score from examiner	/5		
Total score	/28		

SCENARIO 15.2: CARDIOVASCULAR EXAMINATION

A 69-year-old retired builder presents to the emergency department with a 3-week history of shortness of breath and ankle swelling. Carry out a cardiovascular examination and present your findings. You are not expected to take a history.

SUGGESTED APPROACH

It is essential that you have a well-rehearsed routine that is fluent. This can only come with practice, and you should take the opportunity to spend some time in a cardiothoracic/cardiology outpatient clinic, since there will be an opportunity to listen to heart murmurs. At this stage in your career, you should have your own examination system and you should use the following approach to augment your own technique.

Your assessment should start by introducing yourself and obtaining verbal consent to examine the patient. A quick explanation of what you are proposing will help to establish a good rapport.

Clarify with the examiner whether they want you present as you go along or at the end. It is easier to present as you go along, because you will pick up marks as you go; if you present at the end and run out of time, you will miss marks.

Verbalize your actions so that the examiner does not miss a crucial part of your examination: 'I am looking for ...', 'I am listening for ...'.

Ask the patient to undress above the waist, and ensure that you maintain their dignity at all times. Position the patient so that they are lying down at 45°.

General inspection should be conducted from the end of the bed, and you should note whether the patient appears comfortable and whether they are pale, emaciated or oedematous. In addition, you may be able to hear the ticking of a mechanical valve. It is likely that the patient used for the OSCE will be stable and comfortable at rest – if you find that they are not, you should inform the examiner that you would make them more comfortable.

Examine the face for mitral facies, marfanoid features and Down's syndrome.

Look at the chest for the presence of scars. Those that are relevant to a cardiovascular examination include a median sternotomy scar, left-sided subclavicular scar indicative of an implantable device, and valvotomy scars.

Look for gynaecomastia from digoxin or spironolactone use.

Look around the bed for any clues (oxygen or GTN spray)

Examine the hands, looking for:

- cyanosis
- clubbing of the distal fingertips
- splinter haemorrhages in the fingernails (associated with infective endocarditis)
- nicotine staining of the fingers, possibly indicating heavy smoking, which is linked with ischaemic heart disease.

Make a note of whether the hands are cold or warm, dry or sweaty.

Palpate the radial pulse, noting rate and rhythm. Examine for a collapsing pulse (aortic regurgitation).

Suggest that you would like to measure the blood pressure. A wide pulse pressure may be a clue to aortic regurgitation and a narrow pulse pressure may indicate the presence of aortic stenosis.

Examine the conjunctivae for anaemia. The presence of a xanthelasma or a corneal arcus may be suggestive of hypercholesterolaemia.

Examine the oral cavity for:

- central cyanosis of the lips/tongue
- poor dentition, which may represent a risk factor for endocarditis
- a smooth red tongue, which may indicate anaemia
- a high arched palate, which is associated with Marfan's syndrome and aortic regurgitation

Ask the patient to turn their head to the left. Examine the jugular venous pulse (JVP); you may be asked how to distinguish this from the carotid pulse. The main differences between the two are as follows:

- The JVP is biphasic, whereas the carotid pulse is monophasic.
- The JVP is non-palpable and can be occluded in the neck by compressing the internal jugular vein. In contrast, the carotid pulse is easily palpated and is not easily occluded.
- The JVP can identified by the hepatojugular reflux (not reflex) manoeuvre, whereby gently compressing the abdomen over the liver for approximately 30 seconds will increase the venous return to the heart and result in an increase in the JVP. This test will have no effect on the carotid pulse.

Identify and palpate the carotid pulse, commenting on its volume and character.

Palpate for the apex of the heart (5th intercostal space in the midclavicular line):

- Is it displaced? Measure the exact surface anatomy of the apex.
- Make a note of the character of the apex. A tapping character to the apex beat is associated with mitral stenosis and a heaving apex is associated with left ventricular hypertrophy or aortic stenosis.
- Palpate for heaves and thrills

Auscultation is a difficult skill to perfect, and it is important that a methodical approach be taken. Divide auscultation into two phases: simple auscultation of all four cardiac areas, followed by manoeuvres that assist in confirming the diagnosis. It is vital to palpate the carotid pulse during auscultation, so that any murmurs that are elicited can be timed appropriately. It is also useful to warm the head of your stethoscope before you auscultate and ensure that you use both the bell and diaphragm.

- Phase 1: Auscultate in all four areas:
  - ○ Begin in the mitral area, using the bell. Focus on the first heart sound, noting whether it is loud, quiet or metallic. Listen for murmurs, and check whether they are accentuated in expiration.
  - ○ In the tricuspid area, focus on listening for a murmur. If a murmur is elicited, check whether it becomes louder on inspiration, indicating tricuspid regurgitation.
  - ○ In the pulmonary area, listen for the second heart sound. Comment on how loud it is, whether it is metallic or if it is split.
  - ○ In the aortic area, listen for any murmurs and how they vary with respiration.

- Phase 2: Special manoeuvres:
  - ○ Listen in the axilla for radiation of a pansystolic murmur of mitral regurgitation.
  - ○ Turn the patient into the left lateral position, and, using the bell, auscultate over the apex in expiration. The mid-diastolic murmur of mitral stenosis is best heard in this position.
  - ○ Listen over the carotids for radiation of the ejection systolic murmur of aortic stenosis.
  - ○ Sit the patient forward and listen over the left sternal edge in expiration for the early diastolic murmur of aortic regurgitation.

Following auscultation, you should proceed to look for signs of heart failure:

- With the patient sitting up, listen to the lung bases.
- Palpate the liver edge for a pulsatile liver or hepatomegaly.
- Examine the legs for signs of pitting oedema.

As the scenario specifically asks for you to examine the cardiovascular system, you should suggest to the examiner that you would like to perform an examination of the vascular system; this is discussed in detail in Chapter 7. It is very unlikely that you would be asked to perform a vascular examination in the time frame given, but there may be a mark for suggesting it.

Conclude your examination by asking to see the patient's ECG and for the urine to be dipped to look for protein or blood. Do not forget to thank the patient, and help them get dressed.

You should get into the habit of summarizing your findings in no more than two or three sentences and you should outline any appropriate investigations, such as an ECG, blood tests, chest X-ray or an echocardiogram.

Scenarios that may be encountered in the OSCE

For the purposes of the examination, you are likely to get a stable patient who has probably been primed by the examiners on what they can and cannot divulge. These patients are carefully selected in terms of their clinical signs. Do not be put off if you have a normal patient. Ensure that you examine the patient systematically as suggested and present what you find, and do not be tempted to make up signs. The following is a list of some of the cases that you may encounter in the examination. This list is only a guide and is not exhaustive.

Aortic stenosis

A loud ejection systolic murmur is heard in the upper right sternal border, radiating to the carotids.

Clinical markers of severity that should be presented include:

- narrow pulse pressure
- soft second heart sound (S_2)
- slowly rising carotid pulse
- evidence of heart failure (displaced apex and pulmonary oedema)

In the emergency setting, avoid GTN and ACE inhibitors in patients presenting with angina.

Aortic regurgitation

There is a wide pulse pressure, a collapsing pulse and an early diastolic murmur

Markers of severity include:

- quiet S_2
- evidence of pulmonary oedema
- Austin Flint murmur: a regurgitant jet of blood hitting the mitral valve apparatus may result in a mid-diastolic murmur

Pulmonary stenosis

There is an ejection systolic murmur, radiating from the upper left sternal edge towards the left clavicle. S_2 may be widely split and may vary with respiration.

Mitral stenosis

There is a mid-diastolic murmur that is best heard at the apex with the patient lying on their left side. A tapping sound is heard at the apex and there is an opening snap. The murmur does not radiate.

Mitral stenosis is often associated with atrial fibrillation.

Mitral regurgitation

There is a pansystolic murmur, radiating from the apex to the axilla.

Mitral regurgitation is associated with atrial fibrillation and a third heart sound (S_3) may be present.

Ischaemic heart disease and connective tissue disorders are strongly associated with mitral regurgitation.

Ventricular septal defect

A pansystolic murmur is present that is best heard at the left sternal edge, radiating across the chest.

A ventricular septal defect may be associated with Eisenmenger's syndrome (a left-to-right shunt resulting in pulmonary hypertension).

Ventricular septal defects often present with a diastolic murmur over the mitral area due to increased blood flow across the mitral valve.

Valve replacement

This is a common case that frequently appears in postgraduate examinations.

The presence of a midline sternotomy scar should alert you to this diagnosis. Other differentials for a midline sternotomy scar include surgical intervention for congenital heart disease, previous coronary artery bypass graft and cardiac transplantation.

A metallic S_1 implies a mitral valve replacement and a metallic S_2 implies an aortic valve replacement. Tissue valves often sound very loud, and should be suggested as a differential diagnosis in a patient with normal heart sounds and a midline stenotomy scar.

Clinical complications of valve replacement

- Look for features of infective endocarditis.
- A regurgitant murmur suggests valve incompetence or a paravalvular leak. In this instance, an urgent echocardiogram will be required to evaluate the extent of valve dysfunction.
- The presence of jaundice in a patient with a valve replacement should alert the clinician to the possibility of microangiopathic haemolytic anaemia (MAHA).
- Identify any signs of over- or under-anticoagulation (e.g. bruising).

Scoring Scenario 15.2: Cardiovascular examination

	Inadequate/ not done	Adequate	Good
Appropriate introduction	0	1	—
Establishes rapport and ensures patient's comfort	0	1	—
Exposes patient appropriately, maintaining their dignity	0	1	—
Appropriate general inspection: • Identifies any paraphernalia of cardiovascular disease • Identifies scars	0	1	—
Examines hands: • peripheral cyanosis • finger clubbing • nicotine staining • splinter haemorrhages	0	1	—
Examines eyes: • anaemia • corneal arcus • xanthelasma (2 out of 3)	0	1	—
Examines mouth: • central cyanosis • poor dentition • pale smooth tongue (anaemia) • high arched palate (Marfan's syndrome) (2 out of 4)	0	1	—
Palpates the radial pulse (noting rate and rhythm and identifying the presence of a collapsing pulse)	0	1	—
Offers to measure blood pressure	0	1	—
Examines carotid pulse	0	1	—
Examines JVP and distinguishes from carotid pulse: • JVP is a bifid pulse • JVP is collapsible compared with carotid pulse • JVP rises with the hepatojugular reflux	0	1	2
Examines apex (correctly identifying landmarks)	0	1	—
Examines for heaves and thrills	0	1	—
Palpates a central pulse at all times during auscultation	0	1	—
Auscultates in all four cardiac areas with bell and diaphragm	0	1	—

Continued

Scoring Scenario 15.2 *Continued*

	Inadequate/ not done	Adequate	Good
Auscultates in axilla	0	1	—
Auscultates over apex, with patient in left lateral position and holding their breath in expiration	0	1	—
Auscultates over carotid arteries	0	1	—
Auscultates over lower left sternal edge, with patient sitting forwards and holding their breath in expiration	0	1	—
Auscultates lung bases	0	1	—
Palpates abdomen for hepatomegaly	0	1	—
Identifies presence of pedal/sacral oedema	0	1	—
Suggests appropriate bedside tests: • urine dipstick • ECG	0	1	—
Asks to perform vascular examination	0	1	—
Summarizes findings clearly and suggests differential diagnosis	0	1	2
Score from patient	/5		
Global score from examiner	/5		
Total score	/37		

SCENARIO 15.3: ARRHYTHMIA (I)

A 32-year-old woman presents to the emergency department with a 2-hour history of feeling dizzy and light-headed. She complains that her heart is racing and thumping in her chest – and that she has had a 2-day history of diarrhoea and vomiting.

Her observations are:

BP 134/70 mmHg
Oxygen saturation 98% on air
Pulse 160 bpm
Blood glucose 5.6 mmol L^{-1}
Temperature 36.8 °C

A rhythm strip taken in lead II by the ambulance crew is shown in Figure 15.2.

Take a focused history and outline your management. You are not expected to examine the patient.

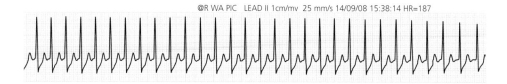

@R WA PIC   LEAD II 1cm/mv 25 mm/s 14/09/08 15:38:14 HR=187

Figure 15.2 Rhythm strip taken in lead II from the patient in Scenario 15.3.

This scenario is frequently encountered in the emergency department. Palpitations are often non-specific, and only 10% of patients will have an underlying arrhythmia diagnosed.

SUGGESTED APPROACH

Ensure that the patient is placed in a monitored cubicle – preferably in the resuscitation room. You should identify the need for resuscitation, by assessing the airway, breathing and circulation, before proceeding to take the history. Your immediate management should include:

- high-flow oxygen according to BTS guidelines
- full cardiac monitoring
- securing intravenous access and checking a venous gas to identify electrolyte disturbances

History

Determine exactly what the patient means by 'palpitations'. Characterize the nature of the palpitations by asking the patient if they are regular or irregular. Enquire about the temporal pattern of the palpitations by asking about their frequency and mode of onset, and identify the duration of each episode. It is useful to ask the patient to tap out the palpitations.

Ask about associated symptoms, particularly fatigue, light-headedness, chest discomfort, dyspnoea, pre-syncope and syncope (which is rarer: 15% of cases).

Ask about a history of congenital heart disease or murmurs as a child, since arrhythmias are more common in patients with structural heart disease

Look for any precipitants. In this case, you are told that the patient has had a 2-day history of diarrhoea and vomiting, which may have resulted in an electrolyte disturbance that triggered the arrhythmia.

Enquire about previous episodes and ask if the patient has an old ECG with them. Many patients will carry old ECGs of their underlying rhythm, which are useful in identifying the arrhythmia.

Enquire about the presence of symptoms suggestive of hyperthyroidism, such as weight loss, heat intolerance, sweating and tremor.

Ask about caffeine and alcohol intake and illicit drug usage (e.g. crystal meth, amphetamines and cocaine).

It is important to ask about other illnesses (e.g. asthma) and, in particular, how previous episodes have been managed.

A detailed drug and allergy history is important, since it may provide clues to the underlying cause and may guide safe medical therapy (e.g. dipyridamole may interact with adenosine, a drug commonly used to treat supraventricular arrhythmias).

Examination

Although an examination of the cardiovascular system is not required, you should mention to the examiner that ideally you would examine the patient, focusing on underlying valvular or structural myocardial disease, in addition to looking specifically for clinical features of anaemia and thyroid disease.

Chest X-ray

Assess cardiac dimensions and assess the lung fields for evidence of pulmonary oedema or cardiomegaly. Note that pulmonary pathology may potentially precipitate palpitations.

Bloods

These should include electrolytes (including magnesium and calcium) and inflammatory markers. It is mandatory to assess thyroid function.

ECG

The management of this patient will depend not only upon clinical considerations but also on the accurate interpretation of the ECG. You may be faced with a variety of ECGs, and you should make sure that you are familiar with the management of the common tachyarrhythmias.

It is best to consider arrhythmias as narrow or broad complex by measuring the duration of the QRS complex. The ECG is key to deciding the management of this patient, and potential scenarios are discussed below.

Differential diagnosis of a narrow complex tachycardia (heart rate >100 bpm and QRS < 120 ms)

This group comprises the following.

Sinus tachycardia

This is a physiological response to illness or stress (pain, dehydration, shock, pulmonary embolus, sepsis, etc.). P waves are of normal shape and axis and the PR interval is normal. The P waves may be difficult to see when the rate is high. Sinus tachycardia should be managed by treating the underlying cause.

Atrioventricular nodal reentrant tachycardia (AVNRT)

AVNRT is the most common form of reentrant tachycardia, and is caused by reentry circuits within the AV node. There are usually no underlying structural abnormalities. It is usually seen as a narrow complex tachycardia unless there is an associated bundle branch block (BBB) – such cases are sometimes confused with ventricular tachycardia (VT).

If no P waves are apparent and the RR interval is regular then AVNRT is very likely. P-wave activity in AVNRT may be partially hidden within the QRS complex and may deform the QRS to give a pseudo-R wave in lead V1 and/or a pseudo-S wave in inferior leads.

Atrioventricular reentrant tachycardia (AVRT)

This type of supraventricular tachycardia (SVT) is associated with the presence of an accessory pathway between the atria and the ventricles that is outside the AV node. The most common example is Wolff–Parkinson–White (WPW) syndrome, which is a congenital condition characterized by an accessory pathway (bundle of Kent) between the atria and the ventricles. The classical ECG findings of WPW syndrome include (Figure 15.3):

- a δ wave, characterized by a slurred upstroke to the QRS complex
- a short PR interval (<0.12 s)

Two variants of WPW syndrome are recognized:

- **type A**, in which there is a left-sided pathway, with an upright δ wave in V1 (common)
- **type B**, in which there is a right-sided pathway, with a negative δ wave in V1

The presence of an accessory pathway predisposes to AVRT as well as atrial fibrillation (AF).

During an episode of AVRT, reentry circuits are formed between the AV node and the accessory pathway. Antegrade conduction (from atria to ventricles) of electrical impulses leads to a narrow complex tachycardia, while retrograde conduction (from ventricles to atria) manifests as a wide complex tachycardia. During episodes of tachycardia, P waves and δ waves are lost.

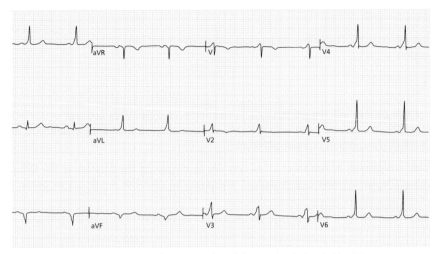

Figure 15.3 WPW syndrome, demonstrating delta waves in leads V4–V6.

AVRTs are managed as for any other SVT, with vagal manoeuvres and AV blockade with adenosine, calcium-channel blockers or digoxin. However, AF in the context of WPW syndrome should not be treated with drugs that block the AV node. In this instance, AV blockade causes preferential conduction of cardiac impulses down the accessory pathway, which can result in progression to ventricular fibrillation (VF).

Atrial tachycardia

This is also referred to as 'focal' atrial tachycardia, and results from activity in localized areas such as the pulmonary veins in the left atrium and the crista terminalis in the right atrium. These regions can fire off at a rate greater than the sinoatrial (SA) node.

The P waves have an abnormal shape. The PR interval is often prolonged, although it may be normal. The QRS complex, however, is normal in shape.

Atrial tachycardia may be associated with structural heart disease or due to underlying infection.

Junctional (AV nodal) tachycardia

This is rare, but may be seen in patients who present with an SVT. There are two forms:

- Automatic junctional tachycardia (AJT) arises as an automatic tachycardia from around the AV node and is associated with drug toxicity (digoxin).
- Permanent junctional reentrant tachycardia (PJRT) is caused by an accessory pathway close to the AV node and may be associated with a reversible cardiomyopathy.

The P waves are often very close to the QRS complexes, which are normal in shape. Occasionally, the P waves may also be buried within the QRS complexes.

Junctional tachycardia is also known to be associated with digoxin toxicity.

Atrial fibrillation/flutter

This is discussed in detail in Scenario 15.4, but you should be aware of the management of pre-excitatory AF associated with WPW syndrom, where the use of drugs such as adenosine and verapamil may induce VF.

Differential diagnosis for broad complex tachycardias (QRS > 120 ms)

These comprise:

- VT
- SVT with aberrant conduction

It is often difficult to distinguish between VT and a broad complex SVT; if in doubt, it is best to treat as a VT rather than an SVT. Some of the discriminating features between the two are shown in Table 15.2.

Table 15.2 Features that can be used to differentiate ventricular tachycardia (VT) from supraventricular tachycardia (SVT) with aberrant conduction

	SVT with aberrant conduction	VT
ECG features		
QRS duration	<140 ms	>160 ms
QRS axis	Normal	Extreme
V-lead polarity	Discordant	Concordant
AV dissociation (fusion/capture beats)	Absent	Possible (Figure 15.4)
ECG pattern	RBBB	RBBB/LBBB
Clinical features		
Vagal manoeuvres	Effective	Ineffective
Cannon waves	Absent	Present
First heart sound	Normal	Variable

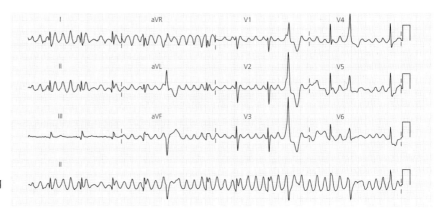

Figure 15.4 VT demonstrating fusion and capture beats.

Management of SVT

DC cardioversion is an appropriate strategy in patients who are haemodynamically compromised.

In regular narrow complex tachycardia, vagal manoeuvres should be initiated in the first instance to terminate the arrhythmia or to modify AV conduction:

- Valsalva manoeuvre
- carotid massage (exclude carotid artery thrombotic disease first by listening for carotid artery bruits)
- facial immersion in cold water

If vagal manoeuvres are ineffective then intravenous antiarrhythmic drugs should be administered.

The first-line drug is adenosine (Figure 15.5). This is a short-acting medication that functions by causing a transient AV block and thereby terminating the tachycardia (AVRT or AVNRT). Although adenosine may not terminate atrial flutter, the slowing of the rhythm may make the flutter waves easier to diagnose.

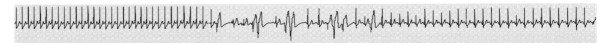

Figure 15.5 Chemical cardioversion of an SVT with adenosine.

Adenosine is contraindicated in patients with second- and third-degree heart block, with pre-excitatory AF in the setting of WPW syndrome. It is also contraindicated in patients who are severe asthmatics.

The recommended dose is a rapid 6 mg bolus while the patient is monitored on a rhythm strip. It is common for the patient to complain of tightness in their chest as well as marked flushing, but this is usually short-lived and you should warn the patient beforehand. If the initial dose is not successful at restoring sinus rhythm, you should give a further 12 mg (18 mg in larger patients). The dose may be increased in patients on theophylline, since methylxanthines prevent binding of adenosine at receptor sites. The dose is often decreased in patients on dipyridamole and diazepam, because adenosine potentiates the effects of these drugs.

Methylxanthines, such as caffeine and theophylline, are competitive antagonists of adenosine.

Rate-limiting calcium-channel blockers are effective treatments for terminating SVTs. Verapamil (5–10 mg intravenously) is a useful second-line agent.

Resistant cases may warrant DC cardioversion.

Management of VT

Correction of potentially causative or aggravating conditions such as electrolyte disturbances and ischaemia is an early priority.

The management is dependent upon how stable the patient is – if they are haemodynamically compromised then urgent DC cardioversion with appropriate anaesthetic cover is indicated.

It is useful to consider whether the VT is monomorphic or polymorphic (torsades de pointes) when planning management options.

Sustained monomorphic VT

Determine the QT interval. If it is normal, consider ischaemia and manage accordingly.

DC electrical cardioversion under sedation with appropriate anaesthetic cover is required if the patient is haemodynamically unstable.

Amiodarone should be considered the first-line treatment in stable patients with VT. This must be administered in a large vein, as a bolus of 150 mg over a period of 15 minutes, followed by a 23-hour infusion.

If the patient is haemodynamically stable, you can consider intravenous 50 mg lidocaine every 5 minutes up to a maximum dose of 200 mg.

Treat any underlying cause and correct any electrolyte disturbances (potassium and magnesium).

Overdrive pacing may be used to treat refractory cases of VT, but as this requires the placement of a transvenous pacing wire into the right ventricle, it will require specialist cardiology intervention.

Polymorphic VT (torsades de pointes)

This is seen when there is a 'beat-to-beat' variation in the shape of the QRS complexes (Figure 15.6). When this is associated with a prolonged QT interval, the complexes may be seen to twist along the horizontal axis (hence the term 'torsades de pointes').

The causes of polymorphic VT include:

- long QT syndrome
- drugs such as tricyclic antidepressants
- electrolyte disturbances (especially potassium and magnesium).

Treat with intravenous magnesium sulphate 2–4 g immediately. An infusion of isoprenaline can be considered while awaiting overdrive cardiac pacing for resistant arrhythmia.

Follow-up

All patients presenting to the emergency department with arrhythmias should have a cardiology follow-up as well as a 24-hour ECG monitoring and an echocardiogram to look for structural abnormalities. Some patients may also undergo electrophysiological studies (EPS) and may go on to have any aberrant foci radioablated. If you discharge a patient, it is important that you give them a copy of their ECG, since this will help diagnosis and management if there are any subsequent attendances.

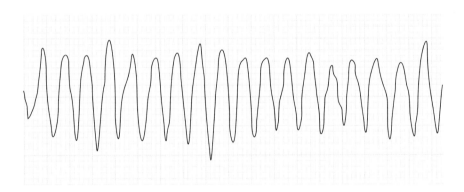

Figure 15.6 Polymorphic VT (torsades de pointes).

Scoring Scenario 15.3: Arrhythmia (I)

	Inadequate/ not done	Adequate	Good
Appropriate introduction	0	1	—
Institutes immediate management: • transfers patient to resuscitation • supplemental oxygen • full cardiac monitoring • 12-lead ECG • intravenous access	0	1	2
Bloods: electrolytes (including magnesium) and thyroid function tests	0	1	—
Asks about symptoms: • chest pain • shortness of breath • palpitations: character and frequency • syncope • previous episodes of arrhythmias/palpitations • precipitating factors: electrolyte disturbances, infection, stress, caffeine • takes focused medical history: asthma, thyroid disorders, congenital heart disease • drugs and allergies	0	1	2
Makes rapid assessment of ECG and interprets rhythm correctly: SVT/VT/AF with pre-excitation	0	1	2
Ascertains that patient is cardiovascularly stable	0	1	—
Able to differentiate between VT and SVT (when prompted by examiner)	0	1	2
Correctly interprets patient's old ECG as WPW syndrome and identifies delta waves correctly	0	1	—
Does not recommend treating with antiarrhythmics such as adenosine or verapamil. Recommends treating with flecainide	0	1	—
Monitors patient continuously on a rhythm strip	0	1	—
Requests a portable chest X-ray once the patient is stable	0	1	—
Suggests appropriate cardiology follow-up for further investigations and management: • 24-hour tape • echocardiogram • EPS studies (radiofrequency ablation) • oral antiarrhythmics	0	1	2
Suggests urgent DC cardioversion if the patient becomes unstable	0	1	—
Score from patient	/5		
Global score from examiner	/5		
Total score	/28		

SCENARIO 15.4: ARRHYTHMIA (II)

A 68-year-old woman presents to the emergency department with a 3-hour history of feeling dizzy and chest pain.

Her observations are:

BP 85/60 mmHg
Pulse 180 bpm
Oxygen saturation 96% on air
Her ECG at triage is shown in Figure 15.7.

Take a history and outline your management using the appropriate equipment. You have an ALS-trained nurse to help you.

SUGGESTED APPROACH

You should immediately identify that this patient is in atrial fibrillation (AF) and that she exhibits evidence of haemodynamic compromise.

Markers of haemodynamic compromise are:

- systolic BP < 90 mmHg
- chest pain
- reduced GCS
- clinical evidence of heart failure

You should suggest to the examiner that you would arrange to perform an urgent DC cardioversion for this patient under appropriate anaesthetic cover and meanwhile you would institute immediate treatment:

- high-flow oxygen
- full cardiac monitoring
- intravenous access
- bloods: electrolytes (including magnesium), thyroid function tests and sepsis screen
- venous blood gas, which can be useful in rapidly screening for electrolyte disturbances
- a portable chest X-ray (looking for signs of heart failure)

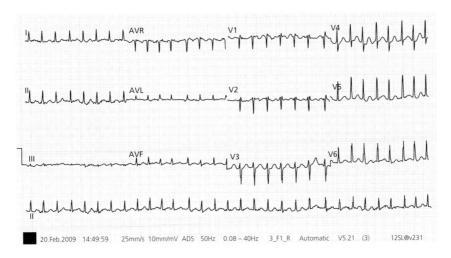

Figure 15.7 ECG of the patient in Scenario 15.4.

History

In a haemodynamically stable patient, it is important to know whether the duration of AF is greater or less than 48 hours, since this dictates whether the patient is suitable for cardioversion.

Identify features in the history that may indicate the underlying cause of AF (sepsis, lung pathology, thyrotoxicosis, electrolyte imbalance following the use of diuretics, or ischaemic heart disease).

A detailed drug and medical history is helpful to identify patients who are at risk of thromboembolic events and in deciding their suitability for long-term anticoagulation.

Ask specifically if the patient has had any adverse affects to a general anaesthetic or has been sedated before with morphine or midazolam. You should also ascertain when they last ate or drank.

Examination

A thorough cardiovascular examination is important; you should look for signs of heart failure, which support management with DC cardioversion and avoidance of beta-blockers.

DC cardioversion

This procedure can be safely performed in the emergency department, and you should ensure that it carried out by appropriately trained staff. The options include cardioversion using anaesthetic agents such as propofol or a combination of morphine and midazolam. In either situation, there should be full anaesthetic back-up and the procedure should be performed in a resuscitation room with full cardiac monitoring and resuscitation support. If the patient is unstable, the on-call anaesthetist should be called to secure the airway before you perform the cardioversion procedure.

Alternatively, if the patient is stable, a senior emergency department clinician who is skilled in advanced airway management and who is able to intubate the patient if required should manage the airway while a second clinician administers sedation (morphine/midazolam) and performs the cardioversion. You should prepare the airway trolley in case emergency intubation is required.

The paddles should be placed appropriately in the anterolateral postion as shown in Figure 15.8. Alternatively, you can place them in an anteroposterior position – studies have shown that neither configuration has any particular advantage over the other in terms of successful cardioversion. All metallic items such as bras should be removed to prevent burns to the skin.

Ensure that you synchronize the cardioversion; this is done by pressing the 'synch' button on the defibrillator.

In this OSCE, you will be marked on your ability to deliver one or more shocks safely. Ensure that you make your checks and remove oxygen before delivering the shock. If you are not successful after the first shock (100–150 kJ), you should increase the voltage by 50 kJ and try again. Alternatively, the paddle position can be changed to the anteroposterior position.

Following successful cardioversion, the patient should be referred to the on-call medical team for further management, as well as treatment of the underlying cause (e.g. infection or ischaemia).

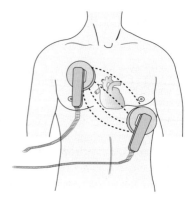

Figure 15.8 Paddle placement.

Classification of AF

You should be aware of the 2006 NICE guideline on AF (see below). AF is commonly classified as follows.

Paroxysmal AF

Each episode comes on suddenly, but will stop without any treatment within 7 days (usually within 2 days). Patients who are able to recognize the onset of their symptoms and are able to take appropriate treatment as soon as the AF develops may be appropriate for a 'pill in pocket' strategy.

Persistent AF

This is AF that lasts longer than 7 days and is unlikely to revert back to sinus rhythm without treatment. However, the heart rhythm can be cardioverted back to sinus through electrical and pharmacological interventions.

Permanent AF

Most people with AF have permanent AF. It is present long-term and the heartbeat cannot be reverted back to sinus rhythm.

People with permanent AF are best treated using a rate-controlling strategy.

Assess bleeding risk as part of clinical assessment before starting a patient on anticoagulation therapy.

Pay particular attention to patients who:

- are aged over 75
- are on multiple other drug treatments, particularly those taking antiplatelet drugs (e.g. aspirin or clopidogrel), non-steroidal anti-inflammatory drugs and antiepilepsy drugs
- have a history of multiple falls
- have a history of excess alcohol consumption
- have uncontrolled hypertension
- have a history of bleeding (e.g. peptic ulcer or cerebral haemorrhage)

The CHAD 2 score is a useful tool to stratify patients into those who need formal anticoagulation with warfarin and those who may be managed with antiplatelet therapy:

    Congestive heart failure

    Hypertension

    Age greater than 75

    Diabetes mellitus

    2 = previous transient ischaemic attack (TIA) or stroke

Patients get 1 point for each criterion; however, a history of TIA or stroke scores 2 points.

- A patient who scores 0 or 1 on the CHAD2 score is at low risk of future embolic events and may be adequately managed with aspirin.
- Patients who score greater than 2 are at an increased risk of future cerebrovascular events, and formal anticoagulation with warfarin reduces the incidence of future adverse events.
- A score of 2 identifies a patient within the grey area of risk for thromboembolic events, and in this instance clinical judgement is required to balance the risks of anticoagulation with warfarin against the detrimental effects of a cerebral infarct secondary to a cardiac thrombus embolizing to the brain.

Management

There are two strategies that may be employed in the management of AF:

- rate control
- rhythm control

The exact clinical indications for a particular approach are not clearly defined, but NICE guidelines suggest that a rhythm-controlling strategy is preferable in patients who:

- are young and symptomatic
- present with lone AF for the first time
- present in acute heart failure
- present with AF secondary to a known or treated precipitant

The results of the AFFIRM (Atrial Fibrillation Follow-up Investigation of Rhythm Management) study indicate that a rate-controlling strategy is preferable in elderly patients, since no advantage is gained through cardioversion (owing mainly to the adverse side-effect profile of the drugs commonly employed).

It is important to note that rate- and rhythm-control measures are not mutually exclusive, and in the event of failure of an initial strategy, the other should be attempted.

Rate control

This employs:

- beta-blockers
- rate-limiting calcium-channel blockers, such as diltiazem and verapamil; note that verapamil causes profound AV blockade and should be avoided in patients with underlying Wolff–Parkinson–White (WPW) syndrome, since it increases the flow of electrical impulses down the accessory pathway (bundle of Kent), which may precipitate VT or VF.
- digoxin

Rhythm control plus antiarrythmic drugs

Pharmacological cardioversion employs:

- amiodarone in patients with evidence of structural heart disease
- flecainide in those with no evidence of heart disease

It is important to determine the time of onset of symptoms in those cases where electrical cardioversion is an appropriate mode of treatment:

- If less than 48 hours, heparinize and consider DC cardioversion.
- If over 48 hours, anticoagulate for at least 3 weeks and consider a transoesophageal echocardiogram to exclude the presence of an intracardiac thrombus.
- If there is a high risk of failure, give 4 weeks of sotalol/amiodarone. Anticoagulate for 4 weeks post cardioversion and consider long-term anticoagulation as determined by the stroke risk stratification algorithm.

NICE guideline on AF

National Collaborating Centre for Chronic Conditions. *Atrial Fibrillation. National Clinical Guideline for Management in Primary and Secondary Care* (NICE Clinical Guideline 36). London: Royal College of Physicians, 2006. Available at: http://guidance.nice.org.uk/CG36.

Scoring Scenario 15.4: Atrial fibrillation

	Inadequate/ not done	Adequate	Good
Appropriate introduction	0	1	—
Transfers the patient to resuscitation and asks assistant to arrange: • full cardiac monitoring • high-flow oxygen • 12-lead ECG • IV access: bloods to exclude sepsis, electrolyte disturbances and thyroid disorders • portable chest X-ray	0	1	2
Identifies ECG rhythm as AF with fast ventricular rate	0	1	—
Suggests that patient is haemodynamically compromised and needs urgent DC cardioversion	0	1	—
Ascertains time of onset < 48 hours	0	1	—
Asks about symptoms: • chest pain • shortness of breath • palpitations • pre-syncope • syncope	0	1	2
Establishes presence of cardiac risk factors.	0	1	—
Asks about other risk factors for AF: e.g. thyrotoxicosis, alcohol, sepsis and lung pathology (at least 4)	0	1	—
Takes a focused drug/allergy history	0	1	—
Prepares for DC cardioversion in the emergency department: • Calls senior colleague/anaesthetist to manage airway • Enquires about any previous adverse reactions to sedation • Ascertains time of last meal • Assesses airway • Prepares airway trolley	0	1	2
Performs DC cardioversion safely: • Uses correct paddle placement • Sedates patient with morphine/midazolam and titrates dose • Uses defibrillator safely (removes oxygen and performs check) • Selects synchronized shock button • Selects appropriate energy level and delivers shock • Checks rhythm post cardioversion	0	1	2
Arranges follow-up: anticoagulation with warfarin and echocardiography	0	1	—
Score from patient	/5		
Global score from examiner	/5		
Total score	/26		

SCENARIO 15.5: ARRHYTHMIA (III)

You are asked to review a 60-year-old man who presents to the emergency department following a collapse at home. The triage nurse hands you his ECG (Figure 15.9).

His observations are:

BP 88/66 mmHg
Pulse 29 bpm
GCS 14
Oxygen saturation 96% on air
Temperature 36.8 °C

Outline your management using the manikin and equipment provided. You are not expected to take a history or examine the patient.

SUGGESTED APPROACH

This is another ALS-type practical scenario where you will be required to manage an arrhythmia. The ECG shows complete (third-degree) heart block, and you would be expected to perform emergency external pacing on the manikin using a defibrillator.

After introducing yourself to the patient, you should ask for them to be transferred to the resuscitation room and be placed on high-flow oxygen and full cardiac monitoring. Immediate management should include:

- securing intravenous access
- full blood count (FBC)
- urea and electrolytes (U&E)
- a venous blood sample to rapidly screen for electrolyte disturbances
- 12-lead ECG
- portable chest X-ray

Although you are not expected to take a history, you should ask about any previous illnesses and features suggesting that the patient has had a recent ischaemic event. Ask about medications such as calcium-channel blockers and beta-blockers, since these can cause complete heart block if taken in overdose.

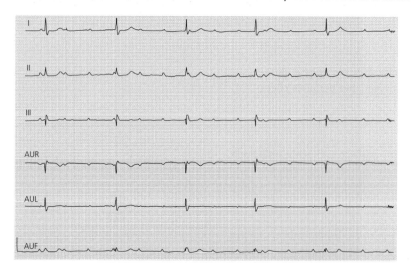

Figure 15.9 ECG of the patient in Scenario 15.5.

Ischaemia is a common precipitant of complete heart block, and you should look for features of myocardial infarction, which may also need to be managed. In addition, look for signs of heart failure or shock.

Atropine 0.5 mg can be given intravenously every 5 minutes up to a maximum dose of 3 mg. It can take up to 5 minutes to take effect and has a half-life of approximately 2–3 hours. If you suspect that the patient has taken an overdose of a beta-blocker or calcium-channel blocker, glucagon is the antidote.

If this is not successful, you should proceed to transcutaneous external pacing. Percussion pacing can be attempted as an emergency measure, with gentle blows to the lower left sternal edge with a closed fist; however, electrical pacing should be organized as soon as possible.

Transcutaneous pacing

Explain to the patient that because their heart is beating very slowly, you will have to control their heart rate using an electronic pacing machine. It is important to explain what the process involves and that you will give them appropriate analgesia. If you are planning to perform this under sedation, you should ask for a second senior emergency department colleague or an anaesthetist to monitor the airway.

Procedure

- Shave the chest if appropriate and attach the pacing pads one anteriorly and one in the left lateral position as shown in Figure 15.8. You should also apply the additional rhythm leads and connect them separately to the defibrillator. It is important that these are not too close to the paddles, since there is a risk of arcing if the paddles are required to defibrillate the patient.
- Select demand mode on the defibrillator and adjust the ECG gain to ensure that intrinsic QRS complexes are being sensed.
- Select an appropriate pacing rate of 60–90 bpm.
- Set the pacing current as low as possible and turn on the pacemaker. Increase the current until *electrical capture* has occurred. This is signified by the presence of a wide QRS complex and T wave following a pacing spike on the ECG. The current required is usually 50–100 mA.
- Once electrical capture has been achieved, you should check the patient's pulse to assess for cardiac output (*mechanical capture*). If there is no pulse, CPR should be commenced. You should inform the examiner that there is no contraindication to touching a patient who is being externally paced.
- Analgesia and sedation should be given to keep the patient comfortable.
- Call for expert help and plan for a transvenous temporary pacemaker to be inserted as soon as the patient has been stabilized. It is important that any underlying cause is also treated appropriately.

Indications

Transcutaneous pacing is appropriate for haemodynamically significant bradyarrhythmias unresponsive to atropine and associated with the following adverse signs:

- hypotension: systolic blood pressure < 90 mmHg
- heart rate < 40 bpm
- pulmonary oedema
- ventricular arrhythmias requiring suppression

In the absence of adverse signs, assess the risk of asystole. This is increased in patients with:

- recent asystolic cardiac arrest
- Mobitz type 2 second-degree heart block
- third-degree heart block with wide QRS complexes
- ventricular pauses greater than 3 seconds

Complications

There may be a failure to recognize VF (which is treatable with defibrillation) owing to the size of the pacing artefact on the ECG screen. You should frequently reassess the patient and the rhythm; defibrillation is indicated immediately if VF occurs.

Other dysrhythmias may be induced.

Soft tissue discomfort may result from pacing. Ensure adequate analgesia and sedation.

There is a potential for local cutaneous injury with prolonged transcutaneous pacing.

Scoring Scenario 15.5: External pacing

	Inadequate/ not done	Adequate	Good
Introduction	0	1	—
Transfers patient to resuscitation area	0	1	—
Initiates immediate management: • high-flow oxygen • full cardiac monitoring • IV access • bloods: FBC and U&E • 12-lead ECG	0	1	2
Identifies complete heart block on ECG	0	1	—
Gives atropine 0.5 mg up to maximum 3 mg	0	1	—
Looks for potential causes: • ischaemia/myocardial infarction • beta-blockers • calcium-channel blockers Considers treatment with glucagon	0	1	2
Explains external pacing to patient	0	1	—
Appropriately attaches pacing pads and monitoring leads. Keeps 2 cm distance between lead and pads to prevent arcing	0	1	—
Selects demand mode on defibrillator	0	1	—
Selects an appropriate pacing rate of 60–90 bpm	0	1	—
Provides suitable sedation and analgesia, with additional anaesthetic/ senior cover	0	1	—
Sets pacing current as low as possible and increases it until electrical capture (50–100 mA)	0	1	—
Checks pulse for mechanical capture	0	1	—
Is aware that there is no electrical hazard in touching patient during pacing	0	1	—
Arranges an urgent cardiology referral for transvenous pacing	0	1	—
Global score from examiner		/5	
Total score		/22	

16
Neurological Emergencies
KATHERINE I M HENDERSON AND CHETAN R TRIVEDY

CORE TOPICS

Causes of headache presenting to the emergency department

- Subarachnoid haemorrhage, arteriovenous malformation
- Meningitis, encephalitis
- Glaucoma
- Raised intracranial pressure
- Temporal arteritis
- Migraine and cluster headaches
- Sinusitis

Status epilepticus

- Appropriate use of pharmacological agents
- Algorithm for status epilepticus, and its complications and side-effects
- Indications for general anaesthetic
- Causes and complications

Coma

- Assessment, including GCS
- Causes and treatment
- Indications for intubation and ventilation
- Indications for imaging

Meningitis, encephalitis and brain abscess

- Clinical features, antiviral and antimicrobial therapy, complications
- Prognosis and differential diagnosis
- Predisposing conditions: HIV etc.

Cerebrovascular disease

- NICE guidelines for management of stroke and transient ischaemic attack (TIA)

- Aetiology of stroke, TIA and stroke syndromes
- Subarachnoid haemorrhage
- Carotid artery dissection
- Venous sinus thrombosis

Cranial nerve lesions (I–XII)

- Anatomical basis for clinical effects of cranial nerve lesions

---

SCENARIO 16.1: HEADACHE HISTORY

A 28-year-old man presents to the emergency department complaining of a severe right-sided headache. He has had similar but milder headaches before. Take a history from the patient and outline your management in the emergency department. You are not expected to examine the patient.

SUGGESTED APPROACH

Headache is a common presentation, and, while the vast majority of headaches are benign, the job of the emergency physician is to identify the potentially life-threatening cases (<1%). This is likely to be the focus of the skill station.

The 'patient' in this scenario will have a set of instructions and a scripted history. You are being examined on your ability to elicit information in a logical, organized way, follow up on clues, process the information that you have obtained, and be able to summarize the history and suggest a plan of action for the patient.

You will also be being examined on your ability to gain the patient's confidence in you as a doctor. It is essential to greet the patient, introduce yourself and then use open questions to encourage the patient to tell you what the problem is. There may be important psychological factors contributing to the complaint of a headache, so be prepared to explore this area.

Know the list of serious causes of headache thoroughly so that you can recognize both 'classical' and classic 'atypical' presentations of these conditions (Tables 16.1 and 16.2).

Ask about analgesia and if the patient would like some painkillers.

The important questions to cover in the history are:

- When did the headache start? Is it continual or episodic?
- Did the headache come on suddenly?
- Was it the worst headache they have ever had and can they score it (10 being the worst headache they have ever had). Some patients may describe a subarachnoid haemorrhage as if they had been hit on the back of the head with a baseball bat.
- What were they doing when the headache started (e.g. exertion, sneezing, bending forward or sexual intercourse)?
- Is this a new headache or have they had problem headaches before?
- If it is an old or chronic headache, what has happened today to make them come to hospital?
- What is the pain like? Is it throbbing, generalized or stabbing? Does it interfere with their normal activities?
- Have they noticed anything else that occurs with or before the headache? Are there any associated features such as an aura, vomiting or photophobia?
- Where is the headache? Is it unilateral or bilateral, behind the eye, or felt over the temporal area?
- Has any treatment (analgesia or antiemetic) or action (lying in a dark room or leaving the location) helped?
- Are there any current medical problems that might be relevant (e.g. cough, colds, earache, dental problems or head trauma)?

- Have there been any previous investigations?
- Is there any important past medical history (e.g. cancer or HIV)?
- Are there any lifestyle factors that may be important (e.g. working or family life, stress and anxiety, alcohol, drug ingestion, or use of sildenafil (which may be associated with SAH))?
- Are they concerned about any particular diagnosis or cause of a headache? Is there any family history of headaches?

Table 16.1 'Classical' presentations of headaches

Type of headache	Clinical features
Subarachnoid haemorrhage (SAH)	Sudden-onset, 'worst ever', 'like a blow', usually occipital. Associated with vomiting. May be preceded by a warning headache days to weeks earlier
Migraine	Throbbing unilateral headache, so severe as to limit activity and made worse by light and noise (photo- and phonophobia). Is a recurrent headache. Associated with nausea/vomiting. Frequently, but not always, preceded by an aura. Builds to a crescendo over about 60 minutes. May last 12–72 hours
Cluster headache	Severe unilateral headache focused around the eye. 'Stabbed in the eye'. Eye may be bloodshot and water. Recurrent, lasting 30–120 minutes, with no aura and no vomiting. Occur in clusters that can last several weeks
Meningitis	Generalized headache in an unwell/drowsy patient. Neck stiffness and photophobia. Rash (meningococcal)
Headache associated with sexual activity – coital cephalgia	Explosive headache indistinguishable from SAH – more common in men (85%).
Brain tumour/space-occupying lesion	Aching headache that gets worse relentlessly. Worse in the morning and on coughing/bending. Personality change/seizures. Patient may have history of cancer
Temporal arteritis	Throbbing headache, scalp tenderness, jaw claudication, tender temporal artery with reduced pulsation

Table 16.2 Additional causes of headaches

Type of headache	Clinical features
Acute glaucoma	Unilateral, associated nausea and vomiting, cloudy cornea with mid-dilated unreactive pupil.
Carbon monoxide poisoning	Headache that improves when the patient leaves the environment!
Tension headache	Bilateral, band-like or squeezing, no vomiting and usually does not prevent normal activities
Sinusitis	Patients complain of a heaviness in the maxillary region and a frontal headache, which is positional
Dental/temporomandibular joint pain	Pain from the jaw joint and maxillary teeth may be referred to the temporal region

Classification system

Primary headaches

- Migraine
- Tension-type headache
- Cluster headache
- Benign exertional, cough- or sexual activity-related headaches

Secondary headaches

- Infectious – including sinusitis and meningitis
- Vascular – including SAH and cavernous sinus thrombosis
- Space-occupying lesions – including brain tumours and subdural haematomas
- Headaches associated with substances or their withdrawal – including caffeine, analgesics and nitrates

Investigations and management

Although a large proportion of the marks in the examination will be for taking a focused clinical history and arriving at a differential diagnosis, there may also be marks for any appropriate investigations and management. You should suggest that you would perform a detailed neurological examination as a part of your assessment.

Any investigations and subsequent management will depend upon the clinical scenario. In the majority of cases, no imaging is required in the emergency department. However, if the scenario suggests that the patient has a SAH, you should suggest to the examiner that you would arrange an urgent CT scan and if this was found to be normal you would perform a lumbar puncture (LP) to exclude a bleed. You should also be able to interpret CT scan imaging as well as LP results. The LP cerebrospinal fluid (CSF) findings in SAH are as follows:

- raised opening pressure
- xanthochromia
- clear or bloody tap
- increased number of red blood cells (RBC > 50 mm^{-3})
- elevated protein
- white cells may occasionally be slightly elevated
- normal glucose
- normal Gram stain

An SAH confirmed with either CT or LP should be referred for a neurosurgical intervention and should be managed in the resuscitation department with appropriate monitoring and necessary medical treatment as outlined in Scenario 2.4.

Alternatively, you may be faced with a situation where the patient has a benign headache and requests a CT scan of the head. In this type of scenario, you may be tested on your negotiation skills and ability to explain to an anxious patient why an urgent CT scan is not indicated. You should avoid being dismissive or confrontational and should explore the patient's underlying concerns and fears.

You should make sure that the patient leaves with appropriate follow-up.

An alternative scenario may involve performing an LP or teaching how to perform an LP to a junior colleague. The procedure is described in Scenario 31.12. You should be prepared to demonstrate the landmarks on an actor and the procedure on a model. You may also be faced with the results of an LP to interpret and act on.

Scoring Scenario 16.1: Headache history

	Inadequate/ not done	Adequate	Good
Appropriate introduction	0	1	—
Establishes patient's presenting complaint of sudden-onset, worst-ever headache	0	1	—
Establishes character of headache: • site • radiation • exacerbating/relieving factors • activity at time of onset (ascertains that headache was postcoital) • impact of analgesia • history of previous headaches	0	1	2
Asks about associated symptoms: • nausea/vomiting • dizziness • collapse • photophobia • visual disturbance • neurological deficit	0	1	2
Takes a focused medical history	0	1	2
Medications (antihypertensives, sildenafil)	0	1	—
Takes a social history/family history of headaches	0	1	—
States intention to examine the patient (does not have to do)	0	1	—
Able to give a differential diagnosis and that SAH is most likely	0	1	—
Suggests urgent CT and LP if CT is negative	0	1	—
Suggests that LP should be performed 12 hours after onset of headache	0	1	—
Correctly identifies positive features of LP CSF interpretation in SAH: • increased opening pressure • xanthochromia • RBC > 50 mm^{-3} • normal Gram stain	0	1	2
Correctly identifies SAH on CT scan	0	1	—
Suggests monitoring patient in resuscitation department: • invasive monitoring • medical treatment for raised intracranial pressure	0	1	—
Arranges urgent referral to neurosurgeons	0	1	—
Explains treatment plan to patient	0	1	—
Score from patient	/5		
Global score from examiner	/5		
Total score	/30		

NEUROLOGICAL EXAMINATION OSCEs

These are designed to examine your skill at performing an important element of your clinical assessment. Often the neurological examination is done poorly in real life as well as in examinations because it is done incompletely. It is essential that you have practised all neurological examination 'set pieces' thoroughly so that your performance is slick. However, be careful to make it clear that you understand what you are examining and not just going through the motions.

Examples

- Examine this patient's cranial nerves.
- Examine this patient's eyes.
- Look at this patient's face and carry out a focused neurological examination.
- Examine this man's lower legs.
- This patient complains of hand tingling and numbness. Carry out a neurological examination of her arm and hand.

POTENTIAL CLINICAL SCENARIOS

Assessment of the cranial nerves (II–VI)

- Pupil abnormalities;
  - ○ Small: Horner's syndrome; Argyll Robertson pupils; age-related; drugs (opiates and pilocarpine)
  - ○ Large: third-nerve palsy; Holmes–Adie syndrome; trauma; drugs (tropicamide, atropine, cocaine, amphetamines and alcohol)
- Fundoscopic abnormalities: diabetic retinopathy
- Visual field abnormalities
- Ptosis

Assessment of the facial (VIIth cranial) nerve

- Lower motor neuron (LMN) facial nerve (Bell's) palsy
- Upper motor neuron (UMN) facial nerve palsy: cerebrovascular accident (CVA)

Examination of the cerebellar system

- Cerebellar stroke
- Cerebellopontine angle tumour
- Dysarthria (patient presenting with abnormal speech)

Examination of the peripheral nervous system (PNS)

- Peripheral neuropathy: diabetes; vitamin B_{12} deficiency
- Wound to arm, hand or leg
- Carpal tunnel syndrome
- Axillary nerve injury
- Paresis as part of a stroke syndrome
- Radial nerve palsy
- Peroneal nerve palsy

SCENARIO 16.2: NEUROLOGICAL EXAMINATION OF THE UPPER LIMB

A 44-year-old woman presents to the emergency department with a complaint of numbness and tingling in her right arm following a fall a week ago. Perform a neurological examination of her upper limbs and outline your differential diagnosis and management plan. You are not expected to take a history.

SUGGESTED APPROACH

You have been asked to conduct a neurological examination, so do not waste time taking a lengthy history. Not only will this not score you marks, it will also eat into the time that you have to perform the examination, present your findings and have a discussion with the examiner. Some examiners will stop you if you start to take a history, but others will let you run on and you may find yourself unable to complete the station. Also make sure that you read the question clearly, since often the examiner may only want an examination of the sensory or motor component and will mark you accordingly.

Introduce yourself to the patient, confirm that she has a problem with her arm and explain what you are going to do. Obtain verbal consent to the examination and ensure that the patient is comfortable and not in pain. Ideally, you should completely expose both arms from shoulder to fingertips so that you can look for asymmetry and muscle wasting.

Ask more specifically where the patient has numbness or loss of sensation. While doing this, examine the patient's arms, looking for scars, wasting of muscles and any deformity. Check whether there is any history of neck problems, in case the problem is higher up. Beware of missing a cervical radiculopathy. Check hand dominance and the patient's occupation, as well as any hobbies.

Then proceed to carry out a neurological examination of both arms, unless you are specifically asked to examine only the affected arm. The brief history of where the numbness is will hopefully make it clear that there is damage over the 'regimental badge' area on the upper arm, suggesting an axillary nerve injury following the patient's fall.

Often candidates are unsure whether they should examine in silence and present at the end or talk through their examinations. We believe that it is better to talk through the examination as you go along, since, first, this will show the examiner that you know what you are doing and, second, if you run out of time, you will have picked up marks on the way. Another approach is to ask the examiner if they have a preference.

The neurological assessment of the upper limbs includes assessment of the following components:

- tone
- power of major muscle groups
- sensation
- reflexes
- coordination
- joint position sense

Although this may appear to be a formidable task to perform in 7 minutes, it is only the assessments of power and sensation that are time-consuming, and time invested in developing a slick examination routine will pay dividends in the OSCE. Ideally, you should examine both arms to look for subtle differences, although the examiner may prompt you to examine just the affected limb. If in doubt, ask the examiner before you start.

Tone

The tone can be easily assessed by clasping the patient's hand as if you were going to shake it. Roll the hand at the wrist and check for resistance in pronation and supination as well as during flexion and extension at the elbow joint.

Look for the following:

Increased tone:

- spasticity (increased tone that may be due to an upper motor neuron lesion)
- cogwheel rigidity (an intermittent increase in tone giving the impression of turning a cogwheel)
- lead pipe rigidity (consistently increased tone throughout the limb)
- myotonia (slow relaxation of the muscle group following movement, e.g. myotonic dystrophy)
- dystonia (the limb fails to relax after movement and both the extensor and flexor muscle remain contracted)
- paratonia (the patient resists your attempts to move their arm)

Decreased tone:

- flaccidity (loss in tone that may be due to a lower motor neuron lesion)

Power

Although testing the power in the limbs is straightforward, many candidates struggle in the OSCE for the following reasons:

- a lack of clear instructions to the patient on what they want them to do – try to demonstrate the movements
- a lack of understanding what muscle group and nerves they are testing – learn the nerve roots
- a lack of appreciation that the patient may be frail, in pain or may have neurology that may affect their ability to perform a movement – be gentle

It is essential that you practise your examination and at least learn the muscles and nerve roots supplying them. This will not only impress the examiner but also allow you localize lesions anatomically.

You should use the Medical Research Council (MRC) scoring system:

5	normal power
4+	suboptimal movement against resistance
4	moderate movement against resistance
4–	slight movement against resistance
3	movement against gravity but not against resistance
2	movement with gravity eliminated
1	flicker of movement
0	no movement

It is important you use this classification, since actors/patients may be primed to have a specific grade of weakness that you will be required to elicit in your examination. A guide to assessing the major movements in the upper limb is summarized in Table 16.3.

Sensation

It is important that sensation be tested using two modalities, such as light touch with cotton wool and with a pin. Both arms should be tested and compared simultaneously to look for any subtle sensory losses. Again it is crucial that you explain to the patient what you are doing and, more importantly, what you want them to do, and you must check that they understand the test. You should dab with the cotton wool and not stroke the skin with it, since these latter tests pain and not touch. The major sensory dermatomes are shown in Figure 16.1. You should mention to the examiner that ideally you would also test for loss of temperature sensation using a cold tuning fork.

In this scenario, the patient has an axillary nerve injury in the right arm and may present with numbness over the C5 (regimental badge area) dermatome as well as a weakness in shoulder abduction.

Table 16.3 Assessment of motor function in the upper limb

Test	Instructions	Muscle(s)	Nerve(s)	Root
Shoulder abduction	Ask the patient to put their elbows out to each side like wings and keep them there while you push down	Deltoid	Axillary	C5
Elbow flexion	Support the wrist and elbow with the forearm supinated and ask the patient to bend their elbow so that their palm reaches for the ipsilateral shoulder tip while you apply resistance at the wrist	Biceps Brachioradialis	Musculo-cutaneous Radial	C5/6 C6
Elbow extension	Support the wrist and elbow and, with the elbow flexed, ask the patient to straighten their arm against resistance	Triceps	Radial	C7
Foream pronation	Ask the patient to pronate their arm from a supinated position against resistance as if they were turning a key in a lock	Pronator teres	Median	C6
Wrist extension	With the forearm pronated, ask the patient to make a fist and cock their wrists downwards and push them up against resistance (as if they were revving the throttle on a imaginary motorbike)	Extensor carpi radialis longus	Radial	C6
Wrist flexion	With the arm in the supinated position, ask the patient to make a fist and abduct the hand at the wrist against resistance	Flexor carpi radialis	Median	C7
Finger extension	Ask the patient to hold their hands out with their fingers straight and palms facing down. Support the wrist with one hand while you push down on the fingers with the ulnar border of your other hand. The patient should be instructed to keep their fingers straight	Extensor digitorum	Radial	C7
Finger flexion	Place the palmar aspect of your fingers on the corresponding palmar surface of the patient's fingers. Ask the patient to make a fist so that your fingers interlock. The patient's resistance to you opening their grip is a test of finger flexion	Flexor digitorum superficialis Flexor digitorum profundus	Ulnar and median	C8
Finger abduction	Ask the patient to spread their fingers out and keep them straight. Support the middle, ring and little finger while you try overcome their resistance by pushing on the lateral border of the index finger	First dorsal interosseous Abductor pollicis brevis	Ulnar and median	T1
Intrinsic muscles of the hand supplied by the median nerve **(LOAF)**	The opponens pollicis is assessed by asking the patient to make a circle by touching the tips of their thumb and little finger together while you try to break the circle with your index finger. The abductor pollicis is assessed by asking the patient to place their hands flat with the palm up and with the thumb pointing up to the ceiling while you try to push it down with your index finger. The flexor pollicis brevis can be tested by asking the patient to lay their thumb on their palm while you try to push it outwards. The lumbricals can be tested by asking the patient to pinch their thumb and index fingers together. The lumbricals are responsible for the 'pulp-to-pulp' pinch.	Lateral lumbricals Opponens pollicis Abductor pollicis brevis Flexor pollicis brevis	Median	T1

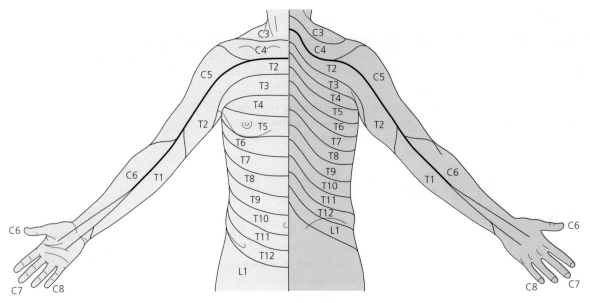

Figure 16.1 Sensory dermatomes in the upper limb (front and back).

Important sensory dermatomal landmarks in the upper limb include:

C5: regimental badge area
C6: thumb
C7: middle finger
C8: little finger
T1: medial aspect of elbow
T2: medial aspect of upper arm

You should specifically examine for sensory loss in the distribution of the three main nerves that supply the hand:

- median nerve (sensory loss over the palmar aspect of the thumb and index finger)
- ulnar nerve (sensory loss over the palmar aspect of the little finger)
- radial nerve (sensory loss over the anatomical snuffbox on the dorsum of the hand)

Reflexes

No neurological examination can be complete without the use of the tendon hammer. The main reflexes in the upper limb that should be tested are:

- biceps reflex (C5/C6)
- triceps reflex (C7)
- supinator (brachioradialis) reflex (C5/C6)

As with power, you should score reflexes accordingly and use the correct nomenclature when you present your findings:

0   absent
±   present with reinforcement
1+   present but depressed
2+   normal
3+   increased
4+   clonus

Coordination

This can be tested by asking the patient to perform a series of tasks such as the following:

- Ask the patient to close their eyes and put their arms out straight ahead of them. Look for drift or marked swinging when either arm is pushed.
- Finger–nose test: ask the patient to touch your finger, which should be an arm's breadth from the patient's finger, and then to touch their nose as quickly and accurately as possible.
- Ask the patient to make rapid alternating movements of the hands (tests for dysdiadochokinesia).

Joint position sense and proprioception

You should complete your examination by informing the examiner that you would check proprioception with a 128 Hz tuning fork and assess joint position sense.

By the time of the examination, you should have a fair idea of where the injury is anatomically and whether the injury is in the hand or at a higher level. Table 16.4 summarizes the characteristics of the major injuries affecting the upper limb. There may also be marks for suggesting a differential diagnosis based on your findings, as well as any investigations that you might arrange in the emergency department.

Management in the emergency department

This patient, who has an isolated axillary nerve injury, may require a shoulder X-ray to look for an underlying injury to the humeral head, and you should suggest referring them for orthopaedic follow-up.

Table 16.4 Differential diagnosis of isolated nerve injuries in the upper limb

Nerve root affected	Motor deficit/weakness	Sensory deficit	Impaired reflex
Level of injury in arm:			
C5 root	• Shoulder abduction • External rotation • Elbow flexion	• Outer aspect of upper arm	• Biceps
Axillary nerve	• Shoulder abduction	• Regimental badge	—
C6 root	• Elbow flexion • Pronation		• Supinator
C7 root	• Elbow and wrist extension	• Middle finger	• Triceps
C8 root	• Finger flexion	• Little finger	• Finger
T1 root	• Wasting of the small muscles of the hand	• Medial aspect of forearm	
Injury in hand:			
Median nerve	• Thenar eminence wasting • LOAF muscles	• Thumb, index and medial border of middle finger	—
Radial nerve	• Wrist extension • Finger extension	• Localized over anatomical snuffbox	• Supinator • Triceps (if injury is high)
Ulnar nerve	• Wasting of muscles except LOAF • Weakness of finger abduction	• Lateral half of ring finger and little finger	—

Scoring Scenario 16.2: Neurological examination of the upper limb

	Inadequate/ not done	Adequate	Good
Appropriate introduction	0	1	—
Establishes patient's presenting symptoms	0	1	—
Obtains consent for examination	0	1	—
Exposes both arms fully and looks for: • posturing • scars • wasting	0	1	2
Performs motor assessment: • shoulder abduction • elbow flexion • elbow extension • wrist extension • wrist flexion • finger extension • finger abduction	0	1	2
Identifies weakness in shoulder abduction on right side	0	1	—
Specifically assesses motor function: • median nerve • ulnar nerve • radial nerve	0	1	2
Performs sensory assessment and names the dermatomes being tested	0	1	2
Identifies sensory loss over regimental badge area	0	1	—
Tests reflexes: • biceps • supinator • reflexes	0	1	—
States intention to test: • coordination • temperature • proprioception/vibration	0	1	—
Differential diagnosis of axillary nerve damage	0	1	—
Arranges shoulder X-ray and orthopaedic follow-up	0	1	—
Carries out examination in systematic and logical manner	0	1	—
Score from patient	/5		
Global score from examiner	/5		
Total score	/28		

SCENARIO 16.3: CRANIAL NERVE EXAMINATION

A 60-year-old woman presents to the emergency department after noticing a weakness on the left side of her face. Examine her cranial nerves with the exception of I, II and VIII and give your differential diagnosis and management plan. You are not expected to take a history.

SUGGESTED APPROACH

Although it may seem obvious, it is vital that you read the instructions very carefully and only examine the cranial nerves that you are asked to look at. Hence, in this scenario, the examination of the visual fields and optic nerve will not score any marks and will waste valuable time. Examination of the IInd cranial (optic) nerve is discussed in detail in Scenario 10.1.

The key to this OSCE scenario is a slick and fluent examination technique that should end with a differential diagnosis relating to the facial weakness. For convenience, the examination of the face can be divided into four parts:

1. General inspection
2. Examination of the IIIrd, IVth and VIth cranial nerves
3. Examination of the Vth and VIIth cranial nerves
4. Examination of the IXth–XIIth cranial nerves

General inspection

As you introduce yourself to the patient, establish how long they have had the facial weakness and ask briefly if they have noticed any weakness in their arms or legs. Listen to the patient's speech to see if there is any obvious slurring. Look at the face for any asymmetry or the presence of a rash or conjunctivitis, which may indicate herpes zoster (HZ) as a potential cause.

Look behind the ear, and if you suspect HZ as a cause then suggest performing an examination of the auditory canal for vesicles, which would suggest Ramsay Hunt syndrome.

Although you are not required to test the hearing formally, you should ask if the patient has noticed any recent change in their hearing, as hyperacusis is associated with a VIIth nerve palsy as a result of the loss of the dampening effects of the stapedius muscle.

Explain to the patient what you are doing and look carefully at their face for any evidence of asymmetry. Check that this is really a unilateral problem – bilateral facial weakness is easy to miss but is unlikely to be in the OSCE. Look for any masses or the presence of surgical scars over the parotid gland, which would suggest a lower motor neuron palsy involving the VIIth nerve as it passes through the parotid gland.

Examination of the eyes (IIIrd, IVth and VIth cranial nerves)

These cranial nerves essentially control eye movements, and you should check the gaze in all directions, not forgetting to make the patient to look downwards and inwards. When examining these nerves, you should consider the anatomical basis of your examination.

IVth cranial (trochlear) nerve

The IVth cranial nerve supplies only the superior oblique muscle. In a IVth nerve lesion, the patient typically complains of double vision when they attempt to look downwards and inwards, for example when they are reading or going down the stairs.

VIth cranial (abducent) nerve

The VIth cranial nerve supplies only the lateral rectus. A VIth nerve palsy is characterized by lack of a lateral (outward) gaze in the affected eye.

IIIrd cranial (oculomotor) nerve

The IIIrd cranial nerve supplies all of the other rectus muscles, as well as the levator palpebrae muscles that lift the eyelid. A IIIrd nerve lesion is sometimes referred to as a 'lazy vagabond' lesion: when the 'lazy' eyelid (ptosis) on the affected side is lifted, the eye is found to be in a 'down and out' position with a dilated pupil that does not respond to light or accommodation because of the disruption to the parasympathetic fibres that travel with the IIIrd nerve.

Examination of the face (Vth and VIIth cranial nerves)

These two nerves both have a motor and a sensory component, as well as reflexes that need to be tested.

Vth cranial (trigeminal) nerve

The Vth cranial nerve supplies the muscles of mastication (masseter and temporalis), as well as sensation on the face. You should initially look for any weakness in the masticatory muscles by asking the patient to open and close their mouth against resistance. You should also look for deviation of the jaw during opening and closing. The sensory component of this nerve can be divided into three branches:

- the ophthalmic branch, which supplies sensation in the forehead
- the maxillary branch, which supplies the skin on the cheek
- the mandibular branch, which supplies the skin over the mandible (excluding the angle of the jaw)

You should test fine touch and pin-prick on both sides of the face simultaneously, looking for subtle differences in sensation. Perform the 'jaw-jerk' reflex by asking the patient to open their mouth slightly and placing two fingers on the centre of the chin, which can be percussed with a tendon hammer.

VIIth cranial (facial) nerve

The motor component of the VIIth cranial nerve supplies the muscles of facial expression, which can be tested by asking the patient to:

- smile
- show you their teeth
- blow out their cheeks against resistance
- whistle
- raise their eyebrows
- screw up their eyes tightly while you try to open them

It also supplies the stapedius muscle, which dampens the hearing, so ask the patient if their hearing is louder on one side than on the other. You should make it clear to the examiner that you are not testing the VIIIth nerve but looking for loss of stapedius function.

The sensory component of the facial nerve can be assessed by testing the sensation of taste in the anterior two-thirds of the tongue. It is unlikely that the examiner will request you to do this. You should also ask if there have been any problems with tear production, since the facial nerve also carries parasympathetic fibres to the lacrimal gland. It is not recommended that you actually test this in the examination.

The corneal reflex is a mixed reflex that has a Vth sensory component and a VIIth motor component. What you are eliciting is the ability of the patient to blink by touching the cornea with a wisp of cotton wool. You should suggest testing the corneal reflex; again it is unlikely that you would have to actually do it.

Upper motor neuron (UMN) or lower motor neuron disorder (LMN)

It is important not only to be able to distinguish a UMN lesion from an LMN lesion (Box 16.1), but also to know some of the common causes of facial nerve weakness (Box 16.2).

Box 16.1 Differentiating upper and lower motor neuron (UMN and LMN) facial weaknesses

UMN weakness	LMN weakness
• Central lesion in facial nerve nucleus in pons • Upper third of face receives supranuclear innervation from both hemispheres (bilateral innervation) • Upper third of face is spared • May be associated with speech and swallowing difficulties, as well as visual field defects and limb weakness • Usually arises as a result of a cerebrovascular accident, a demyelinating disorder or a brainstem lesion	• Peripheral nerve lesion distal to nucleus • Lower part of face receives innervation only from contralateral hemisphere (unilateral innervation) • Weakness affects whole of one side of face • Loss of wrinkle lines on forehead • Patient is unable to raise eyebrow on affected side • Loss of nasolabial fold on affected side • Patient may demonstrate Bell's phenomenon: the eye rolls up when patient attempts to close it

Box 16.2 Causes of LMN facial nerve weakness

Bell's palsy
This is the most common cause of facial palsy. By definition, it is idiopathic, possibly viral in origin (60% of patients have a viral prodrome). There is a higher incident in those with diabetes – this may really be a diabetic mononeuropathy. It is bilateral in less than 1% of patients.

Herpes zoster
Herpes zoster, or Ramsay Hunt syndrome, is the second most common cause of facial paralysis, representing 3–12% of such patients. Patients may have pain over the face and ear that is out of proportion to the physical examination. They may note vertigo, hearing loss (sensorineural) from involvement of the VIIIth cranial nerve, tinnitus, rapid onset of facial paralysis and decreased salivation, and taste is often affected.

Parotid gland disease
As the facial nerve passes through the body of the parotid gland, infections, trauma or tumour affecting the gland may cause facial nerve weakness.

Cerebellopontine angle tumours
Acoustic neuromas or meningiomas arising in the triangle between the cerebellum, the lateral pons and the petrous bone can compress cranial nerves V–VIII as they emerge into this triangle from the pons. The clinical features include loss of corneal reflex (often an early sign), facial sensory loss, later facial weakness and sensorineural deafness.

Bilateral LMN weakness
Systemic conditions such as sarcoidosis and Guillain–Barré syndrome can present with bilateral facial nerve weakness.

Examination of the lower cranial nerves IX–XII

You should complete your assessment of the cranial nerves by examining the four lower cranial nerves.

IXth cranial (glossopharyngeal) nerve

The IXth cranial nerve is mainly a sensory nerve supplying the posterior third of the tongue and pharyngeal mucosa. This nerve also forms the afferent limb of the gag reflex.

Xth cranial (vagus) nerve

The Xth cranial nerve is essentially a motor nerve supplying the muscles of the palate, larynx and pharynx. However, it does have a small sensory supply to the external auditory canal and the tympanic membrane. It forms the efferent limb of the gag reflex.

Use a tongue spatula and a pen torch to visualize the uvula and for displacement when the patient says 'ahh'. Mention to the examiner that you would also test the patient's swallow and the gag reflex, although this should not be attempted in the OSCE.

XIth cranial (accessory) nerve

The XIth cranial nerve is a motor nerve that supplies the sternocleidomastoid and the trapezius. It can be tested by asking the patient to turn their head laterally or shrug their shoulders up against resistance.

XIIth cranial (hypoglossal) nerve

The XIIth cranial nerve is a purely motor nerve, supplying the intrinsic muscles of the tongue. It is tested easily by asking the patient to stick their tongue out and move it from side to side. Any deviation of the tongue during protrusion may be suggestive of a hypoglossal nerve lesion; the direction of deviation points to the side of the lesion. You should also look for muscle wasting and fasciculations.

Management

At the end of your examination, you will be asked for a differential diagnosis and your proposed management of the patient. In this scenario, the patient has Bell's palsy, and you should tell the examiner your management plan, which should include the following:

- You should explain the diagnosis to the patient, reassuring them they have not had a stroke and that they will make a recovery.
- The eye should be protected with an eye patch and artificial tears.
- High-dose steroids are recommended. The use of antiviral drugs is controversial unless you suspect Ramsay Hunt syndrome.
- Routine bloods are usually not necessary in the emergency department unless the patient is immunosuppressed.
- All patients should be followed up by the ear, nose and throat team.

Scoring Scenario 16.3: Cranial nerve examination

	Inadequate/ not done	Adequate	Good
Appropriate introduction	0	1	—
Explains examination to patient	0	1	—
Carries out a general inspection: • asymmetry • scars • swelling • assesses speech	0	1	2
Examines IIIrd, IVth and VIth cranial nerves: • Checks eye movements • Checks pupil and accommodation reflex • Looks for ptosis • Asks about double vision	0	1	2
Examines Vth cranial nerve: • Assesses motor component to muscles of mastication • Assesses sensory component in ophthalmic/maxillary/mandibular region (light touch and pin-prick) • Performs jaw-jerk reflex	0	1	2
Examines VIIth cranial nerve: • Assesses motor function • Suggests testing taste on anterior two-thirds of tongue • Suggests testing stapedius	0	1	2
Suggests testing corneal reflex involving Vth and VIIth nerves	0	1	—
Checks for deviation of uvula	0	1	—
Suggests checking gag reflex and swallow	0	1	—
Tests XIth cranial nerve (sternocleidomastoid and trapezius)	0	1	—
Assesses XIIth cranial nerve for tongue protrusion, fasciculation and muscle wasting	0	1	—
Summarizes findings	0	1	—
Makes a differential diagnosis of LMN facial weakness: • Bell's palsy • Ramsay Hunt syndrome	0	1	2
Suggests management in emergency department: • eye patch • artificial tears • steroids • discusses use of antivirals if herpesvirus implicated • ENT follow-up	0	1	2
Score from patient	/5		
Global score from examiner	/5		
Total score	/30		

SCENARIO 16.4: NEUROLOGICAL EXAMINATION OF THE LOWER LIMB

A 28-year-old man attends the emergency department with weakness in his right leg after being hit by a car bumper while crossing the road. Carry out a neurological examination of his legs. You are not expected to take a history.

SUGGESTED APPROACH

You should approach this scenario in the same way as was described for Scenario 16.2. Although you are not asked to take a history, you should ask the patient if they have any pain, numbness or weakness in their legs. The patient may have been primed not to give anything away.

Start your examination by exposing the patient so that you can see both limbs, while maintaining the patient's dignity.

Look for abnormal posturing, muscle wasting, muscle fasciculation or scars.

You should move swiftly onto your examination, assessing:

- tone
- power
- sensation
- reflexes
- coordination
- joint position/vibration sense
- gait

Tone

Check the tone in the lower limbs by rolling each leg in turn and then suddenly lifting the leg at the level of the knee.

Power

You should check the power in the major muscle groups in the lower limbs as outlined in Table 16.5. Ideally, you should examine both legs while the patient is lying flat in the supine position.

Sensation

Sensation should be assessed in the major dermatomes in the lower limb using fine touch with a cotton-wool pledget and pin-prick sensation. Compare both limbs simultaneously to map out any areas of sensory loss. You are strongly advised to learn the approximate distribution of the dermatomes as shown in Figure 16.2.

Reflexes

Lower limb reflexes include the:

- knee jerk (femoral nerve L3/L4)
- ankle jerk (tibial nerve S1/S2)

You should also check the plantar response (Babinski sign) when the sole of the foot is scratched with an orange stick. The normal response is for the toes to flex, which is a negative Babinski sign. If the big toe extends with the toes spreading, this is a positive Babinski sign and may indicate a UMN lesion.

Table 16.5 Assessment of motor function in the lower limb

Movement	Instruction to patient	Muscle group	Nerve	Root
Hip flexion	Ask the patient to bend their knee and then bring it towards their chest while you place a hand above their knee to overcome their efforts	Iliopsoas	Lumbar sacral plexus	L1/L2
Hip extension	With the leg flat on the bed, place one hand under the ankle and ask the patient to push down on your hand while you try to lift the leg off the bed	Gluteus maximus	Sciatic	L5/S1
Knee flexion	Ask the patient to bend their knee so that the heel is bought towards their bottom and keep it there while you try to straighten it. The patient should resist your efforts	Hamstrings	Sciatic	L5/S1
Knee extension	With the patient's knee bent at 90°, place one of your hands under the knee and the other hand in front of the ankle. Ask the patient to straighten the knee while you offer resistance at the ankle	Quadriceps	Femoral	L3/L4
Dorsiflexion of ankle	Ask the patient to cock their foot up towards their head against your hand while you offer resistance	Tibialis anterior	Deep peroneal	L4
Plantarflexion of ankle	Ask the patient to point their foot down as if they were pushing on the pedal of a car while you offer resistance	Gastrocnemius	Posterior tibial	S1
Ankle eversion	Ask the patient to turn their ankle outwards against resistance	Peronei	Superficial peroneal	L5/S1
Extension of big toe	Ask the patient to bring their big toe towards their face while you try to push the toe downwards	Extensor hallucis longus	Deep peroneal	L5

Coordination

Lower limb coordination can be tested by asking the patient to put the heel of one leg on the knee of the other leg and to run it down the shin in a straight line and then back up the shin from the ankle.

Joint position sense (JPS) and vibration sense

It is important to test these modalities when you suspect that the patient has a neuropathy. Patients with conditions such as diabetes, nutritional deficiencies and Charcot–Marie–Tooth disease may present with a loss of JPS. JPS is tested by holding the big toe on its medial and later aspects and moving it either 'up' or 'down' while the patient has their eyes shut. You should first brief the patient as to what movement is 'up' or 'down'. If the patient fails to identify the movements correctly, you can repeat the process using the ankle instead. Vibration sense can be tested by placing a 128 Hz tuning fork on bony landmarks such as the malleoli.

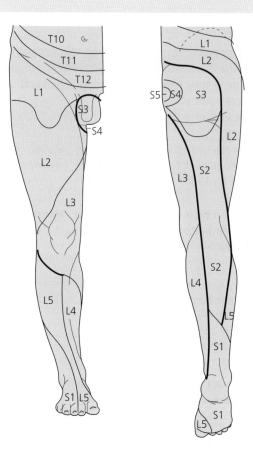

Figure 16.2 Sensory dermatomes in the lower limb.

Gait

If the patient is able to stand, you should attempt to test their gait by asking them to walk a few steps. The following gaits may observed:

- shuffling gait – Parkinson's disease and basal ganglion disorder
- scissoring gait – cerebral palsy and multiple sclerosis
- ataxic gait – cerebellar disease, where the patient may lean to one side
- hemiplegic gait – where one leg is swung out secondary to a UMN lesion (CVA)
- foot drop – a high-stepping gait where the affected foot has to be lifted off the ground, secondary to a common peroneal nerve palsy or an L5 lesion

Differential diagnosis

The patient in this scenario is likely to have a common peroneal nerve injury, which classically presents after a person has been struck by a car bumper at a level below the knee. The features of this type of injury include:

- weakness in dorsiflexion and foot eversion
- sensory loss over the dorsum of the foot and the outside of the shin

Management

You should complete your assessment by summarizing your findings to the examiner and arranging an X-ray of the leg if you suspect that there may be an underlying bony injury. The patient should also have an urgent orthopaedic referral for further investigation and management.

Scoring Scenario 16.4: Neurological examination of the lower limb

	Inadequate/ not done	Adequate	Good
Appropriate introduction	0	1	—
Inspects patient's legs from end of the bed, looking for: • muscle wasting • abnormal posture • limb deformity	0	1	—
Checks with patient whether their legs are painful before examination. Offers analgesia	0	1	—
Assesses tone in both limbs	0	1	—
Assesses power in: • hip flexion (L1/L2) • hip extension (L5/S1) • knee flexion (S1) • knee extension (L3/L4) • foot dorsiflexion (L4) • foot plantarflexion (S1/S2) • ankle eversion (L5/S1) • big toe extension (L5) Extra marks for knowing nerve roots	0	1	2
Tests reflexes using correct technique: • knee jerk (L3/L4) • ankle jerk (S1/S2) • plantar (Babinski response)	0	1	2
Assesses light touch in both limbs	0	1	—
Assess pin-prick sensation in both limbs	0	1	—
Assesses vibration sense in both limbs	0	1	—
Assesses proprioception in both limbs	0	1	—
Tests coordination and either walks the patient to assess gait or expresses desire to do so	0	1	—
Summarizes findings: • foot drop • weakness in ankle eversion • sensory loss over dorsum of foot and lateral aspect of leg	0	1	2
Suggests differential diagnosis and likely diagnosis of common peroneal nerve palsy	0	1	—
Suggests orthopaedic referral	0	1	—
Score from patient	/5		
Total score from examiner	/5		
Total score	/27		

SCENARIO 16.5: MANAGEMENT OF TIA

An 80-year-old man presents to the emergency department after having had a collapse at home 4 hours ago. His wife, who is with him, reports that he fell in the kitchen, following which he appeared to be confused, and slurred his speech for a couple of hours. He has now made a complete recovery, and he is sorry that he has wasted your time.

His observations are:

BP 160/90 mmHg
Pulse 90bpm, irregular
Oxygen saturation 96% on air
Temperature 36.2 °C
Blood glucose 7.2 mmol L^{-1} (random)

Take a focused history and outline your management plan.

SUGGESTED APPROACH

It is clear from the scenario that this patient has had some sort of cerebral event, and the fact that he has now made a full recovery is strongly suggestive of a transient ischaemic attack (TIA). You should start by taking an accurate history from the patient, as well as corroborative history from his wife. This OSCE also tests your ability to take a psychosocial geriatric history and incorporate it into your management plan

History

Timing

Ask the following questions about the event:

- When did it start?
- How long did the symptoms last before resolution?
- Was the onset sudden or gradual?

Type of symptoms

Ask about the following symptoms:

- slurred speech
- limb weakness (specify its distribution)
- facial weakness
- numbness in limbs or face
- difficulty in swallowing
- confusion
- visual disturbances
- headache
- nausea/vomiting
- any period of loss of consciousness
- dizziness
- loss of balance

Focused medical history

Ask about:

- previous stroke/CVA
- atrial fibrillation
- high blood pressure
- diabetes
- family history of CVA
- previous operations
- medications and allergies
- any contraindications for anticoagulation
- social history: smoking, alcohol and type of accommodation

You should also enquire about the patient's activities of daily living (ADL). This is to gauge the impact that a cerebral event may have on the patient. ADL include:

- mobility
- washing
- dressing
- cleaning
- feeding
- shopping
- financial support

As the patient has presented with a history of confusion, you should tell the examiner that you would like to perform a mini-mental state examination (MMSE). It is unlikely that you would be expected to take a history as well as perform an MMSE in the OSCE, but you can mention that it is something you would do under the circumstances.

Risk stratification and management

From the patient's history, it should be clearly evident that he has had a TIA. You should be aware of validated scoring tools that can be used by emergency department physicians either to identify a stroke (e.g. the Recognition of Stroke in the Emergency Room (ROSIER) scoring system, shown in Table 16.6) or to predict the risk of a TIA progressing to a stroke (e.g. the $ABCD^2$ scoring system shown in Table 16.7). These are easy to use: Tables 16.6 and 16.7 also illustrate their use in this scenario.

A ROSIER score greater than zero is suggestive of an acute stroke, whereas an $ABCD^2$ score greater than 4 suggests that the patient is at a high risk of developing a stroke. In this scenario, the patient has a ROSIER score of zero and a $ABCD^2$ score of 5, suggesting that he has had a TIA and is at a high risk of progressing to a stroke.

It is also important that you are at least aware of the 2008 NICE guidelines on the diagnosis and acute managment of strokes and TIAs. These guidelines suggest that patients with an $ABCD^2$ score greater than 4 should be immediately started on aspirin and be seen by a specialist within 24 hours. In addition, such patients should have brain imaging within 24 hours and should have secondary prevention by optimizing their blood pressure and blood sugar control. Early carotid artery imaging is also indicated. It is possible that the patient in this scenario may have undiagnosed diabetes, since he has a random blood sugar of 7.2 mmol L^{-1}, which should prompt further investigation.

Patients who present with an $ABCD^2$ score less than 4 should also be started on aspirin and have imaging and follow-up with a specialist within a week, as well as having secondary prevention as described above.

Interestingly, the NICE guidelines do not recommend supplemental oxygen for patients with acute stroke unless their oxygen saturation drops below 95%, and oxygen should be given according to the 2008 British Thoracic Society (BTS) guidelines (see Scenario 14.1).

Table 16.6 The ROSIER scoring system for identifying acute stroke in the emergency department. The scores for the patient in Scenario 16.5 are underlined

| | Score | |
	Yes	No
Loss of consciousness or syncope	−1	0
Seizure activity	−1	0
New acute onset of asymmetrical weakness in:		
Face	1	0
Arms	1	0
Legs	1	0
Speech disturbance	1	0
Visual disturbance	1	0
Total score range	−2 to 5	
Total score for this patient	0 (−1 + 1)	

Table 16.7 The ABCD^2 scoring system for predicting the risk of TIA progression to stroke. The scores for the patient in Scenario 16.5 are underlined

	Score
Age > 60	1
BP systolic > 140/90 mm/Hg	1
Clinical features:	
Unilateral weakness	2
Speech disturbance without weakness	1
(maximum of 2 marks)	
Duration:	
>60 minutes	2
10–60 minutes	1
<10 minutes	0
Diabetes	1
Total score range	0–7
Total score for this patient	5 (1+1+1+2)

You should also be prepared for a potential scenario where the patient has an acute confirmed stroke, for which the guidelines suggest prompt imaging within the hour. You should also mention that some units are now thrombolysing acute stroke patients who have presented within 3 hours of onset of their symptoms. This is not yet routine practice, but you should be aware of it as a potential option and you should inform the examiner that you would discuss the case with the on-call stroke team.

With this information in mind, you should suggest to the patient that he has a high risk of progressing to a stroke and should be admitted under the medical team so that he can be followed up by a specialist and have any appropriate imaging. You should recommend that he be started on aspirin with proton pump inhibitor cover. You may find that you have to spend time trying to convince the patient that he needs to come in to hospital and you may be tested on your negotiation skills.

Scoring Scenario 16.5: Management of TIA

	Inadequate/ not done	Adequate	Good
Appropriate introduction	0	1	—
Elicits features of event: • accurate timing of TIA (2 hours) • limb weakness • slurring of speech • dizziness • nausea/vomiting • headache	0	1	2
Takes focused medical history: • high blood pressure • diabetes • atrial fibrillation • previous CVA/TIA • medications • allergies • contraindications to anticoagulation	0	1	2
Takes social history: • smoking • alcohol • ADL	0	1	—
States intention to perform MMSE (does not have to do)	0	1	—
Calculates ROSIER score 0 (low risk for acute CVA)	0	1	2
Calulates ABCD² score of 5. Suggests that patient is at high risk for developing a CVA	0	1	2
Suggests management: • aspirin • specialist review in 24 hours • CT scan in 24 hours • secondary prevention	0	1	2
Explains management plan to patient and recommends admission	0	1	—
Score from patient	/5		
Global score from examiner	/5		
Total score	/24		

USEFUL RESOURCES

Aids to the Examination of the Peripheral Nervous System, 4th edn. London: *Brain*/WB Saunders, 2000.

Fuller G. *Neurological Examination Made Easy*, 3rd edn. Edinburgh: Churchill Livingstone, 2004.

National Collaborating Centre for Chronic Conditions. *Stroke. National Clinical Guideline for Diagnosis and Initial Management of Acute Stroke and Transient Ischaemic Attack (TIA)*. (NICE Clinical Guideline 68). London: Royal College of Physicians, 2008. Available at: http://guidance.nice.org.uk/CG68.

17
Acid–Base Disorders
BETH CHRISTIAN

CORE TOPICS

- Interpretation of blood gas results
- Alveolar gas equation and Aa gradient
- Metabolic acidosis, including lactic acidosis
- Acute respiratory acidosis
- Chronic respiratory acidosis
- Respiratory alkalosis
- Metabolic alkalosis
- Anion gap
- Osmolal gap
- Sodium bicarbonate and its role as a therapeutic agent

Respiratory failure and acute fluid and electrolyte disorders are common presenting conditions in the acutely unwell emergency department patient.

It is vital that all emergency medicine trainees and specialists be capable of analysing blood gases and patient biochemistry in order to competently institute early management. For the purposes of the CEM OSCE, the most likely scenario would involve teaching a student on how to interpret an arterial blood gas (ABG). This not only requires you to interpret the ABG yourself but also to teach the student on how you arrived at your analysis.

This chapter will focus on the interpretation of blood gases.

ACID-BASE DISORDERS

Interpreting blood gases can be complicated and may distract from the primary intention of assessing a patient's physiological state.

When applying the rules for blood gas analysis, it is easiest to ask yourself a series of questions:

- Is the pH normal?
    - Is it between 7.35 and 7.45 (i.e. normal)?
    - If not, is it <7.35 or >7.45.
- If the pH is abnormal, what is the primary disturbance?
    - If pH < 7.35 then acidosis must be present.
    - If pH > 7.45 then alkalosis must be present.

○ If $7.35 \leq$ pH ≤ 7.45 then there is no acid–base disorder or there has been an attempt at compensation or there may be a mixed disorder with an acidosis and an alkalosis.
- What is the pattern of arterial partial pressure of carbon dioxide ($PaCO_2$) and bicarbonate (HCO_3^-)?
  ○ If $PaCO_2$ and HCO_3^- are both low then this indicates metabolic acidosis or respiratory alkalosis, with or without a mixed disorder.
  ○ If $PaCO_2$ and HCO_3^- are both high then this suggests respiratory acidosis or metabolic alkalosis, with or without a mixed disorder.
  ○ If $PaCO_2$ and HCO_3^- are both abnormal but one is high and the other is low then a mixed disorder is present.
- In respiratory acidosis, is the process acute or chronic?
- Is there any attempt at compensation?
- What is the alveolar–arterial (Aa) gradient?

Look for additional electrolyte disturbances, such as:

- raised glucose (with ketones and acidosis: diabetic ketoacidosis, DKA)
- raised anion gap (metabolic acidosis)
- hypokalaemia and hypochloraemia (metabolic alkalosis)
- hyperchloraemia (normal-anion-gap acidosis)
- acidosis with raised urea and creatinine (may suggest hypovolaemia or renal failure)

BLOOD GAS ANALYSIS GUIDELINES

While normal ranges are known for each of the blood gas components, it is essential that you assume the midpoint of the range as 'normal' for the purpose of analysis. It is also vital that the estimated fraction of inspired oxygen (FiO_2) be known, depending upon what prescribed oxygen therapy is being given to your patient.

Normal values

- pH = 7.40
- Arterial partial pressure of carbon dioxide, $PaCO_2$ = 5 kPa (40 mmHg)
- Arterial partial pressure of oxygen, PaO_2 = 12 kPa (100 mmHg)
- Bicarbonate, HCO_3^- = 24 mmol L^{-1}

Anion gap

This is defined as follows:

$$\text{anion gap (AG)} = Na^+ + K^+ - (Cl^- + HCO_3^-)$$

The AG is a useful indicator of the aetiology of a metabolic acidosis:

- An AG < 18 mmol L^{-1} is considered to be normal.
- An AG in the range of 20–30 mmol L^{-1} is highly suggestive of metabolic acidosis.
- An AG > 30 mmol L^{-1} confirms metabolic acidosis.

Actual and expected values for $Paco_2$ and HCO_3^-

These calculations are useful for determining whether the disturbance is acute or chronic and what the degree of compensation is:

corrected HCO_3^- = measured HCO_3^- + (anion gap − 18)
expected $Paco_2$ = (0.2 × serum HCO^{3-}) + 1 (Winters' formula)

- Expect HCO_3^- to rise 1.5 mmol L^{-1} per 1 kPa rise in $Paco_2$ acutely
- Expect HCO_3^- to rise 3.0 mmol L^{-1} per 1 kPa rise in $Paco_2$ chronically

Estimation of Fio_2

When uncontrolled oxygen is being given to a patient (i.e. via a nasal cannula, a Hudson mask or a non-rebreathing reservoir mask), you will need to estimate Fio_2 from the following formula:

$$Fio_2 = [\text{L min}^{-1}\ 100\%\ O_2 + (MV - \text{L min}^{-1}\ 100\%\ O_2) \times 0.21]/MV$$

where MV is the minute volume, given by respiratory rate (RR) × tidal volume (TV).

$Paco_2$

Assume that the alveolar partial pressure of CO_2 ($Paco_2$) is equal to the measured $Paco_2$.

Alveolar (A)–arterial (a) gradient

This is defined as follows:

$$\text{Aa gradient} = Pao_2 - Pao_2$$

where Pao_2 is measured and Pao_2 is calculated as follows:

$$Pao_2 = Fio_2 \times 95 - (Paco_2/0.8)$$

The Aa gradient increases with the patient's age from less than 2 kPa in the young to up to 5 kPa in the elderly.

It is useful in distinguishing whether hypoxia is due to a ventilation/perfusion ($\dot{V}/\dot{Q}$) mismatch or to a shunting (perfusion without ventilation). It is particularly useful when you suspect a pulmonary embolism.

Note

There is a single scoring table for Scenarios 17.1–17.4 at the end of the chapter.

SCENARIO 17.1 ACUTE RESPIRATORY ACIDOSIS

A 53-year-old man with acute breathlessness is brought into the emergency department by ambulance. The ambulance personnel state that the patient has a past medical history of asthma and that he has been 'taking his puffers all day' without effect. The patient is unable to speak to you.

His vital signs are:

HR 110 bpm
RR 36 breaths min^{-1}
BP 180/100 mmHg
Oxygen saturation 95% on 15 L min^{-1} O_2 and salbutamol nebulizers

His ABG on 15 L min^{-1} O_2 are:

pH   7.12
$PaCO_2$ 12.8 kPa
HCO_3^- 35 mmol L^{-1}
PaO_2 19.3 kPa
Base excess −1.0 mmol L^{-1}

Teach the F2 how to interpret the ABG.

Interpretation of ABG can be tested in all components of the CEM examinations. However, testing of this topic is more suited to the basic science and data interpretation components of the examinations (Parts A and B). One possible OSCE scenario involves teaching the interpretation of an ABG to a medical student or an F2, as here.

SUGGESTED APPROACH

You should appreciate from the outset that this is a teaching OSCE, and so even if the interpretation of blood gases is not your forte, you can still score well on the teaching aspects.

After introducing yourself, ask the F2 how much they know about the interpretation of ABG. Define the objectives of the teaching session as identifying the components of the ABG, interpreting the ABG and applying the findings to the clinical scenario.

Confirm that the blood gas is arterial and whether it is on air or on oxygen, and document the percentage on the gas. The gas should be clearly labelled with the patient's details and should also show the time that it was taken, so that it can be compared with subsequent gases.

Talk the student through the components of the ABG (pH, $PaCO_2$, PaO_2 and HCO_3^-) and introduce them to the terms base excess, anion gap and Aa gradient. Confirm their understanding of the interpretation of the ABG.

The interpretation of the ABG in this scenario is as follows:

- pH is low, indicating severe acidaemia.
- $PaCO_2$ is high, confirming respiratory acidosis as the primary disturbance.
- HCO_3^- is consistent with an acute rise in CO_2.

In summary, these findings show that this patient has severe respiratory acidosis, which is consistent with type II acute respiratory failure.

Inform the student about books or Internet sites on the interpretation of blood gases to which they can refer. You should also suggest that they bring any interesting gases with them to the next session. Encourage any questions and feedback. Agree a time to meet for further teaching.

This approach can be used to interpret any ABG. The following scenarios are additional examples of potential OSCE scenarios.

SCENARIO 17.2 CHRONIC COMPENSATED RESPIRATORY ACIDOSIS

A 63-year-old woman complaining of breathlessness is brought to the emergency department by ambulance. She has a long history of chronic obstructive airways disease and has home oxygen 2 L min^{-1} for 16 hours per day.

Her vital signs are:

RR 14 breaths min^{-1}
BP 160/95 mmHg
HR 87 bpm
Oxygen saturation 91% on 2 L min^{-1} O_2

She is afebrile

Her ABG on 2 L min^{-1} O_2 are:

pH   7.38
Pa_{CO_2} 8 kPa
HCO_3^- 33 mmol L^{-1}
Pa_{O_2} 8 kPa

Interpret these observations.

The interpretation of the ABG in this case is as follows:

- pH is normal.
- Pa_{CO_2} is elevated (3 kPa higher than normal), implying respiratory acidosis.
- HCO_3^- is elevated (9 mmol L^{-1} higher than normal), implying metabolic alkalosis as compensation.

This scenario demonstrates fully compensated chronic respiratory acidosis with type II respiratory failure.

It is useful to calculate the Aa gradient. Estimate the inspired oxygen concentration:

$$\text{estimated MV} = 14 \text{ breaths min}^{-1} \times 500 \text{ mL}$$

$$= 7 \text{ L min}^{-1}$$

and so

$$F_{iO_2} = [2 + (7 - 2) \times 0.21]/7$$

$$= 0.44 \ (44\%)$$

Pa_{O_2} = 8 kPa on the estimated F_{iO_2} of 44%, and PA_{O_2} is calculated as

$$PA_{O_2} = F_{iO_2} \times 95 - (Pa_{CO_2}/0.8)$$

$$= 0.44 \times 95 - (8/0.8)$$

$$= 32 \text{ kPa}$$

Therefore the Aa gradient = 32 kPa − 8 kPa = 24 kPa, which is more than expected.

SCENARIO 17.3 METABOLIC ACIDOSIS WITH A NORMAL ANION GAP

A 27-year-old woman presents to the emergency department with lethargy.

Her vital signs are:

BP 90/50 mmHg
RR 12 breaths min^{-1}
Oxygen saturation 94% on air
GCS 15

A venous blood gas is taken:

pH	7.14
Pv_{CO_2}	4.5 kPa
Pv_{O_2}	3.0 kPa
HCO_3^-	12 mmol L^{-1}
Na^+	137 mmol L^{-1}
K^+	5.4 mmol L^{-1}
Cl^-	113 mmol L^{-1}
Glucose	4 mmol L^{-1}

Analyse these gases and calculate the anion gap.

Blood gas analysis

pH is low, indicating acidaemia.

HCO_3^- is low, and therefore a metabolic acidosis is the primary disturbance.

Pv_{CO_2} and Pv_{O_2} cannot be commented upon, since this is a venous blood sample and hence they are not accurately reflective of the arterial circulation.

Arterial versus venous blood gas analysis

Venous blood gas analysis will provide a pH and an HCO_3^- that are reliable.

The mean differences between arterial and venous values are:

pH	0.03 pH units
HCO_3^-	0.52 mmol L^{-1}
lactate	0.08 mmol L^{-1}
base excess	0.19 mmol L^{-1}

In respiratory failure, a low pH, i.e. acidaemia and a normal to high HCO_3^-, would indicate that the acidosis was respiratory in origin, and treatment could start for the patient without having to perform an arterial sample. The oxygen saturation will provide an estimate of the degree of hypoxaemia. Once the patient has been stabilized, an arterial line can be inserted for accurate monitoring of invasive blood pressure and blood gases.

Anion gap (AG)

Calculation of the AG is helpful is the analysis of metabolic acidosis. The AG is equal to the difference between the plasma concentrations of the measured cations (Na^+ and K^+) and the measured anions (HCO_3^- and Cl^-). The traditional normal range is 12–20 mmol L^{-1}.

AG calculation helps to determine the aetiology of the metabolic acidosis:

$$AG = Na^+ + K^+ - (HCO_3^- + Cl^-)$$
$$= 137 + 5.4 - (12 + 113) \text{ mmol } L^{-1}$$
$$= 17.4 \text{ mmol } L^{-1}$$

As AG < 18 mmol L^{-1}, this case represents a metabolic acidosis with a normal AG and hyperchloraemia.

High-AG metabolic acidosis

High-AG metabolic acidosis is associated with the *addition* of endogenous or exogenous acids. The mnemonic 'MUDPILES' is useful:

Methanol
Uraemia
Diabetic and alcoholic ketoacidosis
Paraldehyde, phenformin
Isoniazid, iron
Lactic acidosis (including carbon monoxide and cyanide poisoning)
Ethylene glycol and other ethanols
Salicylates

Normal-AG metabolic acidosis

Normal-AG metabolic acidosis is associated with *loss* of HCO_3^- or a failure to excrete H^+ ions from the body. It typically includes hyperchloraemia. It may be due to:

- gastrointestinal tract loss of HCO_3^- as a result of diarrhoea or of pancreatic or intestinal fistulae
- renal loss of HCO_3^- i.e. type 2 proximal renal tubular acidosis
- renal dysfunction and/or failure
- hypoaldosteronism, i.e. type 4 renal tubular acidosis
- ingestion of ammonium chloride, acetazolamide or hyperalimentation fluids
- some cases of ketoacidosis

Osmolal gap (OG)

The OG is the plasma osmolality measured in the laboratory minus the calculated osmolality.

Serum osmolality is composed of all osmotically active substances, including both ionic and non-ionic substances, such as serum ions, glucose and urea. The calculated osmolality (in mosmol kg^{-1}) is given by:

$$\text{calculated osmolality} = (1.86 \times Na^+) + \text{glucose} + \text{urea} + 9$$

where Na^+, glucose and urea are in mmol L^{-1}.

The normal OG < 10 mosmol kg^{-1}

Metabolic acidosis with increased OG indicates methanol or ethylene glycol ingestion.

SCENARIO 17.4 METABOLIC ACIDOSIS WITH A HIGH ANION GAP

A 19-year-old man is brought to the emergency department feeling unwell.

His vital signs are:

HR 120 bpm
BP 90/40 mmHg
Oxygen saturation 93% on room air

His ABG on air are:

pH	7.22
Pa_{CO_2}	3.5 kPa
HCO_3^-	11.0 mmol L^{-1}
Pa_{O_2}	16.2 kPa
Base excess	−31 mmol L^{-1}
Na$^+$	144 mmol L^{-1}
K$^+$	3.2 mmol L^{-1}
Cl$^-$	107 mmol L^{-1}
Glucose	19 mmol L^{-1}
Lactate	1.0 mmol L^{-1}

Blood gas analysis

The pH is very low, indicating severe acidaemia.

Pa_{CO_2} is low – there is profound respiratory alkalosis in an attempt at respiratory compensation. To check whether there is adequate respiratory compensation, the predicted Pa_{CO_2} can be calculated using Winters' formula:

$$\text{expected } Pa_{CO_2} = (0.2 \times \text{serum } HCO_3^-) + 1$$
$$= (0.2 \times 11) + 1$$
$$= 3.2 \text{ kPa}$$

The actual Pa_{CO_2} is 3.5 kPa, so there is an appropriate attempt at respiratory compensation.

HCO_3^- is very low, indicating profound metabolic acidosis.

The anion gap is given by:

$$AG = Na^+ + K^+ - (HCO_3^- + Cl^-)$$
$$= 144 + 3.2 - (11 + 107) \text{ mmol L}^{-1}$$
$$= 29.2 \text{ mmol L}^{-1} \text{ (large-AG metabolic acidosis)}$$

For every molecule of unmeasured anion, one molecule of HCO_3^- is lost. If the unmeasured anion concentration (i.e. the anion gap over 18), is added to the HCO_3^- concentration, this should equal a normal HCO_3^-:

$$\text{corrected } HCO_3^- = \text{measured } HCO_3^- + (AG - 18)$$
$$= 11 + (29 - 18) \text{ mmol L}^{-1}$$
$$= 22 \text{ mmol L}^{-1}$$

Note that if the corrected HCO_3^- is less than normal then there are additional anions contributing to the metabolic acidosis. These anions should come from the normal-AG group of disorders.

This scenario is an example of uncompensated severe high-AG metabolic acidosis with adequate oxygenation. This patient was a newly diagnosed diabetic and had large ketonuria. The diagnosis was made of diabetic ketoacidosis.

SUMMARY

Table 17.1 summarizes the changes in ABG components in acid–base disorders.

Table 17.1 ABG changes in acid–base disorders

Disorder	pH	Pa_{CO_2}	HCO_3^-	Examples
Respiratory acidosis	↓	↑	↑	CNS depression Neuromuscular disease Impaired lung ventilation Acute airway obstruction
Respiratory acidosis with renal compensation	↓/N	↑	↑↑	As above
Respiratory alkalosis	↑	↓	↓	Hyperventilation Increased CNS drive CNS infection Medications (salicylate, aminophylline) Fever Sepsis Carbon monoxide poisoning Hyperthyroidism Liver failure
Respiratory alkalosis with renal compensation	↓/N	↓	↓↓	As above
Metabolic acidosis	↓	N	↓	**Raised-anion-gap acidosis** Ketoacidosis (diabetes, alcohol or starvation) Lactic acidosis (reduced perfusion/sepsis) Methanol Ethylene glycol Salicylate **Normal-anion-gap acidosis (hyperchloraemic acidosis)** Renal tubular acidosis Severe diarrhoea Blocked ileal conduit Small-bowel fistula
Metabolic acidosis with respiratory compensation	↓/N	↓	↓	As above
Metabolic alkalosis	↑	N	↑	Bicarbonate infusion Hepatic metabolism of citrate and lactate to bicarbonate Massive blood transfusion Milk–alkali syndrome Loss of H+ from stomach during vomiting (pyloric stenosis) Loss of H+ as a result of diuretics Potassium-depletion disorders
Metabolic alkalosis with respiratory compensation	↑/N	↑	↑	As above

Scoring Scenarios 17.1–17.4

	Inadequate/ not done	Adequate	Good
Introduces themselves to F2	0	1	—
Asks F2 how much they know about interpreting blood gases	0	1	—
Outlines teaching objectives	0	1	2
Ensures that: • The ABG is labelled with patient details • The amount of O_2 the patient is on is noted • It is confirmed whether the sample is arterial or venous • The time the gas was taken is recorded	0	1	2
Has a structured approach to interpretation. Comments on: • pH • CO_2 • HCO_3^- • O_2 • lactate • base excess	0	1	2
Knows normal reference ranges for the above	0	1	—
Correctly interprets ABG and correlates with clinical findings	0	1	—
Encourages questions and summarizes findings	0	1	2
Plans for next session	0	1	—
Communicates effectively	0	1	—
Score from F2	/5		
Global score from examiner	/5		
Total score	/24		

18
Toxicological Emergencies
SIMON F J CLARKE AND NICK PAYNE

CORE TOPICS

- Assessment and initial management of patients presenting with toxicological problems
- Recognition of the common toxidromes
- Understanding the role of antidotes
- Ability to access poisons information
- Working knowledge of legal, psychiatric and social aspects of overdose
- Understanding the pharmacology of common poisons
- Specific paediatric objectives:
    - Understanding the epidemiology and ability to identify the major types of ingestions by age
    - Understanding management of the adolescent refusing treatment for a life-threatening overdose
    - Awareness of overdose as a self-harm presentation and knowledge that repeated ingestions may be a presentation of neglect

Although much of the knowledge of toxicology and poisoning required for the MCEM examination is assessed by the Part 1 MCQs and particularly the Part 2 SAQs, there is much more to the poisoned patient than just applying that knowledge, so there are a number of aspects of the emergency management of the poisoned patient that might be examined in OSCE scenarios.

It is necessary to be able to take a focused history from the patient to identify potential toxicological causes of the presentation, including asking about drugs taken in overdose, illicit drugs, possible accidental overdose of prescribed medication and potential drug interactions leading to harmful consequences. The physical examination should look for signs providing clues to the cause of poisoning and particularly evidence of any of the classic toxidromes. Demonstrating how you would access expert advice and information on specific poisonings from sources such as TOXBASE or the National Poisons Information Service (NPIS) may also be required by examiners. Finally, a sympathetic, non-judgemental and supportive attitude towards patients who have deliberately overdosed is important and will likely gain marks.

- National Poisons Information Service (NPIS) Website: www.npis.org.
- TOXBASE Website: www.toxbase.org.

Scoring Scenario 18.1: Paracetamol overdose

	Inadequate/ not done	Adequate	Good
Appropriate introduction	0	1	—
Physical symptoms	0	1	—
Medical history of overdose: • type of tablets taken • packets with patient • time of overdose • number of tablets • single or staggered • other drugs taken	0	1	2
Patient's weight	0	1	—
Past medical history: epilepsy, liver disease, eating disorders	0	1	2
Drug history: antiepileptics, rifampicin, St John's wort, psychiatric medication	0	1	—
Alcohol and drug use	0	1	—
Psychiatric history of overdose: • precautions against discovery • attempt to get help • preparation, including suicide note • purpose of attempt • estimate of lethality/fatality • degree of premeditation	0	1	2
Past psychiatric history	0	1	—
Social situation and support	0	1	—
Full-time education	0	1	—
Medical management: • activated charcoal • 4-hour blood tests • treatment nomogram • NAC	0	1	2
Psychiatric management: • appropriate for interview • offer CAMHS/adult psychiatry	0	1	—
Score from patient		/5	
Global score from examiner		/5	
Total score		/27	

SCENARIO 18.2: TRICYCLIC ANTIDEPRESSANT POISONING

A 32-year-old man has been brought to the emergency department 1 hour after ingesting 45 dosulepin tablets (75 mg strength). He denies taking any other medications and the paramedics confirm that they found only an empty bottle of dosulepin, with no other pill packets at the scene. The patient appears to be depressed, but is otherwise calm and cooperative.

Examine the patient, with a particular emphasis on looking for the signs of dosulepin toxicity; explain to the examiner what features you are looking for. What investigations may help you to determine the prognosis of this patient? Outline your initial management. You are not expected to take a psychiatric history.

SUGGESTED APPROACH

Dosulepin (formerly known as dothiepin) is a tricyclic antidepressant (TCA). TCAs are thought to block the reuptake of noradrenaline both centrally and peripherally and possibly inhibit reuptake of serotonin in the brain. They have an anticholinergic effect and block sodium channels in the myocardium and nerve axons, leading to a membrane-stabilizing effect similar to that of the class Ia antiarrhythmics. The clinical features of TCA toxicity are outlined in Box 18.1.

Box 18.1 Acute clinical features of TCA toxicity

Anticholinergic effects
- Warm, dry skin
- Hyperthermia
- Tachycardia
- Respiratory depression
- Delayed gastric emptying, paralytic ileus
- Urinary retention
- Blurred vision, dilated pupils, divergent squint
- Agitation, hallucinations

Reduced conscious level

Seizures or myoclonus

Arrhythmias
- Tachycardias: sinus tachycardia, supraventricular and ventricular arrhythmias
- Bradycardias: all types of heart block may occur, but are uncommon and tend to indicate severe poisoning
- Hypotension

Pulmonary oedema

Death usually occurs owing to ventricular fibrillation, intractable fits or haemodynamic collapse.

Examination

First look at the general condition of the patient:

- Check the GCS. The patient may be agitated. Are there also signs of confusion?
- If the patient is obtunded, are they protecting their airway?
- Take the patient's temperature – hyperthermia may be present owing to anticholinergic excess.
- The skin and oral mucosa may be dry owing to an anticholinergic effect.
- Mention to the examiner that you would ask for the patient to be weighed; ingested doses greater than 10 mg per kg body weight are likely to cause significant toxicity.

Next examine each system systematically, with particular attention to the following:

- Take the pulse. TCAs can cause both tachy- and bradyarrhythmias.
- Ask to measure the blood pressure. This may be raised if the patient is agitated, or low owing to arrhythmias or direct myocardial depression.
- Count the respiratory rate. The onset of a metabolic acidosis will increase respiration, while severe overdose with impaired consciousness may lead to hypoventilation.
- Auscultate the lungs for evidence of pulmonary oedema or aspiration pneumonitis.
- Examine the abdomen for any sign of paralytic ileus or distended bladder.
- Neurological examination may reveal dilated pupils, reduced visual acuity or divergent squint (rare), while limb tone may be increased or reduced with brisk reflexes and, in more severe poisoning, extensor plantars.

Investigations

The ECG and arterial blood gases (ABG) are important investigations in TCA overdose, both to guide treatment and to assess prognosis.

TCAs can cause a wide range of ECG abnormalities (Box 18.2), but there are two particular changes that have prognostic significance:

- QRS prolongation:
  - >100 ms, associated with an increased risk of fits, coma, hypotension and need for intubation
  - >160 ms, associated with an increased risk of ventricular arrhythmias
- aVR: R wave ≥ 3 mm or R/S ratio ≥ 0.7 has the same sensitivity as QRS > 100 ms.

A metabolic acidosis on the ABG is an indicator of severe toxicity.

Box 18.2 ECG abnormalities associated with TCA poisoning

Conduction blocks
- Widening of the QRS complex
- Lengthening of the PR interval
- QT prolongation
- Atrioventricular block (all types) in severe poisoning

Tachyarrhythmias
- A sinus tachycardia is the most common abnormality
- Supraventricular tachycardia (SVT)
- Broad complex tachycardia:
- Sinus tachycardia/SVT with aberrant conduction
- Ventricular tachycardia: both monomorphic and torsades de pointes

Cardiac arrest
- Ventricular tachycardia/ventricular fibrillation
- Asystole

Management

The management of any patient who has been poisoned with pharmaceuticals should follow the same pattern:

- preventing absorption of ingested drug – 'gut decontamination'
- symptomatic and supportive treatment
- promoting elimination of absorbed drug – 'enhanced elimination techniques'
- specific treatments – 'antidotes'

This translates into the following actions for a patient poisoned with TCAs.

Gut decontamination

Activated charcoal (1 g kg^{-1}) should be given if the patient presents within 2 hours of ingestion. TCAs slow gastric emptying; therefore activated charcoal may be effective for longer than most other types of overdose.

Symptomatic and supportive care

This should follow the standard ABC format and is the mainstay of treatment for any poisoned patient:

- The airway should be protected if necessary.
- Adequate oxygenation, ventilation and hydration should be provided.
- Vital signs (pulse, blood pressure, oxygen saturation, respiratory rate and Glasgow Coma Scale) and serum electrolytes and acid–base status should be closely monitored.
- Cardiac monitoring is mandatory.

Enhanced elimination techniques

- Optimizing the patient's fluid balance will increase the glomerular filtration rate.
- Extracorporeal techniques such as dialysis are ineffective.

Antidotes

Sodium bicarbonate is a specific antidote to TCA poisoning. More important than its effect on pH is the fact that bicarbonate provides a sodium load to overcome the sodium-channel-blocking effects of the TCA. Sodium bicarbonate is indicated in TCA overdose where there is any QRS prolongation, arrhythmia or hypotension, regardless of whether or not the pH is low. Treatment with sodium bicarbonate is as follows:

- A bolus of 1–2 mmol kg^{-1} (1–2 mL kg^{-1} of 8.4%) bicarbonate is given over 15 minutes.
- An infusion of 500–1000 mL isotonic (1.26% or 1.4%) bicarbonate over 4 hours can be considered for ongoing toxicity. It is recommended that the NPIS should be consulted in these instances of severe poisoning.
- *If an infusion is given, the patient's serum potassium should be checked hourly* and hypokalaemia should be treated.
- The pH should be kept between 7.45 and 7.55.

Scoring Scenario 18.2: Tricyclic antidepressant poisoning

	Inadequate/ not done	Adequate	Good
Appropriate introduction	0	1	—
Examination: • Asks for temperature • Looks at oral mucosa • Pulse rate *and* rhythm • Asks for BP • Respiratory rate • Auscultates lung fields • Examines abdomen for distended bladder and paralytic ileus • Measures GCS • Looks for dilated pupils • Neurological examination: tone, reflexes and plantars	0	1	2
ECG interpretation: • wide QRS • QRS >100 ms: risk of fits • QRS >160 ms: risk of arrhythmias • aVR: R wave	0	1	2
ABG: metabolic acidosis as a poor prognostic marker	0	1	—
Immediate management: • activated charcoal • symptomatic and supportive care ABCs • bicarbonate as antidote – must mention checking potassium regularly • contact NPIS	0	1	2
Score from patient	/5		
Global score from examiner	/5		
Total score	/18		

SCENARIO 18.3: ETHYLENE GLYCOL POISONING

You have been called to the resuscitation room to see a 64-year-old man found collapsed at his allotment with a bottle thought to have contained antifreeze next to him. On arrival in the emergency department, the patient is drowsy and appears intoxicated, but does not smell of alcohol.

His basic observations are as follows:

Pulse 120 bpm, regular
BP 170/110 mmHg
RR 32 breaths min^{-1}
Oxygen saturation 98% on air
Temperature 36.5 °C
Blood glucose 5.2 mmol L^{-1}

The patient is poorly cooperative with history taking and refuses to give details. The ambulance crew are still present and you have one experienced nurse to help you.

Make an assessment and formulate a management plan, including any particular investigations.

SUGGESTED APPROACH

The toxic alcohols are rapidly absorbed following ingestion, and then *slowly* metabolized by alcohol dehydrogenase to either glycolaldehyde (in the case of ethylene glycol) or formaldehyde (in the case of methanol). The aldehydes are then *rapidly* metabolized further by aldehyde dehydrogenase and other enzymes – the secondary metabolites are predominantly acids and are responsible for the toxic effects. Both of the antidotes (ethanol and fomepizole) act on the initial rate-limiting step as competitive inhibitors of alcohol dehydrogenase to prevent the development of the toxic metabolites. Since ethylene glycol requires metabolism before the toxic effects develop, the clinical presentation can vary with time from ingestion:

- Early (<12 hours): inebriation, mild depression in consciousness, nausea and vomiting, focal fits, ataxia, nystagmus, and decreased tone and reflexes
- Middle (12–24 hours): tachycardia, tachypnoea, hypertension and cardiac failure
- Late (>24 hours): renal failure and hyperkalaemia, abdominal pain, tetany, convulsions, coma, hypocalcaemia, arrhythmias, and hypomagnesaemia

This is basically a moulage on dealing with a patient who has a decreased level of consciousness where limited information is available. However, the information that has been given should direct you along the lines of considering poisoning with ethylene glycol as the cause in this patient.

Clinical assessment

This should follow the standard ABCDE approach:

- Ensure a patent airway (provide adjuncts as necessary).
- Provide supplemental oxygen as per BTS guidelines (see Scenario 14.1).
- Assess breathing, including respiration rate and auscultation for equal air entry and added sounds. Attach pulse oximetry.
- Take the pulse, measure the blood pressure and look for signs of shock. Apply cardiac monitoring and request a 12-lead ECG. Obtain intravenous access.
- Obtain a blood glucose.
- Assess the formal GCS.
- Expose the patient but maintain a comfortable environment. Check for any signs of obvious injury, especially to

the head. Look for any alert badges and signs of chronic disease (e.g. liver disease, intravenous drug use and sites of insulin injection).
- Perform a brief neurological examination, including pupils, eye movements, reflexes and plantars.

Find out more information from the sources available:

- Talk to the ambulance crew about the circumstances. Ask particularly about the bottle found with the patient for any clues as to its contents or the amount ingested.
- Check the patient's pockets and any bags.
- Try to contact any witnesses or family members. When was the patient last seen?

Investigations

- Take blood for a full blood count (FBC), U&E, LFT, calcium, magnesium and albumin. Consider paracetamol levels.
- Perform ABG. Patients presenting late with ethylene glycol poisoning have a raised-anion-gap metabolic acidosis that is due to the metabolism of the parent alcohol to a number of organic acids. This is not specific for ethylene glycol poisoning; the causes of raised-anion-gap metabolic acidosis ('MUDPILES') are given in Box 18.3.
- Calculate the osmolal gap OG as the difference between the measured and calculated serum osmolalities, i.e.

$$OG = \text{measured osmolality} - \text{calculated osmolality}$$

(all in mosmol kg^{-1}), where the calculated osmolality is given by:

$$\text{calculated osmolality} = (1.86 \times Na^+) + \text{glucose} + \text{urea} + 9$$

with Na^+, glucose and urea in mmol L^{-1}. An OG > 10 mosmol kg^{-1} is a strong indicator for toxic alcohol ingestion. Other causes of a raised OG ('ME DIE O') are given in Box 18.4.
- Measurement of ethylene glycol in the serum is rarely performed in practice.
- The presence of calcium oxalate crystals in the urine is diagnostic for ethylene glycol poisoning.
- Ethylene glycol has no specific cardiac effects and the ECG will likely show a sinus tachycardia.
- Request a chest X-ray to look for signs of aspiration.

Box 18.3 Causes of raised-anion-gap metabolic acidosis: 'MUDPILES'

Methanol
Uraemia
Diabetic ketoacidosis
Paraldehyde
Isoniazid, iron
Lactic acidosis
Ethanol, ethylene glycol
Salicylate, starvation, solvents

Box 18.4 Causes of raised osmolal gap: 'ME DIE O'

Methanol
Ethylene glycol
Diuretics (mannitol)
Isopropanol
Ethanol
Other (ketoacidosis, multiple organ failure)

Management

The management of ethylene glycol poisoning should follow the standard pattern for any toxicological emergency as described in Scenario 18.2. Always mention the benefit of using TOXBASE.

Gut decontamination

- Gastric lavage may be considered if ingestion may have been within the last hour.
- Activated charcoal is of no benefit, because it does not adsorb alcohols.

Symptomatic and supportive

- This is along the ABCDE lines as detailed above.
- Control seizures with intravenous lorazepam.
- Rehydrate with intravenous fluids.
- Consider bicarbonate to correct the metabolic acidosis. High doses may be required, and U&E and ABG need to be regularly monitored.

Enhanced elimination techniques

Haemodialysis may be used in severe toxic alcohol poisoning (including ethanol).

Antidotes

The specific antidote for use in ethylene glycol poisoning is ethanol. This should be given where there is a strong suspicion of ethylene glycol poisoning and at least two objective indicators:

- pH < 7.3
- serum bicarbonate < 20 mmol L^{-1}
- osmolal gap > 10 mosmol kg^{-1}
- urinary oxalate crystals
- severe symptoms
- ethylene glycol levels > 200 mg L^{-1}

Ethanol may be given orally or intravenously and is commenced as a loading dose equivalent to 800 mg kg^{-1} of 100% ethanol followed by maintenance therapy based on the clinical situation. Full dosing regimens are available on TOXBASE. Serum ethanol levels need to be taken at least every 2 hours; the aim of therapy is to achieve a level of 1–1.5 g L^{-1} (100–150 mg dL^{-1}).

Fomepizole is given intravenously. Although it is more expensive than ethanol, it does not require regular biochemical monitoring. It must be obtained from the NPIS, who will also advise on the dosing regime.

Scoring Scenario 18.3: Ethylene glycol poisoning

	Inadequate/ not done	Adequate	Good
Appropriate introduction	0	1	—
Standard ABCDE approach: • Assesses airway • Gives oxygen, • Assesses breathing • Assesses circulation • Attaches appropriate monitoring • GCS, pupils, gross neurology • Blood glucose • Exposure and environment control	0	1	2
Paramedic history	0	1	—
Questions regarding bottle found with patient: contents and amount potentially ingested	0	1	—
Checks patient's clothes and belongings	0	1	—
Attempts to obtain additional history	0	1	—
Specific investigations: • ABG • osmolal gap • urine for calcium oxalate crystals • ethylene glycol levels • U&E, LFT	0	1	2
Medical management: • IV bicarbonate • ethanol • fomepizole • haemodialysis in severe cases • IV lorazepam • IV fluids	0	1	2
Score from patient	/5		
Global score from examiner	/5		
Total score	/21		

SCENARIO 18.4: DIGOXIN TOXICITY

An 82-year-old man is brought to the emergency department from his nursing home. He has a 3-day history of nausea and malaise and two episodes of loose stool. An ambulance was called when he was unable to get out of bed this morning owing to lethargy and blurred vision. He has not complained of any pain. He completed a course of erythromycin this morning for a chest infection, which seems to have resolved successfully.

His initial observations are:

Pulse 42 bpm, irregular
BP 110/60 mmHg
RR 18 breaths min^{-1}

Take a history from this man. What investigations would you perform? Give a management plan.

SUGGESTED APPROACH

It is common for elderly patients to present to emergency departments with relatively non-specific symptoms. There are, however, a number of clues in this scenario to suggest that the patient is suffering from digoxin toxicity:

- The insidious onset of the symptoms goes against an acute cause.
- Excess digitalis causes bradycardia.
- The irregular heart rate suggests that the patient has atrial fibrillation.
- Macrolide antibiotics such as erythromycin are known to interact with digoxin.

If any patient presents with non-specific symptoms, take a thorough drug history. This should include non-prescribed (OTC) medications and herbal or other traditional remedies. If a patient is taking digoxin, think of the possibility of digoxin toxicity, because the clinical features are non-specific (Box 18.5). A particular risk factor is a recent change in medication, such as starting a drug that may precipitate digoxin toxicity (Box 18.6). In addition, patients who become confused, for example owing to another acute illness, may not take their medication reliably.

Box 18.5 Features of digoxin toxicity

- Early features: nausea, vomiting, diarrhoea
- Headache
- Confusion
- Visual disturbance
- Hyperkalaemia
- Hypotension
- Bradycardia – any form of heart block
- Tachyarrhythmias

History

The presenting complaint is vague, but a systematic history should uncover the relevant further information in this patient.

Further history of the presenting complaints involves asking about the gastrointestinal symptoms, which in this case are in fact quite mild. The visual disturbance rarely involves loss of vision, but rather is described as a generalized blurring along with everything going 'yellow'. Other than that, the patient just feels overwhelmingly tired.

Box 18.6 Drugs that may precipitate digoxin toxicity

• ACE inhibitors: captopril	• Carbenoxolone
• Angiotensin II antagonists: telmisartan	• Ciclosporin
• Antiarrhythmics: amiodarone, propafenone, quinidine	• Corticosteroids
• Antibiotics: gentamicin, macrolides, trimethoprim	• Diuretics
• Antifungals	• Interferon-γ
• Antimalarials	• Non-steroidal anti-inflammatory drugs:
• Antivirals: ritonavir	diclofenac, indometacin, and possibly fenbufen
• Benzodiazepines: alprazolam, diazepam	and ibuprofen
• Beta-agonists	• Opioids: tramadol
• Calcium-channel blockers: verapamil	• Proton-pump inhibitors

A past medical history would uncover a history of chronic atrial fibrillation, as suspected

A thorough review of systems would reveal no other suggestion of infection or acute illness.

A drug history indicates that the patient is on aspirin, digoxin, simvastatin and quinine for cramps. Do not forget to ask about OTC medications, which are quite common in the elderly.

The patient is penicillin-allergic (rash) – hence the prescription for erythromycin for the recent chest infection.

Investigations

Investigations are aimed at supporting the diagnosis of digoxin toxicity, refuting other possible diagnoses and then looking for the complications of digitalis excess:

- An FBC and inflammatory markers help to rule out infectious causes of a non-specific presentation.
- Digoxin levels can be measured in most hospital laboratories to confirm toxicity. Potassium levels should be obtained, since hyperkalaemia is associated with digoxin toxicity and may exacerbate the potential for cardiac dysrhythmia.
- An ECG should be performed to look for digitalis-induced brady- or tachyarrhythmia
- A chest X-ray and urinalysis are needed to rule out potential sources of sepsis.
- Any patient who develops loose stools while taking broad-spectrum antibiotics must have stool samples sent for culture and sensitivities and *Clostridium difficile* toxin.

Management

Chronic digoxin toxicity is most commonly seen with accidental or iatrogenic overdose; digoxin should be stopped until it is safe to resume.

Gut decontamination

Activated charcoal can be used if the patient presents within 1 hour of an acute overdose.

Symptomatic and supportive

Assess and maintain the airway and support breathing with supplemental oxygen.

The circulation may be compromised by bradycardia. Treat along ALS guidelines with intravenous atropine 0.5 mg, repeated up to 3 mg if necessary. Temporary pacing may be required if there is a limited or short-lived response to atropine.

Hyperkalaemia should be treated with standard therapy (insulin–glucose infusion).

Fluid rehydration should be given as required.

Antidotes

Digoxin-specific antibody fragments (Digibind) are the antidote to digoxin poisoning. They should be used where there is:

- bradycardia unresponsive to atropine
- hyperkalaemia (>6 mmol L^{-1}) unresponsive to insulin–glucose
- tachyarrhythmias associated with hypotension

Formulae for determining the dose of Digibind can be found on TOXBASE. Further advice on management on treating digoxin toxicity can be obtained from the NPIS.

Scoring Scenario 18.4: Digoxin toxicity

	Inadequate/ not done	Adequate	Good
Appropriate introduction	0	1	—
History of presenting complaint: • relatively mild GI symptoms • marked fatigue, out of keeping with mild GI symptoms • lack of symptoms on formal systematic enquiry to suggest alternative pathology • timing of onset of symptoms with course of antibiotics • bradycardia	0	1	2
Past medical history: chronic atrial fibrillation	0	1	2
Drug history: • Asks about drugs and doses • Recognizes that macrolides interact with digoxin • Lack of other medication associated with GI upset (e.g. statins) or fatigue (diuretics, beta-blockers, calcium-channel blockers)	0	1	2
Investigations: • U&E • digoxin level • stool sample (culture and sensitivities and *C. difficile* toxin) • FBC, chest X-ray and urinalysis • ECG	0	1	2
Management: • airway, breathing and supplemental oxygen • looks for and treats complications • bradycardia • hyperkalaemia • knowledge of Digibind • IV fluids	0	1	2
Score from patient	/5		
Global score from examiner	/5		
Total score	/21		

19
Renal Emergencies
JOBAN S SEHMI AND AMIT K J MANDAL

CORE TOPICS

- Acute renal failure
- The dialysed patient
- Hyperkalaemia
- Renal colic
- Urinary tract infection
- Rhabdomyolysis

SCENARIO 19.1: ACUTE RENAL FAILURE

A 74-year-old man comes to the emergency department for a repeat blood test. He had gone to the phlebotomy department earlier in the day for routine blood tests, and that evening the GP had telephoned him to tell him to go to the emergency department urgently, since his potassium level was too high.

Take a history from this patient and outline your management plan.

You will be provided with the results of any investigations that you request when you have completed your history:

Na 134 mmol L^{-1}
K 6.9 mmol L^{-1}
urea 34 mmol L^{-1}
creatinine 575 µmol L^{-1}
bilirubin 8 µmol L^{-1}
CRP 26 mg L^{-1}
Hb 9.7 g dL^{-1}
WCC 10.7 × 10^9 L^{-1}

SUGGESTED APPROACH

This is a not uncommon scenario in clinical practice: an elderly person who already has a degree of renal impairment and takes nephrotoxic drugs suffers a further acute insult to the kidneys in the form of dehydration and is tipped into acute renal failure or acute-on-chronic renal failure. In this case, it is the incidental finding of the high potassium that triggers the presentation.

You do not start with much information except that the patient has a high potassium. Common causes of high potassium to be considered are:

- artefact due to haemolysis during blood taking
- oliguric renal failure
- potassium-sparing diuretics (e.g. spironolactone)
- other drugs (e.g. ACE inhibitors)
- Addison's disease
- rhabdomyolysis

After a polite introduction to the patient, the first thing to do is to request that a repeat urea and electrolytes (U&E) measurement be taken, along with an ECG. Patients with known or suspected hyperkalaemia should be placed on a cardiac monitor. The examiner will acknowledge your request and say that it is being dealt with while you continue your history. In addition to checking a repeat laboratory potassium, you should ask to perform a venous blood gas to get a rapid result for the serum potassium.

The scenario then offers a good opportunity to show your skill in taking a systematic history. Starting with open-ended questions on what has brought the patient to the emergency department, you should follow the leads given by asking specific questions to discover that the reason for the routine tests is to monitor his renal function. The degree of chronic renal failure can be roughly gauged by asking whether the patient has ever seen a renal physician, whether he is followed up regularly in a renal clinic, and whether dialysis has ever been discussed (or started!). The patient will also volunteer the information about his recent diarrhoeal illness in response to open-ended questioning.

As part of your systems enquiry, ask about cardiac symptoms that may arise from hyperkalaemia (chest pain, palpitations or light-headedness); rule out rhabdomyolysis by asking about falls or recent injuries. In this OSCE, only when asked about urinary symptoms specifically will the patient tell you that he is, for some reason, passing little urine.

You should now have a fairly good idea that the likely cause of the hyperkalaemia is renal failure. Most acute renal failure in the emergency department is multifactorial, and the common causes should be sought.

In the background medical history, think about:

- diabetes
- hypertension
- heart failure
- myeloma
- systemic lupus erythematosus
- renal scarring from recurrent infection
- glomerulonephritis
- nephrectomy

In the drug history, look for potentially nephrotoxic agents:

- diuretics (loop diuretics, thiazides)
- ACE inhibiters (and angiotensin receptor antagonists)
- non-steroidal anti-inflammatory drugs
- aminoglycosides
- amphotericin

Then ask questions to explore any acute precipitants:

- dehydration
- hypovolaemia
- sepsis
- congestive heart failure
- introduction of a new nephrotoxic drug
- recent use of radio-contrast media

These lists are far from exhaustive, but cover the more common factors in acute or acute-on-chronic renal failure presenting to the emergency department.

The detailed history has now provided a likely scenario to explain the acute renal failure in this patient: on a background of mild renal impairment, he is taking two potentially nephrotoxic agents (a diuretic and an ACE inhibitor), with a third (diclofenac) being added since his last renal check. Finally, a diarrhoeal illness causing dehydration has lead to an acute deterioration in his already precarious renal function, leading to oligouria and hyperkalaemia.

Once you have finished the history, the examiner will present you with the results of the blood tests, confirming your clinical suspicions, along with an ECG demonstrating the tall 'tented' T waves of hyperkalaemia.

Urgent action is required to lower the potassium. Ensure that the patent is monitored and give:

- 10 mL of 10% calcium gluconate in a slow intravenous push
- insulin–glucose infusion (e.g. 10 units Actrapid with 50 mL of 50% glucose over 10 minutes)
- haemodialysis or haemofiltration on HDU/ITU for persistent raised potassium despite emergency therapy or where the patient is anuric

Calcium gluconate is cardioprotective and can be given in 10 mL boluses up to 30 mL or until the ECG improves. Insulin–glucose lowers serum potassium by 1–2 mmol L^{-1} by moving potassium into cells. Nebulized salbutamol may also be used to lower potassium in emergencies. Repeat the ECG at regular intervals.

Treatment of the underlying renal failure will take place over a few days' inpatient stay, but appropriate measures should be initiated in the emergency department:

- Catheterize if there is any possibility of post-renal obstruction as the cause.
- Rehydrate with intravenous fluids at a rate appropriate for the patient and the degree of fluid deficit.
- Stop *all* nephrotoxic drugs.
- Treat any precipitant (e.g. sepsis or vomiting)
- Consider central venous pressure (CVP) monitoring in oliguric renal failure or where there is coexistent cardiac failure.
- Monitor urine output and start a fluid balance chart.
- Initiate investigations of underlying renal disease (e.g. urinalysis, renal ultrasound and vasculitic markers).
- There should be early involvement of the medical team and the HDU/ITU team as appropriate.

If you have not mentioned it already, the examiner will ask for indications for dialysis in acute renal failure:

- pulmonary oedema
- persistent hyperkalaemia
- metabolic acidosis of renal cause (pH < 7.2)
- severe complications of uraemia (e.g. pericarditis)

Scoring Scenario 19.2: Renal colic

	Inadequate/ not done	Adequate	Good
Appropriate introduction	0	1	—
Recognizes and deals with patient's pain as a priority: • Gives diclofenac rectally • Follows with opiates if pain returns	0	1	—
Takes an appropriate pain history: • onset • location • radiation • duration • severity (score pain) • nature: sharp, dull, colicky • exacerbating factors • associated features: fever, nausea/vomiting, sweating • bowel frequency: constipation or diarrhoea • urinary symptoms: dysuria, visible haematuria	0	1	2
Past medical (diabetic) and surgical history	0	1	—
Drugs (metformin) and allergies	0	1	—
Requests initial investigations: • urinalysis • bloods for markers of infection and renal function	0	1	2
Formulates preliminary diagnosis with patient	0	1	—
Requests further imaging: • Knows pros and cons of different imaging modalities • Recognizes implications of IVU for patients taking metformin • Also use of N-acetylcysteine as a chemoprotective agent and stopping metformin prior to IVU • Suggests a plain KUB film followed by the IVU and 20 minutes post-micturition film • Suggests CT-KUB	0	1	2
Considers indicators for admission and that it is not necessary in this case, provided that outpatient follow-up is easily arranged	0	1	—
Summarizes findings and results of investigations and explains diagnosis and management to patient in appropriate terms	0	1	—
Score from patient	/5		
Global score from examiner	/5		
Total score	/23		

SCENARIO 19.3: URINARY TRACT INFECTION

You are asked to see a 69-year-old man who has been unwell for 3 days with fever, nausea/vomiting, dysuria and lower abdominal pain. He is oriented in time and place. Five days ago, he had a transurethral resection of the prostate (TURP) for benign prostatic hypertrophy.

His observations are:

Temperature 38.9 °C
BP 105/70 mmHg
HR 110 bpm
Oxygen saturation 98% on air
GCS 15

MSU shows:

Leukocytes ++
Nitrites +++
Protein +
Blood ++
Ketones +++

Bloods show:

WCC 22.5 × 10^9 L^{-1}
Hb 12.3 g dL^{-1}
Platelets 455 × 10^9 L^{-1}
Neutrophils 18 × 10^9 L^{-1}
Urea 11.9 mmol L^{-1}
Creatinine 96 μmol L^{-1}
Serum lactate 2.2 mmol L^{-1}

Take a history and suggest appropriate investigations and management.

SUGGESTED APPROACH

First introduce yourself, and begin with open-ended questions to establish the duration of the illness and the main symptoms, then focus on what appears to be a urinary tract infection. Attend early to any discomfort that the patient may be experiencing by commencing analgesia, antiemetics or antipyretics as appropriate. Urinary tract infection (UTI) is the term applied to a variety of clinical conditions ranging from asymptomatic presence of bacteria in the urine to severe infection of the kidney with resulting sepsis. A useful clinical approach is to risk-stratify UTIs as either uncomplicated or complicated:

- **Uncomplicated UTIs** include episodes of acute cystitis and acute pyelonephritis that occur in individuals who are otherwise healthy and where there are no factors known to increase the risk of complications or of treatment failure. The organism most commonly implicated in uncomplicated UTI is *Escherichia coli* (80–90%); others include *Staphylococcus saprophyticus* (10%), *Proteus*, *Klebsiella*, *Enterococcus* and *Chlamydia*. Acute uncomplicated pyelonephritis may occur in the absence of typical urinary tract symptoms, and is suggested by flank pain, nausea and vomiting, fever (>38 °C), or renal angle tenderness.

- **Complicated UTIs** (see below) involve a higher risk of systemic illness, sepsis and treatment failure. Such UTIs are often caused by antibiotic-resistant bacteria, including *E. coli*, *Pseudomonas*, *Klebsiella*, *Staphylococcus aureus*, *Enterococcus*, *Serratia* and *Enterobacter*. Complicated UTIs may be exclusively lower urinary tract or may involve ascending infection and pyelonephritis.

Focused history taking from the patient should seek to establish further details of the illness as well as obtaining information that might help to decide whether this is likely to be an uncomplicated or complicated UTI. Ask about:

- urinary tract symptoms (dysuria, frequency and urgency)
- cloudy urine or haematuria
- rigors (a feature of systemic Gram-negative sepsis)
- loin pain
- recent interventions involving the urinary tract (catheterization or instrumentation)
- abnormalities of the urinary tract, either functional (e.g. incomplete voiding) or anatomical (e.g. benign prostate enlargement) – has the patient ever seen a urologist before?
- sudden loin-to-groin pain – could the patient have renal calculi complicated by infection?
- recent antibiotic use
- past medical history – conditions predisposing to infection (e.g. diabetes), conditions that place the patient at increased risk of sepsis (e.g. immunocompromise) and previous UTIs, especially with resistant bacteria
- past surgical history – has the patient ever seen a urologist before?
- medications and allergies

Dipstick urinalysis testing for leukocytes and nitrites is quick and simple and should be used to aid diagnosis. Where there is a need, bacteriuria may be proven with urgent microscopy of a urine specimen, while Gram staining can be used as an initial guide to antibiotic therapy. Urine culture provides the definitive diagnosis, but it takes upward of 24 hours to obtain a culture result along with antibiotic sensitivities. Other investigations include blood tests for electrolytes and renal function, as well as a full blood count (FBC). Febrile (>38.0 °C) and septic patients should have blood cultures taken before starting antibiotics.

A **complicated UTI** is an infection associated with a structural or functional abnormality of the genitourinary tract, or with the presence of an underlying disease that increases the risk of acquiring infection or failing therapy. Two criteria are mandatory to define a complicated UTI: a positive urine culture and one or more of the following clinical features:

- male sex
- hospital-acquired infection
- pregnancy
- indwelling urinary catheter
- recent urinary tract intervention
- functional or anatomical abnormality of the urinary tract
- recent antimicrobial use
- symptoms for >7 days at presentation
- diabetes mellitus
- immunosuppression

The patient in this OSCE scenario is therefore likely to have a complicated UTI following instrumentation of the urinary tract. He is also systemically unwell and has tachycardia and mild hypotension, probably septic. As well as a bedside dipstick, it would be wholly appropriate to request urgent microscopy and Gram stain of the patient's urine to guide empirical treatment. Urine and blood cultures should be sent and the patient started on an empirical intravenous antibiotic regime with good Gram-negative and anti-pseudomonal cover such as a third-generation cephalosporin and once-daily gentamicin. Markers for severe sepsis should be sought (arterial blood gas and serum lactate). A good urine output (≥30 mL h^{-1}) should be maintained with intravenous fluids and the patient should be admitted under the urology team. Any deterioration in clinical parameters (blood pressure, conscious level, acidosis or raised lactate) should prompt an intensive care review.

Management of alternative scenarios involving complicated UTI

Most catheter-associated UTIs are derived from the patient's own colonic flora. The predominant risk factor for development of catheter-associated bacteriuria is the duration of catheterization. Most episodes of short-term catheter-associated bacteriuria are asymptomatic and caused by a single organism. There are two priorities: the catheter system should remain closed and the duration of catheterization should be minimal. Asymptomatic bacteriuria should in general not be treated, since this promotes the emergence of resistant organisms. Usually, after catheter removal, the urinary tract will clear bacteria spontaneously. Parenteral antibiotics should be administered to catheterized patients who are febrile and symptomatic, particularly if the blood culture is positive.

Patients with urosepsis should be diagnosed at an early stage, especially if they have risk factors for a complicated UTI. The systemic inflammatory response syndrome (fever or hypothermia, hyperleukocytosis or leukopenia, tachycardia, and tachypnoea), is recognized as the first event in a cascade that can lead to multiple organ failure if left untreated. Treatment of urosepsis calls for a combination of adequate life-supporting care, appropriate and prompt antibiotic therapy, and adjunctive measures such as inotropes, hydrocortisone, tight blood glucose control and recombinant activated protein C. Drainage of any obstruction in the urinary tract is essential as first-line treatment. Urologists are recommended to treat patients in collaboration with intensive care and infectious diseases specialists.

Antibiotic therapy for UTIs

Table 19.1 provides a summary of antibiotic therapy for UTIs according to the EAU guidelines.

Table 19.1 Antibiotic therapy in urinary tract infection

	Organisms	Empirical antibiotic treatment	Duration of treatment
Uncomplicated UTI	*Escherichia coli* (80%) *Klebsiella* *Proteus* Staphylococci	1. Trimethoprim 2. Nitrofurantoin 3. Amoxicillin 4. Fluoroquinolone (nalidixic acid)	• 3 days for simple cystitis in young women. • 7 days in the elderly
Uncomplicated pyelonephritis	Same as for uncomplicated UTI	1. Cephalosporin 2. Fluoroquinolone (ciprofloxacin) + Gentamicin if unwell and admitted	• 7 days
Complicated UTI	*E. coli* Enterococci *Pseudomonas* Staphylococci	1. Fluoroquinolone (e.g. ciprofloxacin) 2. Cephalosporin 3. Co-amoxiclav + Gentamicin if unwell/septic	• 7 days • Or 3–5 days after control of complicating factor
UTI in pregnancy	Same as for uncomplicated UTI	1. Cephalosporins 2. Amoxicillin	• 7 days
Urosepsis	*E. coli* Enterobacteria After intervention: resistant pathogens such as *Pseudomonas, Proteus, Serratia, Enterobacter*	1. Third-generation anti- pseudomonal cephalosporin IV + gentamicin IV 2. Fluoroquinolone (e.g. ciprofloxacin)	• Convert to oral antibiotics as soon as clinical improvement isseen

Note

The management of UTIs in children is discussed in Scenario 26.5

Scoring Scenario 19.3: Urinary tract infection

	Inadequate/ not done	Adequate	Good
Appropriate introduction	0	1	—
Attends to patient's comfort as indicated by clinical presentation	0	1	—
Starts history with open-ended questions to identify UTI as likely problem	0	1	—
Focuses on UTI with specific questioning, including: • urinary tract symptoms: dysuria, frequency, urgency • cloudy urine or haematuria • rigors (a feature of systemic Gram-negative sepsis) • loin pain	0	1	2
Looks for complicating factors: • catheterization • instrumentation • urinary tract abnormalities • recent antibiotics • medical conditions predisposing to infection or increased risk of sepsis	0	1	2
Requests appropriate investigation: • urine dipstick and culture • urgent microscopy and Gram stain urine • blood cultures • WCC, electrolytes and renal function • markers of severe sepsis	0	1	2
Able to classify UTI appropriately along the lines complicated/ uncomplicated.	0	1	—
Recognizes that this patient has complicated UTI and is systemically unwell/mildly septic	0	1	—
Gives management plan, including: • IV fluid resuscitation • appropriate antibiotics for Gram-negative and pseudomonal cover • admission under urology • initiation of monitoring and triggers for further review	0	1	2
Score from patient	/5		
Global score from examiner	/5		
Total score	/23		

USEFUL RESOURCE

European Association of Urology. *Guidelines on Urological Infections*. March 2009. Available at: www.uroweb.org/nc/professional-resources/guidelines/online.

20
Endocrine Emergencies
ZULFIQUAR MIRZA AND CHETAN R TRIVEDY

CORE TOPICS

- Diabetic ketoacidosis
- Hyperosmolar non-ketotic coma
- Hypoglycaemia
- Acute adrenocortical insufficiency
- Thyroid storm
- Hypothyroidism

Endocrine emergencies are a common presentation to the emergency department, and this topic is frequently tested in the OSCE component of the CEM examinations.

SCENARIO 20.1: DKA HISTORY AND MANAGEMENT

A 26-year-old female trainee bus driver presents with a 2-day history of worsening abdominal pain, vomiting and shortness of breath. She has no significant past medical history. She is alert but clearly unwell at triage.

Her initial observations are:

Temperature 37.4 °C
Pulse 116 bpm
BP 105/70 mmHg
Oxygen saturation 94% on air

A urine dipstick shows:
Protein   +
Blood   –
Glucose +++
WCC   –
Ketones +++
Nitrites –
β-hCG   –

Take a focused history and outline your management. You are not expected to examine the patient.

SUGGESTED APPROACH

First take a moment to interpret the information that you have been given. A history of abdominal pain coupled with urinary glucose and ketones in a young patient strongly suggests diabetic ketoacidosis (DKA). DKA is not infrequently the initial presentation of type 1 diabetes, but is often initially overlooked if the patient is not previously known to be diabetic. DKA may be precipitated by sepsis, recent viral upper respiratory tract infection (URTI), gastroenteritis, pancreatitis or other infection. Poor compliance with insulin treatment in patients with known type 1 diabetes may also result in DKA. The negative urine β human chorionic gonadotropin (β-hCG) result is important since it excludes ectopic pregnancy, a diagnosis that must be considered in any female presenting with abdominal pain.

This patient has abnormal observations, and immediate management should involve initiating cardiac and saturation monitoring, placing on high-flow oxygen, and obtaining a bedside blood glucose measurement. Indicate to the examiner that the patient's pain would also be addressed early.

After introducing yourself, you should take a focused history, asking about:

- duration and onset of symptoms
- history of diabetes (compliance with insulin regime)
- history of polyuria
- history of polydipsia
- recurrent infections (URTI, gastroenteritis, abscesses, thrush)
- recent weight loss
- family history of diabetes or other autoimmune disorders
- past medical history (intercurrent illnesses may precipitate or exacerbate DKA)
- medications (steroids, insulin regime)
- allergies
- occupation (a new diagnosis of diabetes may have a significant impact on some professions)

In this case, the patient's history confirms polyuria and polydipsia, and it seems highly likely that she has newly diagnosed type 1 diabetes. The examiner tells you that the blood glucose reading that you requested was 29 mmol L^{-1}.

The final step in diagnosing DKA is to take an arterial blood gas (ABG). Strictly, the criteria for diagnosing DKA are a metabolic acidosis with pH < 7.30, blood glucose > 11.1 mmol L^{-1}, urinary ketones (2+ or greater) and bicarbonate < 15 mmol L^{-1}. The ABG will also likely show a degree of respiratory compromise. Thus, the investigations that you should request include:

- ABG
- bloods for full blood count (FBC), urea and electrolytes (U&E), liver function tests (LFTs), C-reactive protein (CRP), amylase and clotting screen
- plasma glucose to confirm bedside level
- plasma ketone level
- ECG
- urine culture
- chest X-ray to exclude a chest infection

Despite better understanding, DKA continues to have a high mortality rate (10%), and patients deteriorate rapidly if effective treatment is not delivered as soon as the diagnosis is made. The main causes of death in these patients are hypokalaemia and cerebral oedema. Poor prognosis is usually associated with the following factors, and the presence of one or more should prompt review by the intensive care team:

- pH < 7.3
- shock
- serum osmolarity > 320 mosmol L^{-1}
- plasma ketone level > 5 mmol L^{-1}
- increased age/significant comorbidity
- reduced GCS

Management

Intravenous fluids and insulin are the mainstay of treatment, with careful attention being paid to serum electrolytes. Fluid loss can be significant (5–6 L) by the time of presentation, and aggressive replacement is required to reverse the acidosis. More caution may be needed in the elderly or those with cardiac comorbidity. Fluid and electrolyte replacement go together, and a typical regime is:

- 1 L 0.9% saline over 30 minutes with no added potassium
- 1 L 0.9% saline *with potassium* over 2 hours
- 1 L 0.9% saline *with potassium* over 4 hours
- 1 L 0.9% saline *with potassium* over 6 hours

Change the fluid to 5% glucose with potassium once the blood glucose is less than 14 mmol L^{-1}.

Whole-body potassium is always depleted and requires replacement, but actual serum potassium may be normal, high or low. Therefore, check the blood potassium initially and at 2-hourly intervals, and then supplement the second and subsequent bags of fluid as shown in Table 20.1. Most give an initial intravenous bolus of insulin of between 6 and 10 units Actrapid, followed by an insulin infusion (50 units Actrapid in 50 mL 0.9% saline) according to a sliding scale. Sliding scales vary, but a typical example is given in Table 20.2.

Table 20.1 Potassium supplementation

Plasma potassium (mmol L^{-1})	K$^+$ (mmol) per litre fluid
<3.0	40
<4.0	30
<5.0	20
>5.0	0

Table 20.2 Sliding scale for continuous insulin infusion

Blood glucose (mmol L^{-1})	Insulin (units h^{-1})
<4	0.5
4.1–7	1
7.1–9	2
9.1–11	3
11.1–15	4
>15	6

Other features of management include the following:

- There should be frequent clinical reassessment of GCS, fluid status, acidosis (repeat ABGs), blood glucose and serum electrolytes.
- If pH < 7.0, an infusion of isotonic sodium bicarbonate (1.26%) may be given at a maximum rate of 500 mL h^{-1}.
- Prophylactic low-molecular-weight heparin (LMWH) should be given empirically to prevent venous thrombosis secondary to dehydration and hospitalization.
- Look for and treat any precipitating or coexisting pathologies: infection is the most common, but beware a wider range of disease as age increases (e.g. cardiac ischaemia).
- Both a nasogastric tube (especially if there is a reduced GCS) to prevent aspiration and a urinary catheter should be inserted to monitor output. Invasive monitoring in the form of a central venous line and an arterial line should also be considered.
- There should be an HDU/ITU review where poor prognostic factors are present.

Scoring Scenario 20.1: DKA history and management

	Inadequate/ not done	Adequate	Good
Appropriate introduction	0	1	—
Immediate management of: • monitoring • high-flow oxygen • Blood glucose • pain control	0	1	2
Confirms history and symptoms	0	1	—
Asks if diabetic (type 1)	0	1	—
Elicits features of diabetes: • polyuria • polydipsia • recurrent infections • weight loss • lethargy	0	1	2
Asks about past medical history	0	1	—
Medications and allergies	0	1	—
Makes a working diagnosis of DKA	0	1	—
Plans investigations: • ABG • appropriate blood tests • mentions plasma ketones • septic screen (urine culture and chest X-ray) • ECG	0	1	2
Institutes management: • Describes appropriate fluid regime • Describes appropriate K^+ replacement • Insulin sliding scale • Urinary catheter • Nasogastric tube • Looks for and treats precipitants	0	1	2
Referral to HDU/ITU	0	1	—
Score from patient	/5		
Global score from examiner	/5		
Total score	/25		

SCENARIO 20.2: THYROID EXAMINATION

You are asked to see a 30-year-old woman who presents with palpitations and a swelling of her neck. Examine her neck, paying particular attention to her thyroid status. You are not expected to take a history.

SUGGESTED APPROACH

Start by introducing yourself to the patient and explaining to them that you have been asked to examine their neck and thyroid gland. You should briefly explain what the thyroid gland does and what your examination will entail. Ensure the patient's privacy and ask for a chaperone. You should position the patient sitting on a chair so that you can examine them from behind. The patient's neck and clavicles should be exposed.

Inspect the face, neck and eyes, looking for:

- a goitre
- exophthalmos and lid retraction
- scars (previous surgery)
- lymphadenopathy
- raised jugular venous pulse (JVP) due to the obstruction of the superior vena cava (SVC)
- loss of the outer third of the eyebrows (hypothyroidism)

Look at the hands for:

- thyroid acropachy (painful swelling of the digits)
- tremor
- onycholysis
- palmar erythema
- vitiligo

Take the patient's hand – warm sweaty hands with a resting tremor may be suggestive of hyperthyroidism.

Check the pulse for tachycardia or atrial fibrillation. Ask for a blood pressure

Proceed to palpate the thyroid gland from behind, commenting on its size, shape and consistency. Check for the presence of any nodules.

Ask the patient to stick out their tongue – if the gland moves, this may be indicative of a thyroglossal cyst.

Ask the patient to take a sip of water into their mouth and swallow it as you palpate the gland. You should feel the mass rise up if it arises from the thyroid gland. (Before performing this test, you should ask the patient if they have any swallowing difficulties.)

Palpate the lymph nodes in the neck for any swelling.

Palpate the trachea for midline shift.

Percuss over the sternum – a dullness in the resonance would be suggestive of a retrosternal goitre.

Listen to the swelling for a bruit.

Using a pen torch, check to see if the gland transilluminates, which would be suggestive of a cystic lesion.

Examination of the thyroid status indicates that you would be expected to examine the eyes as well as performing a neurological examination of the limbs:

- Look for other eye signs, including lid lag and lid retraction, and assess extraocular movements as well as visual acuity.
- State that you would like to examine the lower limbs for pre-tibial myxoedema and elicit the reflexes (slow relaxing reflexes are seen in hypothyroidism).
- The skin may also be coarse or have a 'peaches and cream' appearance in hypothyroidism.

The patient has a diffuse midline neck swelling, and the examiner asks for a differential diagnosis and further investigations.

Two questions to ask about a neck swelling are, first, is it focal or diffuse and, second, is it midline or lateral to the midline (Table 20.3)?

Table 20.3 Focal and diffuse, midline and lateral neck swellings

	Midline	Lateral
Focal	Thyroid adenoma Thyroid cyst Thyroglossal cyst Submental lymph nodes	Cervical lymph nodes Hodgkin's lymphoma Carotid artery aneurysm/tumour (pulsatile) Other tumours/metastasis Cystic hygroma Branchial cysts
Diffuse	Non-toxic goitre Graves' disease Subacute thyroiditis	Salivary gland stone or tumour

The presence of palpitations suggests symptomatic hyperthyroidism, and, in combination with a diffuse midline neck swelling, the diagnosis is likely to be Graves' disease or a subacute thyroiditis. Further investigations might include:

- ECG
- blood tests: FBC, U&E, LFTs and erythrocyte sedimentation rate (ESR)
- thyroid function tests (TFTs)
- chest X-ray
- ultrasound of the neck swelling
- iodine radioisotope scan and fine-needle aspiration (FNA) for cytology may be done by specialists

Scoring Scenario 20.2: Thyroid examination

	Inadequate/ not done	Adequate	Good
Appropriate introduction	0	1	—
Ensures privacy, and chaperone if appropriate	0	1	—
Makes sure that patient is comfortable	0	1	—
Exposes neck and shoulders	0	1	—
Inspects head and neck: • position of swelling: midline or lateral • scars • exophthalmos • lid retraction • raised JVP	0	1	2
Inspects hands for: • warmth • tremor • thyroid acropachy • pulse and blood pressure • palmar erythema/vitiligo	0	1	2
Stands behind patient and palpates thyroid gland, commenting on: • size and shape • consistency • nodular, focal or diffuse • tender • mobility	0	1	2
Asks patient to protrude tongue while palpating (thyroglossal cyst)	0	1	—
Asks patient to take a sip of water and swallow as gland is palpated	0	1	—
Palpates trachea for midline shift	0	1	—
Palpates for cervical lymphadenopathy	0	1	—
Listens for a bruit	0	1	—
Percusses sternum for retrosternal goitre	0	1	—
Examines eyes for lid retraction, lid lag, visual acuity	0	1	—
Examines power and reflexes in limbs	0	1	—
Examines skin (pretibial myxoedema)	0	1	—
Offers differential diagnosis: goitre/tumour/cyst	0	1	—
Suggests investigations: bloods (including TFTs), ultrasound, radioisotope scan, FNA and chest X-ray	0	1	2
Arranges appropriate follow-up	0	1	—
Score from patient	/5		
Global score from examiner	/5		
Total score	/33		

Scoring Scenario 20.3: Addisonian crisis

	Inadequate/ not done	Adequate	Good
Appropriate introduction	0	1	—
Acts on observations and suggests immediate management: • monitoring • high-flow oxygen • IV access and fluid resuscitation • checks blood glucose	0	1	2
Reviews history and asks about: • vomiting and diarrhoea • abdominal and back pain • anorexia and weight loss • known endocrine disease • history of malignancy • recent infection (identified in this case as TB) • recent surgery or stress • medications (rifampicin)	0	1	2
Makes a working diagnosis of addisonian crisis	0	1	—
Identifies TB or TB medications as likely cause	0	1	—
Investigations: • electrolytes and blood glucose • Takes blood for cortisol and ACTH • TFTs • Performs septic screen • ECG and ABG • Suggests ultrasound of adrenals	0	1	2
Management: • IV hydrocortisone 100–200 mg immediately • fluid resuscitation/rehydration • treat infection • treat cause and refer to HDU	0	1	2
Score from patient		/5	
Global score from examiner		/5	
Total score		/21	

21
Haematological Emergencies
PETER JAYE AND MATHEW HALL

CORE TOPICS

- Sickle cell crisis
- Disseminated intravascular coagulation (DIC)

Although these may seem rare and unusual topics, this depends very much on the location of your practice. Some departments will see sickle cell patients every day, whereas others may never come across them. This makes predicting the OSCE frequency difficult, but it is wise to review your knowledge of this condition if you practice in an area where it is little encountered. The other topics within the core curriculum are relatively difficult to construct OSCEs for, and are perhaps best tested in the SAQs. We have, however, given an example of how DIC may be tested in the OSCE format.

SCENARIO 21.1: SICKLE CELL CRISIS

A 23-year-old Nigerian man presents with acute left knee pain and chest pain. His left knee is swollen, hot and painful. It became painful 24 hours ago, with no associated trauma. His chest pain is not as severe and has been present for 6 hours. He has had a recent flu-like illness with a non-productive cough. He is in severe pain and is demanding pethidine analgesia. An F2 examined him and found a clear chest. The knee was able to flex 45°. The pain was no worse with movement.

His observations are:

Temperature 37.9 °C
RR 24 breaths min^{-1}
Pulse 100 bpm
BP 130/90 mmHg

The emergency department sister asks you to see the patient, since he is in some discomfort. Take a history, perform a focused examination and institute an appropriate management plan.

SICKLE CELL DISEASE

A clear understanding of sickle cell disease is required for management of this scenario.

Sickle cell anaemia is an autosomal recessive genetic disorder that results from the substitution of valine for glutamic acid at position 6 of the β-globin gene, leading to production of a defective form of haemoglobin, haemoglobin S (HbS). Under physiological stress, deoxygenated HbS polymerizes, deforming the red blood cell (RBC) into the classic sickle shape. The sickled RBCs obstruct the microcirculation, causing tissue hypoxia, which in turn promotes further sickling.

Patients who are homozygous for the HbS gene (HbSS) have full-blown sickle cell anaemia. Milder forms of disease are seen in patients with one HbS allele and a second allele that is also abnormal, for example with haemoglobin C (HbSC) or β-thalassaemia (HbSβ⁺). Heterozygote carriers of the disease are mostly asymptomatic.

The clinical manifestations of sickle cell anaemia are diverse, since any organ system can be affected. They are commonly divided into vaso-occlusive, hematological and infectious crises.

Vaso-occlusive crisis

Vaso-occlusive crisis occurs when sickled RBCs obstruct the microcirculation, causing ischaemic injury to tissues. Pain is the most frequent complaint during these episodes, and it is ischaemic in origin. Most crises of this type last between 3 days and a week.

Bones (e.g. the femur, tibia, humerus and lower vertebrae) are frequently involved, giving rise to the painful 'bone crisis', while involvement of the femoral head may cause avascular necrosis. Vaso-occlusive crisis can involve the joints and soft tissue, and it may present as dactylitis or as hand-and-foot syndrome (painful and swollen hands and/or feet in children).

Acute chest syndrome is a life-threatening complication of vaso-oclusion, with chest pain, fever, hypoxia and pulmonary infiltrates on the chest X-ray. The acute chest syndrome is difficult to diagnose in the emergency department setting, since radiological abnormalities lag symptoms. In one study, half of the patients who developed acute chest syndrome were initially admitted for a pain crisis. Pneumonia may coexist with acute chest syndrome, each condition exacerbating the other.

Vaso-occlusion involving the abdominal organs can mimic an acute abdomen. With repeated episodes, the spleen autoinfarcts, rendering it fibrotic and functionless in most adults with sickle cell anaemia.

Central nervous system (CNS) manifestations of vaso-occlusive crisis are myriad, including cerebral infarction (children), haemorrhage (adults), seizures, transient ischaemic attacks, cranial nerve palsies, meningitis, sensory deficits and acute coma. Cerebrovascular accidents are not uncommon in children, and they tend to be recurrent. These patients are often maintained on hypertransfusion programmes to suppress HbS.

Skin ulceration, especially over bony prominences (malleoli), and retinal haemorrhages frequently complicate sickle cell disease. Finally, vaso-occlusion may involve the corpus cavernosum, preventing blood return from the penis and leading to priapism.

Vaso-occlusive crisis is often precipitated by the following:

- dehydration (especially from exertion or during warm weather)
- cold weather (owing to vasospasm)
- hypoxia (flying in unpressurized aircraft)
- infection
- alcohol
- emotional stress
- pregnancy

Haematological crisis

Haematological crisis is manifested by a sudden exacerbation of anaemia, with a corresponding drop in the haemoglobin level. This can be due to acute splenic sequestration, in which sickled cells block splenic outflow, leading to the pooling of peripheral blood in the engorged spleen (seen in young patients with functioning spleens). Less commonly, it is due to hepatic sequestration.

Haematological crisis can also be caused by aplasia, in which the bone marrow stops producing new RBCs (*aplastic crisis*). This is most commonly seen in patients with parvovirus B19 infection or folic acid deficiency.

Infectious crisis

In most adults with sickle cell anaemia, infectious crisis is due to underlying functional asplenia leading to defective immunity against encapsulated organisms (e.g. *Haemophilus influenzae* and *Streptococcus pneumoniae*).

Individuals with infectious crisis also have lower serum immunoglobulin M (IgM) levels, impaired opsonization and sluggish alternative complement pathway activation. Accordingly, persons with sickle cell anaemia also exhibit increased susceptibility to other common infectious agents, including *Mycoplasma pneumoniae*, *Salmonella typhimurium*, *Staphylococcus aureus* and *Escherichia coli*.

SUGGESTED APPROACH

Introduce yourself to the patient and treat their pain promptly. Most sickle cell patients have been in this situation before – numerous times – and know what works for them. They probably have a regime of home treatment with codeine and non-steroidal anti-inflamatory drugs (NSAIDs) for pain, and only come to hospital when this fails. Hospitals in areas with a significant sickle cell population will have written protocols for pain management; in some places, these may be individualized for frequently attending patients. In the absence of specific guidance, deliver analgesia appropriate to pain scoring and use opiates where required.

Assess the presenting problem and explore the patient's symptoms. Pain is the most common presentation of vaso-occlusive crisis:

- Where is the pain located: extremities, abdomen, back, flank, chest or joints? Is it monoarticular or oligoarticular?
- Ask about its duration and onset (acuity of onset).
- What is its character: migrating, diffuse in the abdomen, or pleuritic in acute chest syndrome?
- Ask about previous similar episodes (painful crises tend to recur in the same pattern).
- What analgesia have they been taking at home? Do they have a regime that they follow?

Look for other complications of sickle cell crisis:

- chest pain, fever and shortness of breath (chest crisis)
- focal neurological symptoms (CNS vaso-occlusion)
- noticeable increase in weakness or pallor (haematological crisis)
- syncope (the most common presentation in acute sequestration crisis)

Look for any precipitants of the current crisis:

- causes of dehydration (exercise, warm weather and not taking in adequate oral fluids)
- infection (fever, coughs, colds, sore throat, urinary symptoms, etc.)
- alcohol
- emotional stress
- trauma

Ask about the background to their sickle cell disease:

- What is the genetic background: HbSS or HbSC? (HbSS is the most severe form.)
- What is the frequency of pain crises? Does it always follow the same pattern?
- Have they ever had a chest crisis?
- What is their normal haemoglobin and have they required blood transfusion in the past?
- Ask about vaccinations: pneumococcal, Hib and hepatitis B.
- Ask about medications. Functionally asplenic patients should be on prophylactic penicillin V and all sickle cell patients should take folic acid daily.

In the OSCE, you are unlikely to have an unwell patient to examine, but the following should be looked for in all sickle cell patients and commented upon:

- Hypotension and tachycardia may be signs of septic shock or sequestration crisis.
- Tachypnoea may be present with pneumonia or the acute chest syndrome. Hypoxia is commonly seen in patients with acute chest syndrome.
- In children, fever suggests infection; however, it is less significant in adults unless it is a high-grade fever.
- Assess hydration status; postural hypotension suggests hypovolaemia
- Observe for pallor, icterus, and erythema or oedema of the extremities or joints.
- Examine the head and neck to look for meningeal signs or possible sources of infection (e.g. otitis media and sinusitis).
- Auscultate the lungs to search for signs of pneumonia or acute chest syndrome
- Palpate for tenderness (abdomen, extremities, back, chest and femoral head) and hepatosplenomegaly.
- Perform a neurological examination to search for focal neurological deficits.
- Examine painful joints

Emergency department care

Investigate with full blood count (FBC) and reticulocyte count (typically 10–15% in sickle cell disease). Haemoglobin electrophoresis for sickle genotype can be performed where this is not known. A chest X-ray should be performed if chest signs are present and a septic screen should be performed if the patient is febrile. Hydration and analgesia are the mainstays of treatment in the emergency department.

Oxygen supplementation is necessary when hypoxia is present.

Well patients with mild sickle cell crisis may be treated with oral fluids and appropriate analgesia. Often, such patients can be discharged from the emergency department once their pain has improved.

More severe sickle cell crises require intravenous fluids, opiate analgesia and admission – preferably under a haematologist. Rehydrate with 3–4 L 0.9% saline over 24 hours or according to clinical assessment, taking care not to fluid-overload.

Antibiotics should be given where there is evidence of infection – broad-spectrum if the source is unclear.

Sickle cell patients typically have haemoglobin levels of 6–8 g dL^{-1}, and in uncomplicated vaso-occlusive crisis, correction of their chronic anaemia is not helpful. However, the haemoglobin may drop substantially during aplastic crisis and acute sequestration crisis, making transfusion in these situations both indicated and lifesaving.

Exchange transfusion consists of replacing the patient's RBCs by normal donor RBCs, decreasing HbS to less than 30%, and can be used when the severe complications of sickle cell disease – acute chest syndrome, sequestration crisis and priapism – do not respond to adequate hydration.

Intubation and mechanical ventilation may be required in patients in whom cerebrovascular accidents have occurred and in patients with respiratory failure due to acute chest syndrome.

Discharged patients should have a pain management plan with escalating oral analgesia and should be counselled on avoiding precipitants – alcohol and other recreational drugs, dehydration, and cold.

Scoring Scenario 21.1: Sickle cell disease

	Inadequate/ not done	Adequate	Good
Appropriate introduction	0	1	—
Immediately addresses patient's pain	0	1	—
Takes an appropriate history of the presenting complaint – pain: • location • duration • previous episodes • analgesia so far	0	1	2
Looks for complications of sickle cell disease; asks about: • chest pain and shortness of breath • neurological symptoms: headache, focal weakness • lethargy/generalized weakness • syncope/collapse	0	1	2
Considers precipitating event; asks about: • causes of dehydration • symptoms of infection • alcohol	0	1	—
Takes background history of patient's sickle cell disease: • genotype: HbSS/HbSC/others • previous crisis • previous severe complications; acute chest syndrome • haematology management • vaccinations and medications	0	1	2
Carries out examination, with attention to: • vital signs, including temperature • hydration status • pallor or jaundice • chest examination • examines affected joints	0	1	2
Proposes appropriate management plan: • investigations: FBC, reticulocytes, septic screen • analgesia • IV rehydration • treats infection • admits • when prompted, is aware of indications for blood transfusion	0	1	2
Score from patient	**/5**		
Global score from examiner	**/5**		
Total score	**/23**		

SCENARIO 21.2: DIC

You have been approached by an F2, who explains that he saw a patient the previous day with suspected meningococcal septicaemia on the basis of fever and a petechial rash. He had treated the patient promptly with fluids and antibiotics and had called ITU. However, the patient began to bleed profusely from their nose, in their urine and from the oropharynx when intubation was attempted by the anaesthetist.

The F2 has a set of the patient's blood tests that he wants to discuss with you since he is worried that he may not have treated the patient fully:

Hb 8.5 g dL^{-1}
WCC 18.6 × 10^9 L^{-1}
Platelets 42 × 10^9 L^{-1}
Na 142 mmol L^{-1}
K 4.8 mmol L^{-1}
Urea 5.6 mmol L^{-1}
Creatinine 153 µmol L^{-1}
Calcium 2.2 mmol L^{-1}
CRP 153 mg L^{-1}
INR 1.6
D-dimer 1230 µg L^{-1}

Discuss the blood results with the F2 and answer any questions that they may have.

DISSEMINATED INTRAVASCULAR COAGULATION

The clinical scenario and blood tests indicate that the patient is suffering from disseminated intravascular coagulation (DIC) as a complication of meningococcal septicaemia. DIC results from pathological overactivation of the coagulation cascade, leading to the consumption of clotting factors as well as of fibrinogen and platelets. It is seen in association with a number of well-defined clinical situations, including sepsis, major trauma, malignancy and obstetric emergencies. The resultant widespread intravascular clotting causes:

- blood vessel occlusion, leading to tissue ischaemia and end-organ damage
- depletion of clotting factors, fibrinogen and platelets, leading to profuse and uncontrollable bleeding
- haemolysis of passing red cells by fibrin strands in the small vessels, leading to a microangiopathic haemolytic anaemia

Clinically, DIC is characterized by bleeding from any site. Bleeding into the skin gives petechiae and/or widespread ecchymoses. Intracranial, pulmonary and gastrointestinal bleeding may be life-threatening. Early evidence of DIC is often seen at sites of iatrogenic trauma: as excessive bleeding from venepuncture sites or from the oropharynx after intubation or as haematuria following catheterization. Despite greater understanding and more aggressive therapy, the mortality from severe DIC remains high, and early recognition and treatment is vital for any chance of survival.

Diagnosis of DIC requires the presence of clinical manifestations of DIC – either haemorrhagic or thrombotic – and the following laboratory investigations:

- thrombocytopenia on the FBC
- raised International Normalized Ratio (INR), prothrombin time (PT) and activated partial thromboplastin time (APTT)
- elevated D-dimer
- reduced fibrinogen
- raised fibrinogen degradation products (FDPs)

SUGGESTED APPROACH

This scenario requires both communication skills to uncover the anxieties of the F2 and knowledge of the subject under discussion. To some degree, a thorough knowledge of DIC will be required to effectively communicate with the F2, particularly where they are anxious for reassurance and will ask some difficult questions!

Start by asking a few questions about the clinical scenario as given, but probing a little deeper to uncover any other information that the F2 is primed to give you. Ask directly about what it is that concerns them – in this case that they did not recognize that the patient with meningococcal septicaemia also had DIC and as a result treatment was delayed, with adverse results. It should become clear to you that it is important to offer reassurance to the F2 – but also that that there is an opportunity to teach and improve their knowledge and understanding of the topic.

Reassure the F2 by pointing out that the most important part of treating DIC is to recognize and treat the underlying cause, in this case the septicaemia, which was performed promptly and correctly. Then ask what they know about DIC and explore their understanding of the pathophysiology of the condition, leading into an explanation of the blood test abnormalities that did indicate that DIC was present.

The actor playing the F2 is primed to ask specifically for an explanation of the blood tests. Remember that the INR (PT) and APTT are raised because of the depletion of clotting factors required for both the extrinsic and intrinsic coagulation pathways. The platelet count is low, owing to consumption of platelets in the myriad blood clots forming throughout the microvasculature. D-dimer is a fibrin degradation product (FDP) that, along with other FDPs, is elevated owing to excess fibrinolysis of the pathological clots. At the end of the clotting cascade, activated thrombin cleaves fibrinogen to give fibrin, which, in polymer form, is the essential molecular ingredient of blood clots; thus, the low fibrinogen level in DIC indicates the pathological overactivity of the clotting cascade. Measurement of fibrinogen and FDPs was not included in the tests initially taken by the F2, but once DIC became clinically suspected, these could have been requested to help confirm the diagnosis.

The F2 asks how DIC can be treated. Emphasize that the cornerstone of DIC management is treatment of the underlying disorder, since this is the only way to halt the overactivation of the clotting cascade. However, once DIC is recognized, aggressive supportive measures are required and, where appropriate, should be initiated in the emergency department:

- Attend to life-threatening issues such as airway compromise or severe haemorrhage requiring resuscitation and aggressive blood transfusion.
- Determine the underlying cause of the patient's DIC and initiate therapy.
- Once DIC is suspected, draw blood for coagulation studies, D-dimer, fibrinogen and FDPs to confirm the diagnosis.
- Cross-match blood in preparation for transfusion.
- Replace platelets with platelet concentrates as guided by platelet counts.
- Replenish clotting factors with fresh frozen plasma (FFP), cryoprecipitate and/or antithrombin III concentrate as guided by a haematologist.
- The patient will certainly need ITU care.
- Involve a haematologist early.

Finally, the F2 asks if he ought to take meningococcal prophylaxis. In general, prophylaxis is only required for close contacts (family members or partners) or, in the case of healthcare workers, where contact with respiratory secretions has occurred. Doctors who have examined and treated a patient with meningococcal disease do not routinely require prophylaxis. However, advice should always be sought from the microbiologist or, in the case of a wider outbreak of meningococcal disease, from the public health consultant responsible. Where recommended, a single dose of ciprofloxacin 500 mg or a 2-day course of rifampicin 600 mg twice daily are acknowledged regimes.

Scoring Scenario 21.2: DIC

	Inadequate/ not done	Adequate	Good
Appropriate introduction	0	1	—
Establishes reason for approach by F2 and identifies their concerns	0	1	2
Explores clinical scenario with the F2 in a non-judgemental manner	0	1	2
Offers appropriate reassurance to F2	0	1	—
Demonstrates knowledge of pathophysiology of DIC	0	1	—
Able to relate pathophysiology to diagnostic investigations. Discusses reasons for (with or without prompting): • thrombocytopenia • raised INR (PT) and APTT • raised D-dimer • low fibrin • raised FDPs	0	1	2
Discusses management, including: • resuscitation along standard lines • treatment of underlying disorder • blood transfusion as appropriate • correction of clotting deficiency with FFP and/or cryoprecipitate and/or antithrombin III • early involvement of haematologist	0	1	2
Answers question about meningococcal prophylaxis: • Demonstrates knowledge of indications • Is aware of when to seek advice • Knows appropriate regimes	0	1	2
Score from F2	/5		
Global score from examiner	/5		
Total score	/23		

22
Infectious Diseases
BETHANY DAVIES AND DUNCAN BOOTLAND

CORE TOPICS

The CEM curriculum highlights a small number of topics under the title 'Infectious diseases', but it is easy to see that knowledge and management of a wider number of potential scenarios may be examined under this banner. These may include the following:

- Malaria
- Tuberculosis
- HIV and AIDS
- Meningitis and meningococcal septicaemia
- Pneumonia
- Sepsis
- Pyrexia of unknown origin
- Fever in the returning traveller
- Needlestick injury
- The febrile child
- Kawasaki's disease

SUGGESTED APPROACH

It is easy to go off on the wrong track here, but you should stop to ask why you are being presented with a fit and healthy young man with an apparent minor viral illness. You are expected to identify the possibility of a sexually transmitted infection (STI) from the limited (but 'classical') history and progress from there. Along with your knowledge of STIs, this station will, in all likelihood, be used to assess your communication skills (see Chapter 30). While these consultations can be challenging, particularly if the actor plays up the awkwardness of the patient, it is most important to ask those difficult questions that are part of a sexual history and then consider and broach the unwanted diagnosis in a professional manner. Failure will result from colluding with the patient to avoid the whole issue of possible STI because it is making the patient uncomfortable.

The differential diagnoses include viral upper respiratory tract infection (URTI), glandular fever or a streptococcal sore throat, and some questions about general symptoms are appropriate, although you should quickly focus your history on the key questions of a sexual history to gain marks. Demonstrate sensitivity as the consultation shifts gear, saying to the patient that you need to ask some more personal questions about their sex life and asking if they are OK with that. Often the patient will already be aware that an STI is a possibility and, although initially reluctant to suggest it to the physician as a diagnosis, they will be relieved that you are going to ask them appropriate questions to get to the heart of their concerns. Ask about:

- When was their last sexual partner/sexual intercourse?
- How many partners have they had in the last 3 months?
- Have they had 'casual sex'?
- Was the sex with men or women, homosexual or heterosexual?
- Did they use protection and, if so, were there any occasions when they did not or any occasions when the protection failed?
- Have they ever had an STI before and, if so, what treatment did they receive?
- Have they got a current partner? And what do they know of their sexual health/history?
- Where appropriate, questions about the consensual nature of the sex and whether rape or abuse has occurred also need to be asked.
- Women should also be asked about contraception and the possibility of pregnancy.

Also enquire about current symptoms of STI, such as genital discharge, pain, sores and itching. Women may have dysuria and symptoms of pelvic inflammatory disease: fever and abdominal pains. Assess for any symptoms of immunocompromise, such as weight loss, chronic diarrhoea or nightsweats.

If you are asked to examine the patient, you should include a thorough examination of the main systems. Equally important is to look in the mouth for ulceration, tonsillar enlargement, bleeding gums and oral candidiasis, and also for the presence of lymphadenopathy. If appropriate (and you may be given a model pelvis in an examination), you should examine the external genitalia for the presence of ulcers (syphilitic chancre), vesicles (herpes) and discharge (gonorrhoea). Ask for the temperature and document the full extent of the rash.

Seroconversion illness often presents with non-specific symptoms. Those at high risk of HIV infection include:

- men who have sex with men
- injecting drug users
- people from countries with a high prevalence of HIV infection (e.g. sub-Saharan Africa, the Caribbean and South-East Asia)
- sexual partners of all of the above

History taking should cover these areas specifically, but a lack of risk factors does not mean that HIV should be excluded as a potential diagnosis.

If asked, investigations should include an FBC, U&E, LFTs, glandular fever screen, monospot test, syphilis serology and HIV serology (remember that patients must be counselled and their consent obtained prior to HIV testing). Genital swabs may be performed in the emergency department by experienced practitioners, but, on the whole, high cervical and male urethral swabs need to be obtained by specialists to be of most diagnostic value. This, coupled with the need for follow-up and treatment of positive swab results, leads most emergency departments to refer patients with likely STIs to local specialist clinics and services. Such STI clinics will also offer HIV counselling and testing, as well as contact tracing and treatment for positive diagnosis of HIV as well as other STIs.

In the scenario above, given the non-specific nature of the presentation and the history of high-risk sexual activity while abroad, coupled with the classical macular rash and otherwise normal examination, the possibility of HIV seroconversion illness should be raised directly with the patient. He should be advised to attend his local STI clinic and provided with information on opening hours and location. He should be reassured regarding confidentiality of his visit and advised of its importance. You should explain the 3-month window period for serocoversion, and so a HIV test that is negative now should be repeated in 3 months from the time of the exposure to confirm the result. Abstinence from unprotected intercourse with others should be advised for the safety of the partner until the seroconversion window has passed. You should ask if he has any questions or whether there is anything else he would like to discuss. Allow time for the response and deal with it sensitively!

Useful resource

British Association for Sexual Health and HIV Guidelines. Available at: www.bashh.org/guidelines.

Scoring Scenario 22.3: HIV seroconversion

	Inadequate/ not done	Adequate	Good
Appropriate introduction	0	1	—
Begins with asking about general symptoms	0	1	2
Obtains patient's permission to take a sexual history	0	1	—
Takes a focused sexual history, including: • genitourinary symptoms: pain, ulcers, discharge, dysuria, abdominal pain • partners: number, sex, etc. • protection used, if any • current partner and their sexual health • weight loss, lymphadenopathy, diarrhoea • specific risk factors for HIV	0	1	2
Gives an appropriate differential diagnosis, including some benign and some STIs: • non-specific viral illness • glandular fever/streptococcal sore throat • syphilis • HIV seroconversion illness	0	1	2
Discusses the possibility of HIV infection with the patient	0	1	—
Asks for appropriate investigations, which should include HIV testing	0	1	—
Understands role of counselling in HIV testing	0	1	—
Gives appropriate information on seroconversion illness, including 3-month seroconversion window	0	1	—
Refers to specialist STI service, either in hospital or community, and gives contact information	0	1	—
Advises abstinence from unprotected intercourse	0	1	—
Score from patient	**/5**		
Global score from examiner	**/5**		
Total score	**/24**		

SCENARIO 22.4: BACTERIAL MENINGITIS

You are asked to review a 23-year-old female student who has been brought in by her boyfriend. He returned from the student union bar to find her confused and unwell. At triage, she was found to have a GCS of 11, and the following observations were obtained:

Temperature 38.2 °C
Pulse 104 bpm
BP 110/65 mmHg
RR 24 breaths min^{-1}
Oxygen saturation 96% on air

Take a brief history from the boyfriend, give a differential diagnosis and outline your management in the emergency department. You are not expected to examine the patient.

On request, the examiner will hand you a card with the examination results as follows:

GCS 11/15 (E3, V3, M5)
Blood glucose 5.9 mmol L^{-1}
Neck stiffness present
No rash visible
Capillary refill time < 2 s
ABG and lactate normal
No significant past medical or travel history and no allergies

The examiner is primed to ask about chemoprophylaxis of meningitis once you have finished giving your management plan.

SUGGESTED APPROACH

The differential diagnosis for this patient at presentation might include:

- acute bacterial meningitis
- other central nervous system (CNS) infection (encephalitis, cerebral abscess, etc.)
- severe sepsis (including meningococcal)
- seizure (seizure thresholds in people with epilepsy are lowered during febrile illness)
- hypoglycaemia and diabetic ketoacidosis (febrile illness may precipitate both)
- recreational drug overdose (e.g. ecstasy)
- deliberate neuroleptic overdose

State to the examiner that you would first assess the patient's airway, breathing and circulation and obtain a bedside blood glucose reading. Provided that these are satisfactory, ask for the patient to be placed on a monitor, give supplemental oxygen and institute regular neurological observations. Never forget the blood glucose in any patient with reduced GCS. Then turning to the boyfriend, introduce yourself, check his relationship to the patient and take a brief focused history to distinguish between the above diagnoses:

- When did he last see her and was she well then?
- Were there any preceding flu-like symptoms or sinus/ear infections (local spread of organisms to the brain)?
- Had she complained of headache, photophobia or nausea?
- Had she been vomiting at all?
- How did he find her when he returned? Was there any evidence of fits?

- Is she taking antibiotics currently for this or another illness that may mask the full severity of disease?
- Has she had any contact with other recent cases of meningitis?
- Could she have taken any drugs either recreationally or in overdose? Reassure the boyfriend about the confidentiality of any information that he gives.
- What does he know of her past medical history, particularly any history of epilepsy, diabetes or immunocompromise?
- Has she been depressed or ever treated for an overdose?
- Is she taking any medications?
- Does she have any allergies?

You may now ask the examiner for the results of the examination, which, together with the history that you have obtained, clearly point to the diagnosis of acute bacterial meningitis. The British Infection Society (BIS)/Meningitis Research Foundation offers a one-page algorithm for the early management of meningococcal disease, and this is worth reviewing and using in both OSCE answers and clinical practice.

You should initiate investigations with FBC, U&E, LFTs, C-reactive protein (CRP), blood glucose, clotting screen and microbiological samples (blood culture and throat swab). If sepsis still needs to be excluded, an ABG and lactate measurement can be performed.

All patients with suspected meningitis should have a lumbar puncture – preferably before antibiotic therapy, in order to maximize the chances of organism culture. However, patients need to be carefully assessed for signs of raised intracranial pressure (ICP); if this is present, antibiotic therapy must be initiated immediately and lumbar puncture deferred. More specifically, the BIS advises immediate antibiotics if performing a lumbar puncture will delay antibiotics for more than 30 minutes (e.g. while awaiting CT) or when there is evidence of:

- marked depressed of conscious level (GCS < 12)
- fluctuating conscious level (fall in GCS > 2)
- persistent seizures
- focal neurology
- papilloedema
- bradycardia and hypertension (Cushing's reflex)
- shock, respiratory failure or acidosis

The patient in this scenario has a GCS of 11 on arrival in the emergency department, and so immediate antibiotics are appropriate in this case.

Causative organisms in adults are mainly *Neisseria meningitides*, *Streptococcus pneumoniae* and *Haemophilus influenzae*, but in those aged over 55 years, *Listeria monocytogenes* becomes more common. The first-line antibiotic to cover these pathogens in the UK is usually 2 g ceftriaxone or 2 g cefotaxime intravenously; if the patient is over 55 years old, add ampicillin to cover *Listeria*. Patients with immunocompromise, penicillin anaphylaxis or recent foreign travel (raising the possibility of resistant pneumococcus) should be discussed with the microbiologist.

Early involvement of senior help and the critical care/ITU team would be appropriate in this case, given the presenting features and the high risk of further deterioration.

A CT scan of the brain, looking for raised ICP, mass lesions and hydrocephalus, should be organized from the emergency department as soon as practical and safe. A normal CT scan does not completely exclude raised ICP, but may provide sufficient reassurance, coupled with clinical judgement, that a lumbar puncture may be safely performed.

For practical reasons, most lumbar punctures are performed by the medical teams on the ward, but being able to perform and interpret the results from an LP is included in the CEM curriculum (see Chapter 31). Once obtained, cerebrospinal fluid (CSF) is urgently sent for microbiology and biochemistry, specifically asking for white cell count, red cell count, protein and glucose (with a contemporaneous serum glucose), Gram stain, and culture.

You should also discuss the use of steroids: these are advised in bacterial meningitis unless the clinician is not confident in the diagosis. If a steroid is to be used then dexamethasone at 0.15 mg per kg body weight four times daily for 4 days is recommended. The first dose must be before – or at least with – the first dose of antimicrobials, thus making this an emergency department decision; therefore discuss promptly with the microbiologist, especially if there is any doubt about the diagnosis.

Meningitis and meningococcal septicaemia are notifiable diseases, and all cases should be reported to the Department of Health (DH). In the case of probable or confirmed meningococcal disease, close contacts (including the boyfriend of the patient in this scenario) will need antibiotic prophylaxis with either rifampicin 600 mg twice daily for 2 days or a single dose of ciprofloxacin 500 mg. Once reported, the DH communicable disease consultant will advise on prophylaxis and do any further contact tracing required.

Useful resources

British Infection Society/Meningitis Research Foundation. *Early Management of Suspected Bacterial Meningitis and Meningococcal Septicaemia in Immunocompetent Adults*, 2nd edn. Available at: www.britishinfectionsociety. org/drupal/guidelines/guidelines and www.meningitis.org/health-professionals/hospital-protocols-adults. See also: Heyderman RS, Lambert HP, O'Sullivan I et al. Early management of suspected bacterial meningitis and meningococcal septicaemia in adults. *J Infection* 2003; **46**: 75–7.

de Gans J, van de Beek D; European Dexamethasone in Adult Bacterial Meningitis Study Investigators. Dexamethasone in adults with bacterial meningitis. *N Engl J Med* 2002; **347**: 1549–56.

Tunkel AR, Hartman BJ, Kaplan SL et al. Practice guidelines for the management of bacterial meningitis. *Clin Infect Dis* 2004; **39**: 1267–84 (Infectious Diseases Society of America guidelines).

Scoring Scenario 22.4: Bacterial meningitis

	Inadequate/ not done	Adequate	Good
ABC approach: asks for oxygen, blood glucose and monitoring	0	1	—
Appropriate introduction to boyfriend	0	1	—

Takes appropriate history:
  • history of presentation
  • symptoms: meningitis headache, photophobia, vomiting,
  • risk factors for acute bacterial meningitis: contacts, local spread, preceding flu-like illness
  • other possibilities: epilepsy, drug overdose
  • past medical history
  • medications and allergies
	0	1	2

Gives appropriate differential diagnosis, including some of:
  • acute bacterial meningitis
  • severe sepsis
  • other forms of CNS infection
  • seizure
  • drug ingestion (recreational/deliberate overdose)
	0	1	2

Recognizes likely diagnosis of meningitis after being given examination results	0	1	—
Plans investigations, including FBC, CRP, glucose and coagulation screen; blood cultures and throat swab	0	1	—
Gives immediate antibiotics and understands reasons for deferment of lumbar puncture (can be prompted by examiner to explain this)	0	1	2
Knows appropriate antibiotic regime with doses	0	1	2
Involves on-call microbiologist/critical care team	0	1	—
Initiates request for CT brain	0	1	—
Indicates that lumbar puncture can be performed once raised ICP ruled out	0	1	—
Understands notifiable nature of disease	0	1	—
Gives appropriate advice regarding prophylaxis of close contacts to boyfriend	0	1	—
Score from boyfriend	/5		
Global score from examiner	/5		
Total score	/27		

SCENARIO 22.5: NEEDLESTICK INJURY

You are asked to see a 28-year-old female healthcare worker (HCW) from a ward who has sustained a needlestick injury on the middle finger.

Take a history and discuss with the ... how you will manage this problem. You are not expected to examine the patient.

[Handwritten notes: BM, Nemod, 4/7, Cnhbiotcs, prop< Rifampican / Ciprofloxacib, Lepar it]

Occupational health departments act as ... site for advice and treatment of occupational needlestick injuries in NHS employees. Many, if not all ... departments will have an appropriate protocol, although this varies between hospitals ... should be seen urgently (i.e. not left in the waiting room) in order that exposure prophylaxis (PEP) where ... indicated, can be started promptly and if possible within 1 hour of the injury.

When considering blood-borne virus (BBV) exposure, we are primarily thinking of hepatitis B, hepatitis C and HIV. For these agents, the risks of transmission after exposure to infected blood are as follows:

- hepatitis B: 30%
- hepatitis C: 3%
- HIV: 0.3% (0.1% for mucous membrane exposure)

In addition, most centres have details of the HIV and hepatitis B/C prevalence in certain local populations, and this can sometimes be used to assess risk of contamination of the donor blood.

Before taking a history, you should ensure that standard immediate management has been performed:

- **Contaminated needlestick, sharps injury, or bite or scratch:** encourage bleeding and wash with soap and running water.
- **Blood or body fluid in eyes or mouth:** irrigate with copious quantities of cold water.
- **Blood or body fluid on broken skin:** encourage bleeding if possible, and wash with soap under running water (but without scrubbing).

To assess and manage a needlestick injury, you must gather information about the recipient (i.e. the HCW), the donor (i.e. the patient on the ward) and the injury or 'stick' itself. You should decide whether the injury is significant, i.e. has the potential to transmit BBVs. Questions to ask are:

- Was the skin punctured, i.e. did the injury site bleed after the stick? Other mechanisms of exposure include through broken skin or via mucous membranes (e.g. the eye).
- Were gloves being worn?
- Was the needle hollow or solid?
- Was the puncture deep or did it involve injection of contaminated material?
- Was the needle visibly contaminated with donor blood?
- What was the immediate management after the injury; for example, was bleeding encouraged?

The most important information needed about the recipient is their hepatitis B immunization status. All NHS employees who perform exposure-prone procedures are required to have had a course of hepatitis B vaccination and should have immunity confirmed with a blood test showing a hepatitis B antibody titre (anti-HBs) greater than 100 mIU L^{-1}. Nevertheless, to be sure, ask the recipient about their status. Staff successfully immunized against hepatitis B will be protected. Currently there are no vaccinations for hepatitis C or HIV, but blood testing for both viruses among clinical staff is currently being rolled out across NHS occupational health departments.

You also need to find out about the donor patient on the ward, particularly whether they are a known carrier of hepatitis B or C or are HIV-positive. Further, where this is not known (as in the majority of cases), a brief assessment of risk should be undertaken by finding out the age of the patient and the reason for their admission and, where appropriate, taking a sexual history and asking about intravenous drug use. This interview should not be performed by the recipient of the needlestick, but you can ask the ward doctor to talk to the patient for you and report back.

Armed with the background knowledge about BBV exposure and with the information gathered about the donor, the recipient and the injury, you can advise on management:

- Take 10 mL clotted blood ⸻ ⸻ ⸻ for baseline HIV testing at a later date if required.
- Take 10 mL clotted blood ⸻ ⸻ hepatitis C testing and HIV testing. Again, the ward ⸻ ⸻ d consent from the patient, particularly for HIV testin⸻
- The stick itself was signifi⸻ ⸻ low needle making transmission of a BBV a p⸻
- In this case, the patient i⸻ ⸻ nized against hepatitis B. No further action is required, ⸻
- Again, the donor is not kn⸻ ⸻ taken at this time.
- The donor patient is elderl⸻ ⸻ fore a low risk for HIV infection. Where the dono⸻ ⸻ HCW can be safely advised that PEP for HIV i⸻ ⸻ then PEP should be started immediately. PEP should al⸻ ⸻ – it can always be stopped once the result of donor bl⸻
- Advise the HCW to attend ⸻ ⸻ or the results of their hepatitis B antibody titre, ⸻ ⸻ pational health team once the result of the donor bloc⸻
- Ensure that the HCW is cov⸻
- Ask the HCW to fill out an incident form.
- The HCW should be counselled appropriately regarding safe sex and not to donate blood while under follow-up.

The actor playing the HCW is primed to test your communication skills also here by showing concern about the risk of HIV infection and requesting PEP, which one of the other HCWs had told them they need in this situation. Take their concerns seriously and present the rationale behind your advice in simple language. The HCW needs to know that PEP is not an entirely benign treatment and has a number of short-term side-effects, such as gastrointestinal disturbance and potentially serious liver dysfunction. You can recommend that they are followed up by occupational health with HIV testing at 6 weeks, 3 months and 6 months after a significant needlestick injury.

If PEP is to be started, you will need to ensure you have gained informed consent – mentioning specifically the unknown efficacy of PEP and the known short-term side-effects. For patients taking PEP, the seroconversion window may be prolonged, and so an HIV test after 6 months will be required to ensure that HIV infection has not occurred. Send them to occupational health the next day for occupational advice and follow-up.

Useful resources

Guidance for Clinical Health Care Workers: Protection against Infection with Blood-Borne Viruses. Available at: www. dh.gov.uk/en/Publicationsandstatistics/Publications/PublicationsPolicyAndGuidance/DH_4002766.

HIV Post-Exposure Prophylaxis: Guidance from the UK Chief Medical Officer's Expert Advisory Group on AIDS. Available at: www.dh.gov.uk/en/Publicationsandstatistics/Publications/PublicationsPolicyAndGuidance/DH_088185.

Needle-Stick Injury (PatientPlus article). Available at: www.patient.co.uk/showdoc/40001843.

Scoring Scenario 22.5: Needlestick injury

	Inadequate/ not done	Adequate	Good
Appropriate introduction	0	1	—
Initiates immediate management of injury	0	1	—
Takes history of the incident: • full skin puncture/other exposure • wearing of gloves • hollow versus solid needle • needle visibly contaminated with blood	0	1	2
Obtains hepatitis B vaccination status from HCW, including antibody titre	0	1	2
Gains information about donor: • hepatitis B/C and HIV status, if known • age and reason for admission • risk factors for BBV/HIV	0	1	2
Correctly assesses stick injury as having potential for BBV transmission	0	1	—
Correctly assesses donor as low risk for BBV carriage (including low risk for HIV infection)	0	1	—
Advises appropriate management plan: • Collects blood from recipient • Collects blood from donor • Advises no action regarding hepatitis B • Advises no action regarding hepatitis C • Advises that PEP is not required • Advises occupational health follow-up next day	0	1	2
Gives adequate explanations for above management, including explaining the risk of transmission of BBV (HBV 30%, HCV 3%, HIV 0.3%) and that donor is low risk for BBV exposure	0	1	2
Deals appropriately with HCW concerns regarding HIV infection and explains side-effects of PEP	0	1	—
Gives appropriate advice on performing exposure-prone procedures until occupational health follow-up	0	1	—
Ensures that HCW is covered for tetanus	0	1	—
Suggests that an incident form should be completed	0	1	—
Score from HCW	/5		
Global score from examiner	/5		
Total score	/28		

23
Dermatological Emergencies
HARITH AL-RAWI

CORE TOPICS

Skills

- Taking a dermatological history
- Examining the skin and mucous membranes

Specific skin diseases

- Eczema/dermatitis
- Impetigo
- Cellulitis
- Psoriasis
- Vesiculobullous lesions of the skin
- Herpes zoster
- Stevens–Johnson syndrome
- Erythroderma
- Urticaria
- Angio-oedema
- Basal cell carcinoma
- Malignant melanoma
- Leg ulceration

Skin problems are a common occurrence in the emergency department. You will often be asked 'How good are you with rashes?' Getting a diagnosis can be quite difficult, even for the specialist, so it is imperative to obtain an adequate history with an accurate description of the rash or lesion in order to reach a differential diagnosis or to convey the details to the dermatologist while referring.

The objective of this chapter is to provide guidance on how to approach patients presenting with skin problems, what questions to ask in taking a dermatological history and how to examine and describe skin lesions. Some common dermatological conditions will be described, but there is no scope to cover the entire field of dermatology in this chapter.

It is unlikely that you will be presented with a patient with a serious skin complaint in the actual OSCE, but you may be asked to take a history from an actor and then be given a photograph to demonstrate that you can correctly describe and diagnose a skin condition.

Scoring Scenario 23.1: Eczema history

	Inadequate/ not done	Adequate	Good
Appropriate introduction	0	1	—
Starts with open-ended questions about the problem	0	1	—
Focuses on an appropriate dermatological history, including: • onset • initial lesions • associated symptoms: itch, pain bleeding, etc. • aggravating factors • treatments	0	1	2
General history, including: • previous skin problems and episodes of rash • other atopic illnesses and family history of atopy • medications and allergies • occupation and possible occupational exposure • social history, looking for possible exposures	0	1	2
Previous episodes and similarity to this episode	0	1	—
Diagnoses likely cause as contact dermatitis due to frequent detergent exposure at restaurant job. Explores impact on lifestyle	0	1	2
Advises appropriately to prevent irritant exposure	0	1	—
Advises on emollient use	0	1	—
Prescribes moderate-strength topical steroid cream	0	1	—
Arranges follow-up with GP	0	1	—
Score from patient		/5	
Global score from examiner		/5	
Total score		/23	

SCENARIO 23.2: EXAMINATION OF A RASH (ERYTHEMA MULTIFORME)

Your F2 has asked you to review a 25-year-old woman with a skin rash (Figure 23.2). The patient had a sore throat 2 weeks ago, which has now cleared, and she is afebrile.

Examine this patient's rash and teach your F2 about describing skin rashes. Discuss possible causes of the rash with the patient.

SUGGESTED APPROACH

After introducing yourself to the F2 as well as the patient, you should start the OSCE by asking the patient if they are comfortable and asking the F2 how experienced they are with examining rashes. Normally in these 'teaching a junior how to …' OSCEs, the junior will have little prior knowledge and you are required to start with the basics. Outline your objective to the F2: 'In this session, I want us to look at this skin rash and then discuss how to examine the skin and describe skin lesions in accurate terms. ' Ask for the patient's permission to use the consultation for teaching purposes as well.

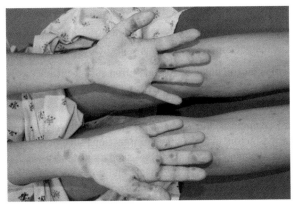

Figure 23.2 The rash in Scenario 23.2. Reproduced with permission from DermAtlas, ©Bernard A Cohen and DermAtlas: www.dermatlas.org.

Adequate exposure of the patient is important, since the skin covers the entire body. In practice, you would ask the patient to undress to their underwear, ensuring adequate privacy and a chaperone. The examiner will let you know what is suitable for the purposes of the OSCE.

The first thing that you note on examination is the distribution of the lesions, making a note of all affected areas. Is the rash generalized or localized or does it affect certain areas such as the extensor or flexor surfaces. Is it symmetrical? Do the lesions occur in crops?

Are all the lesions of the same appearance or do lesions of different ages seem to be present?

Note the colour of the rash. Is it erythematous, silvery, bluish, and do the lesions blanch with pressure?

Then comes the difficult part – describing the morphology of the lesions by both looking and feeling (preferably with gloves). Palpation is important, but some rashes are painful, so, while tenderness should be noted, be gentle! Dermatological terms used for accurate description are listed in Box 23.1.

Box 23.1 Dermatological terms

Macule	Impalpable area of discolouration, <1 cm
Patch	Impalpable area of discolouration, >1 cm
Papule	Raised palpable lesion, <1 cm
Nodule	Raised palpable lesion, >1 cm
Plaque	Raised palpable area with well-defined edges, usually >2 cm
Vesicle	Raised palpable fluid-filled lesion, <0.5 cm
Bulla	Raised palpable fluid-filled lesion, >0.5 cm
Pustule	Pus-filled lesion
Atrophy	Thinning or loss of tissue
Excoriation	Partial or complete loss of epidermis due to scratching
Ulceration	Loss of epidermis and upper dermis, heals with scarring
Erosion	Loss of superficial epidermis, heals without scarring
Fissure	Full-skin-thickness slit
Desquamation	Superficial scales peeling, may follow acute inflammation
Purpura	Discoloration due to bleeding into the skin
Petechia	Purpura, <2 mm
Eccymosis	Purpura, >2 mm
Weal	Raised area of dermal oedema
Scale	Flake of detachable keratin
Crust	Accumulation of dried exudates
Nummular	Coin-like lesion
Annular	Ring-shaped lesion
Reticulate	Net-like lesion

SUGGESTED APPROACH

After introducing yourself, assess whether the child is comfortable and indicate that you would prescribe appropriate analgesia (paracetamol) if needed.

Start with open-ended questions, and then focus on the dermatological history. Ask specifically about:

- onset
- the initial lesions
- associated symptoms (itch/pain/bleeding)
- aggravating factors
- whether it is worsening
- current treatment
- any previous similar skin problems

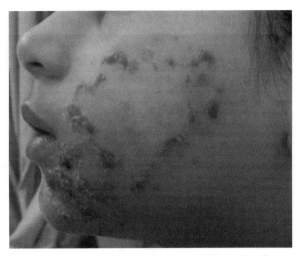

You will have recognized the rash as impetigo. Impetigo is a staphylococcal or streptococcal skin infection and is contagious. Therefore, some further questions are appropriate:

Figure 23.3 The rash in Scenario 23.3. Reproduced with permission from DermAtlas, ©Nasser Altamimi and DermAtlas: www.dermatlas.org.

- Has the child been unwell with the rash? Ask specifically about fevers, feeding and wet nappies.
- Have any other family members had a similar problem recently?
- Ask to see the 'red book'.

Then take a general paediatric history, asking about past medical problems, medications, allergies and vaccinations (see Chapter 26). Impetigo is associated with poor social conditions such as overcrowding and poor hygiene. It is therefore worth tactfully exploring the child's social situation with the parent to see if there may be any concerns.

You have been asked specifically to describe the rash, so a complete examination of the child is not required. The rash has the following characteristics:

- Distribution – it is localized to the facial/periorbital region.
- It occurs in crops.
- Appearance – erythematous lesions with small papules. The lesions burst and exude a yellow–brown honey-coloured crust over affected areas.

Specifically, this is the most common form of impetigo – the non-bullous form – and the appearances in the picture are classical. Causative organisms are *Staphylococcus aureus* and *Streptococcus pyogenes*. Mild impetigo affecting only small areas can be treated with a topical antibiotic cream effective against staphylococcal infections, such as fusidic acid (Fucidin). More widespread infection should be treated with 7 days of systemic antibiotics – flucloxacillin (or erythromycin for penicillin-allergic patients) – as well as topical creams. The infection rarely causes systemic illness, and admission is only required in rare cases where extensive rash has caused dehydration. Parents also need advice on hygiene and to keep the child isolated from other children until the rash has stopped crusting. Separate bedsheets, flannels, bath towels, etc. should be used for the child to prevent spread among the family. Swabs are not normally required for localized lesions, but should be sent in cases of severe disease or if the lesions are not responding to appropriate treatments.

Typically, impetigo resolves over 7 days or so, and the mother should be told to return to her doctor if the infection is still present after a week. Rarely, impetigo may cause more serious complications: cellulitis, scarlet fever and post-streptococcal glomerulonephritis. With regard to the last of these, tell the mother to seek medical help again if the child becomes oedematous ('puffy') or develops dark-brown urine, even if this occurs after the rash has disappeared.

Scoring Scenario 23.3: Examination of a rash (impetigo)

	Inadequate/ not done	Adequate	Good
Appropriate introduction	0	1	—
Focuses on an appropriate dermatological history, including: • onset • initial lesions • associated symptoms: itch, pain, bleeding, etc. • aggravating factors • treatments	0	1	2
Takes a general paediatric history: • past medical history • unwell, fevers, feeding, wet nappies • growth and development	0	1	2
Asks about social circumstances/takes social history	0	1	—
Suggests that would expose patient appropriately with child's and parent's consent	0	1	—
Accurately describes: • distribution of lesions • morphology of lesions • colour of lesions	0	1	2
Identifies rash as impetigo	0	1	—
Gives appropriate management and advice: • swabs and justification for taking/not taking them • topical antibacterial • systemic antibiotics • hygiene advice • isolation advice • advice on complications and when to seek medical help again	0	1	2
Demonstrates good knowledge of condition	0	1	—
Plans appropriate follow-up	0	1	—
Score from patient	/5		
Global score from examiner	/5		
Total score	/24		

ACKNOWLEDGEMENT

We would like to acknowledge Dr Chris Lehmann MD for permission to use photographs from DermAtlas.

USEFUL RESOURCES

Buxton PK, ed. *ABC of Dermatology*, 4th edn. London: BMJ Books, 2003.

DermAtlas. *Dermatology Image Atlas*. Available at: www.dermatlas.org.

Wyatt J, Illingworth R, Graham C et al. *Oxford Handbook of Emergency Medicine*, 3rd edn. Oxford: Oxford University Press, 2006.

24

Oncological Emergencies

ANDREW PARFITT

CORE TOPICS

- Complications related to tumour progression (cord compression)
- Immunosuppression/sepsis secondary to chemotherapy (neutropenic sepsis)
- Biochemical complications (hypercalcaemia)

SCENARIO 24.1: CAUDA EQUINA SYNDROME IN MALIGNANCY

An 89-year-old man attends the emergency department, referred by his GP. He has known prostate carcinoma and has previously been treated for bone metastasis. He has had some falls recently, and appears to have some lower limb weakness and urinary incontinence when examined by the GP. His observations are normal and he is pain-free.

Take a history from this patient and perform the relevant examinations to determine whether further investigation is required to rule out the diagnosis. Briefly discuss investigation and further management.

SUGGESTED APPROACH

Cauda equina syndrome (CES) refers to the symptoms that result from damage or compression of lumbosacral nerve roots within the dura at the distal end of the spinal cord below L2. The cauda equina includes the lower lumbar and all of the sacral nerve roots and provides the sensory supply to the perineal area, the motor supply to the sphincters and parasympathetic innervation of the bladder and bowel, as well as both motor and sensory fibres innervating the lower limbs.

CES as a complex of symptoms consists of lower back pain, unilateral or bilateral sciatica, saddle-area sensory disturbances, and variable lower extremity motor and sensory loss in conjunction with bladder, bowel and erectile dysfunction. Implicit in the diagnosis is the presence of bladder or bowel dysfunction. The onset of these symptoms may be acute or insidious and more chronic. Motor loss may range from mild weakness to flaccid paralysis, while sensory loss typically includes saddle anaesthesia (the sacral and perianal area) and variable sensory loss in the lower extremities. CES can be caused by:

- secondary malignancy, most commonly bone metastasis from prostate carcinoma
- a herniated lumbar intervertebral disc
- primary malignancy of the spinal canal, spine or nerve roots (schwannoma)
- trauma to the lumbar spine
- spinal abscesses

The risk of CES is greater in patients with narrowing of the spinal canal, either congenitally or due to inflammatory processes such as Paget's disease or ankylosing spondylitis.

CES must be excluded as one of the 'red flags' in patients presenting to the emergency department with back pain, incontinence, urinary retention, bowel difficulties, and motor and sensory disturbances affecting the lower limb. Patients suspected of having CES should have emergency MRI of the spine.

Proven CES require urgent surgical decompression to improve clinical outcome. A meta-analysis of cohort study patients showed that there is potential for considerable improvement in sensory, motor and sphincter deficits if surgery is performed within 48 hours. Untreated, CES may progress to permanent disabilities such as paraplegia and permanent urinary and faecal incontinence.

History

The marking scheme for the OSCE will probably allocate as many marks for history as for examination. As always, start by introducing yourself and addressing any immediate needs that the patient may have, such as pain relief. You have read the GP letter and now need to start by asking a few open-ended questions to establish the nature of the problem from the patient's perspective. If not already covered, bring the discussion around to the patient's prostate carcinoma and ask how long he has had the disease and what treatment he has received. The GP letter mentions bone metastasis – establish which bones have been affected and what treatment has been given for this. Ask in particular about palliative radiotherapy to the spine, since this itself can precipitate CES. Move quickly on to the features that would suggest bony involvement of the spine and then ask directly regarding CES symptoms:

- Ask about back pain. Is it a malignant-sounding pain, i.e. non-mechanical, present at rest and keeping him awake at night?
- Explore any urinary or bowel symptoms: incontinence, overflow, leakage, constipation or tenesmus.
- Ask about sensation when passing urine and stool.
- Enquire directly about sciatica and weakness, including foot drag or drop, specifically asking questions targeting the quadriceps, such as whether he has problems climbing stairs or standing from sitting.
- Ask about lack of sensation and numbness of the lower limbs or buttock area, for example lack of sensation of coldness of toilet seats.

Establish the onset of the symptoms and, more importantly, their duration, since the latter clearly affects further imaging prognosis and choice of treatment and the urgency of both. Patients with CES due to malignancy often have a longer non-specific course with intermittent urinary disturbance reported.

A cursory inspection of the spine to look for local tenderness should be performed. Conduct a full neurological examination of the lower limbs, including tone, power and reflexes of all muscle groups (see Chapter 6). Test sensation in the perineal saddle area and ensure that you inform the examiner that you would like to perform a rectal examination to test for anal tone. Watch the patient to ensure that he can walk. Do not forget to screen for a palpable bladder – with ultrasound if necessary. Remember that CES is compression of the lumbosacral nerves after their exit from the spinal column and is therefore associated with lower motor neuron signs – decreased tone, weakness, and reduced reflexes. Any upper motor neuron signs, including upgoing plantar reflexes, will be from another cause!

Plain imaging is of the spine is often unhelpful, but may show sclerotic metastases, bone destruction or pathological fracture. Patients with genuine CES should have MRI of the spine performed as soon as possible, even if this means transfer to a centre with access to MRI. Further treatment depends on the cause as identified post-imaging: malignant CES, as appears to be the case in the patient in this OSCE, is most often treated with steroids and radiotherapy. Urgent involvement of the clinical oncologist and neurology/neurosurgical specialists is critical. Where these specialists are not available locally, the patient should be referred and transferred to a tertiary centre that day.

Scoring Scenario 24.1: Cauda equina syndrome in malignancy

	Inadequate/ not done	Adequate	Good
Appropriate introduction	0	1	—
Ensures patient comfort and gives pain relief if necessary	0	1	—
Begins with open	0	1	—
Establishes nature	0	1	—
Asks specifically • back pain • bowel sym • urinary sy • weakness • saddle ana • duration o	0	1	2
Asks about me	0	1	—
Performs adeq • spine for • tone in l • power in • reflexes i • plantar r • sensation in lower limbs • palpates for bladder fullness • assesses gait • asks to perform rectal examination to check anal tone	0	1	2
Interprets clinical findings correctly as CES and understands need for urgency in making definitive diagnosis	0	1	—
Requests plain films of lumbar spine	0	1	—
Recommends urgent MRI scan	0	1	—
Considers steroids	0	1	—
Obtains specialist input	0	1	—
Score from patient		/5	
Global score from examiner		/5	
Total score		/24	

[Handwritten note overlaid on table:]
Cauda equina
- e rest
- awake e night
- urinary sym
- leg weakness
- saddle anen
- duration syn.
Consider stenoch.

SCENARIO 24.2: HYPERCALCAEMIA IN MALIGNANCY

An F2 has seen a patient with known lung carcinoma who attended the emergency department with pain in his left hip and difficulty mobilizing. A recent skeletal survey showed a metastasis in the femur but was otherwise normal. The oncologists are happy that otherwise his disease is under control. He has been found to have a pathological fracture of his left femoral neck. As part of his workup, the F2 performed liver function tests and a calcium level:

Ca 3.19 mmol L^{-1}
Na 138 mmol L^{-1}
K 4.2 mmol L^{-1}
Creatinine 111 µmol L^{-1}
Albumin 40 g L^{-1}
Bilirubin 2 µmol L^{-1}
Alkaline phosphatase 500 units L^{-1}

Take a focused history and outline your management plan. You are not expected to examine the patient.

SUGGESTED APPROACH

Expect the F2 to be asking questions during the 7 minutes of the examination, but you are not asked to 'teach' the F2, so respond to their questions and include them in a discussion on management rather than turning the OSCE into a teaching session. You should focus on the hypercalcaemia aspect of the patient's management. However, you should briefly ensure that the pathological fracture is being managed correctly and, in particular, that the patient is comfortable, before taking a full history.

Hypercalcaemia is a commonly encountered metabolic disturbance. Two causes predominate: hyperparathyroidism and malignancy. Approximately 10–20% of malignancies are complicated by hypercalcaemia, with multiple myeloma and bone metastasis from lung, breast, thyroid and ovarian tumours being the most frequently associated. Other causes of elevated calcium are less common, and are not usually considered until malignancy and parathyroid disease are ruled out. As indicated in the set of results above, normal or low albumin together with raised alkaline phosphatase strongly suggests metastatic disease as the cause.

First ask the question whether this calcium is really elevated. Hypercalcaemia is defined as a serum calcium concentration above 2.20–2.56 mmol L^{-1}. Roughly 40% of plasma calcium is bound to albumin, and, since it is the unbound free calcium that is metabolically important, the result for total serum calcium must be adjusted for albumin. The calcium level can be corrected to reflect the albumin level as follows:

- If the serum albumin is less than 40 g L^{-1}, increase the measured calcium by 0.10 mmol L^{-1} for every 5 g of albumin below 40 g L^{-1}.
- If the serum albumin is greater than 40 g L^{-1}, reduce the measured calcium by 0.10 mmol L^{-1} for every 5 g of albumin over 40 g L^{-1}.

Alternatively, use the following formula:

corrected calcium (mmol L^{-1}) = measured calcium (mmol L^{-1}) + 0.020 × [40 − measured albumin (g L^{-1})]

In this patient, the calcium is indeed markedly elevated, since he has normal serum albumin (40 g L^{-1}) and so the corrected calcium and measured calcium are identical.

Hypercalcaemia can cause distressing symptoms, serious complications and death. The severity of symptoms is not always related to the degree of hypercalcaemia, but often reflects the rapidity of onset. In other cases, the onset may be insidious. Below is a list of the main features of hypercalcaemia, although not all patients will exhibit all of the features, which need to be looked for in either the history or the examination. If nothing else, remember 'bones, stones, groans and psychic moans'.

- General:
  - ○ dehydration – may lead to pre-renal failure
- Neurological:
  - ○ **easy fatigability**
  - ○ lethargy
  - ○ confusion
  - ○ myopathy
  - ○ hyporeflexia
  - ○ seizures
  - ○ coma

  Note that the most frequent effect of severe hypercalcaemia is delirium.
- Musculoskeletal:
  - ○ weakness
  - ○ **bone pain**
- Gastrointestinal:
  - ○ **abdominal pain**
  - ○ constipation and ileus
  - ○ anorexia
  - ○ nausea and vomiting
- Cardiac:
  - ○ shortened QT interval
  - ○ prolonged PR interval
  - ○ wide T waves
  - ○ ventricular and atrial arrhythmias
  - ○ bradycardia

  Note that arrhythmias, such as bradycardia, can be fatal.
- Renal:
  - ○ polyuria
  - ○ polydipsia
  - ○ dehydration
  - ○ development of **kidney stones**
  - ○ renal failure
- Psychiatric:
  - ○ **psychosis**
  - ○ depression
  - ○ impaired concentration

A past medical history may reveal alternative causes of hypercalcaemia, such as parathyroid disease or sarcoidosis. Enquiry regarding calcium-elevating medications such as lithium, calcitriol, vitamin D and thiazides is also important.

Early diagnosis and hydration followed by specific agents to decrease calcium levels can produce symptomatic improvement and can be lifesaving. The situation may well be different if the underlying malignancy is disseminated and no further treatment is being considered.

Next ask for an ECG. Hypercalcaemia may produce ECG abnormalities related to altered transmembrane potentials that affect conduction time. QT-interval shortening is common, and, in some cases, the PR interval is prolonged. At very high calcium levels, the QRS interval may lengthen, T waves may flatten or invert and a variable degree of heart block may develop. The ECG provided by the examiner is abnormal, with a short QT interval. The patient should be placed on a cardiac monitor.

The most effective management of cancer-associated hypercalcaemia is successful treatment of the underlying malignancy. Until this is achieved, the three primary treatment goals are:

1. Correcting intravascular volume depletion
2. Enhancing renal excretion of calcium
3. Inhibiting accelerated bone resorption

Important general supportive measures include the removal of calcium from parenteral feeding solutions, discontinuation of the use of oral calcium supplements and discontinuation of medications that may independently lead to hypercalcaemia (e.g. lithium, calcitriol, vitamin D and thiazides). Correct other electrolyte imbalances, since potassium and magnesium particularly aid renal excretion of calcium.

Many agents are available to treat acute hypercalcaemia, including 0.9% saline, bisphosphonates, furosemide, glucocorticoids and calcitonin:

- Hydration with intravenous 0.9% saline is the first step in the acute management of hypercalcaemia. Most patients suffering from acute hypercalcaemia are dehydrated, sometimes severely, and the administration of 0.9% saline is therefore important because it expands intracellular volume in addition to increasing renal calcium clearance.
- Bisphosphonates include zoledronic acid, etidronate disodium and pamidronate disodium. They are toxic to osteoclasts and inhibit osteoclast precursors, thereby decreasing osteoclast function. A single intravenous infusion of pamidronate 60 mg will lower plasma calcium over 2–3 days and the effects last for a month.
- Furosemide promotes calcium excretion by the kidneys and can be used to treat hypercalcaemia. Caution must be used, however, as furosemide therapy in the absence of adequate volume expansion may cause a reduction in glomerular filtration rate and therefore of calcium clearance. It should, therefore, only be administered after adequate hydration.
- Glucocorticoids combat hypercalcaemia by increasing urinary calcium excretion and decreasing intestinal calcium. However, they are no longer a blanket treatment for hypercalcaemia of malignancy.
- Calcitonin impairs bone resorption. It has a rapid onset of action, but there is doubt about whether it is helpful in the longer term. Calcitonin has now been largely superseded by bisphosphonates, but can be added in refractory cases.
- Dialysis can be used in severe hypercalcaemia or hypercalcaemia in the setting of oligaemic renal failure.

The patient in this scenario has moderate hypercalcaemia, and a reasonable management plan might be intravenous rehydration and a single dose of 60 mg pamidronate by intravenous infusion. He will need joint care from general medicine and oncology as well as from orthopaedics.

Scoring Scenario 24.2: Hypercalcaemia in malignancy

	Inadequate/ not done	Adequate	Good
Appropriate introduction	0	1	—
Ensures that patient is comfortable and that fracture is managed appropriately	0	1	—
Is aware of need to calculate corrected calcium and that corrected calcium is elevated	0	1	2
Takes history and asks about key features of hypercalcaemia: • tiredness/lethargy • abdominal pain • symptoms of renal colic/known renal calculi • bone pain • polyuria/polydipsia • depression	0	1	2
Examines patient, commenting on: • alertness • degree of dehydration • generalized weakness • abdominal signs • mental state: psychosis, delirium • reflexes for hyporeflexia	0	1	2
Takes past medical history	0	1	—
Asks about medications and allergies	0	1	—
Asks for ECG	0	1	—
Describes features of hypercalcaemia on ECG	0	1	—
Is aware of possible treatment options: • IV fluid rehydration • bisphosphonates • furosemide • calcitonin	0	1	2
Discusses these with F2 as instructed	0	1	—
Initiates appropriate therapy, including IV fluid hydration and single-dose bisphosphonate	0	1	—
Score from patient	/5		
Global score from examiner	/5		
Total score	/26		

25

Rheumat̶ ̶ ̶ ̶ ̶ ̶ ̶es

ALASTAIR NE̶

> *Ensure pt is comfortable & offered analgesia*

CORE TOPICS

- Acute monoarthropathy
- Acute low back pain
- Other topics:
  - Polyarthropathy
  - Crystal arthropathy
  - Osteoarthritis
  - Rheumatoid arthritis
  - Tendonitis/tenosynovitis
  - Bursitis
  - Peripheral nerve syndromes
  - Complications of drugs used in rheumatic diseases
  - Reflex sympathetic dystrophy

SCENARIO 25.1: ACUTE MONOARTHROPATHY

A 56-year-old man presents to the emergency department with a 2-day history of a painful swollen knee with no history of trauma. He has a history of high blood pressure and has taken bendroflumethiazide for the previous 4 years. He is on no other medication.

On examination, the knee is warm to the touch and swollen. There is moderate-sized effusion and generalized tenderness around the joint. The joint has a range of motion of 20–70°. The patient's temperature is 37.5 °C. The rest of the examination is unremarkable.

Discuss the differential diagnosis and relevant investigations with the patient. Demonstrate to the examiner how you would aspirate the knee.

SUGGESTED APPROACH

This is a relatively common presentation to the emergency department. Although the knee is one of the commonly affected joints, any joint in the body can be involved. It is essential to have a good system for examination and a technique for aspiration/injection of each of the commonly affected larger joints (shoulder, elbow, knee and ankle).

The differential diagnosis and subsequent management of this presentation, like many clinical presentations to the emergency department, need to be based on the dual perspective of ruling in one of the most likely causes and ruling out the most serious causes of morbidity and mortality (Box 25.1).

Box 25.1 Differential diagnosis of non-traumatic monoarthropathy

---

Common
- Acute exacerbation of osteoarthritis
- Crystal arthropathy
- Reactive arthropathy
- Exacerbation of inflammatory arthritis (especially psoriatic)

Uncommon
- Spontaneous haemarthrosis (e.g. patients on warfarin)
- Lyme's disease
- Septic arthritis

Non-arthropathic causes of swelling
- Tendonitis
- Bursitis
- Baker's cyst
- Cellulitis

Several aspects of the history, examination or simple laboratory tests may suggest one or other particular diagnosis; however, none of these is specific or sensitive enough to provide a definitive diagnosis. Reasonable initial investigations would include full blood count (FBC), C-reactive protein (CRP) (or erythrocyte sedimentation rate, ESR) and serum urate. X-rays are often performed for this presentation, but will yield little diagnostic information. In the vast majority of cases of acute monoarthropathy, a diagnostic aspiration will be required for correct diagnosis. It is important in the OSCE situation to be able to describe your technique, and the examiner will be looking for you to demonstrate a good rapport with the patient while explaining what you are doing.

Ensure that the patient is comfortable and offer analgesia if needed.

Discuss the possible diagnoses with the patient. Explain that the most likely diagnosis is one of the common causes. Mention the rarer possibility of septic arthritis and the importance of ruling it out.

Discuss other investigations that might be performed (blood tests and X-rays) and their limitations.

Discuss the pros and cons of aspiration, especially the potential adverse effects such as pain and the small risk of introducing infection. Explain the procedure to the patient, including what will happen afterwards (e.g. samples will be sent to the laboratory) and the time until the results are obtained.

Importantly, obtain the patient's verbal consent for the joint aspiration.

It is now necessary to demonstrate to the examiner how you would aspirate a knee. Most often, you will be provided with a model leg, all the instruments that you require and an assistant. Ensure that you use the assistant to facilitate the sterile technique, but ensure their safety from sharps – never draw up the local anaesthetic from a vial held in the assistant's hands!

- Position the patient sitting comfortably with their legs outstretched and the affected knee slightly flexed at 10–15°.

- Demonstrate the anatomy by palpating the patella and identifying a suitable site for aspiration, such as on the lateral side of the knee just beneath the proximal third of the patella.
- Prepare the knee with antiseptic cleaning solution and drapes.
- The procedure is done under strict aseptic conditions. Wash your hands and put on sterile gloves.
- Infiltrate the skin with a small amount of local anaesthetic (1% lidocaine).
- With a 20 mL syringe attached to a green needle, advance through the soft tissues, heading for the space beneath the patella. Lightly draw back on the syringe as you go and until fluid is aspirated.
- Draw 5 mL of fluid into two separate sterile containers – one for urgent microscopy and Gram stain (including microscopy for birefringent crystals) and another for culture.
- Draw off further fluid to provide symptomatic relief.
- Withdraw the needle and cover the entry site with a plaster.
- Dispose of sharps into a sharps container.
- Discuss subsequent management with the patient (analgesia, steroid injection into joint or antibiotics if there is a suspicion of septic arthritis).

Essential background information

Acute crystal arthropathy (gout and pseudogout)

This will account for a large proportion of the cases of true monoarthropathy seen in the emergency department. The age range is usually 40–70 years and risk factors include excess alcohol consumption, male sex, obesity, renal impairment and drugs (low-dose aspirin and diuretics). A raised serum urate level is neither specific nor sensitive enough to assist in the diagnosis, since it is often normal in acute episodes of gout. Other blood tests (FBC and CRP) that are often performed in the emergency department in attempts to differentiate the causes of acute monoarthropathy are equally lacking in sensitivity and specificity. The diagnosis of crystal arthropathy is confirmed by the presence of birefringent crystals viewed on polarized light microscopy. Treatment options in the acute phase include intra-articular steroid injection, non-steroidal anti-inflammatory drugs (NSAIDs) or colchicine.

Reactive arthritis

This usually develops 2–4 weeks after a genitourinary (*Chlamydia*) or gastrointestinal (*Shigella, Salmonella* or *Campylobacter*) infection, although approximately 10% of cases do not have a preceding symptomatic infection. Only a minority of patients will have the classical triad (conjunctivitis, urethritis and arthritis) described by Reiter. The age range is typically 2–40 years. Onset is usually acute and can resemble septic arthritis, but will often affect more than one joint. Elevated white cell count (WCC) and CRP are common, and joint aspiration will be needed to exclude septic arthritis. The disease is self-limiting in 3–12 months, but will require management with NSAIDs or steroids (either systemic or intra-articular).

Septic arthritis

This is relatively rare, but must always be considered, since missed diagnosis has the potential to cause devastating joint destruction (up to 50%). Risk factors include chronic arthritides (especially rheumatoid arthritis), previous surgery (especially prosthetic joints), immunosuppression, extremes of age, diabetes and intravenous drug abuse. Large joints are more commonly affected than small joints and the majority of cases are in the hip or knee. Although patients are often systemically unwell (fever and malaise), this may be absent, and the WCC and CRP may also be normal. Also remember that fever and elevated WCC and CRP can occur in crystal arthropathy. It is essential to have a high index of suspicion, and commence treatment prior to definitive diagnosis. Send fluid for urgent microscopy and Gram stain (as well as looking for crystals) and take blood cultures (positive in up to 50%). Treatment consists of intravenous antibiotics (either broad-spectrum or targeted to the likely causative agent until a culture result is available) and consideration of joint washout by an orthopaedic surgeon.

Scoring Scenario 25.1: Acute monoarthropathy

	Inadequate/ not done	Adequate	Good
Appropriate introduction	0	1	—
Ensures comfort and offers analgesia	0	1	—
Discusses diagnoses, including: • flare-up of osteoarthritis • gout/crystal arthropathies • reactive/inflammatory arthritis • spontaneous haemarthrosis • septic arthritis • non-arthropathic causes	0	1	2
Differentiates between common and uncommon causes	0	1	2
Indicates that septic arthritis must be ruled out	0	1	—
Discusses non-invasive investigations: • bloods • X-rays • clear about limitations in diagnosis	0	1	—
Discusses joint aspiration: • Gives reasons for performing • Mentions complications • Explains procedure in terms that patient can understand • Mentions post-procedure process	0	1	2
Obtains verbal consent for knee aspiration	0	1	—
Performs knee aspiration: • Locates appropriate site for aspiration • Uses aseptic technique • Uses local anaesthetic • Uses appropriate aspiration technique • Sends samples for appropriate investigations • Observes sharps safety	0	1	2
Discusses management options with patient after the procedure	0	1	2
Score from patient	/5		
Global score from examiner	/5		
Total score	/25		

SCENARIO 25.2: BACK PAIN AND 'RED FLAGS'

A 62-year-old man presents to the emergency department with a 3-day history of severe low back pain with no history of trauma.

Take a history from the patient and discuss possible investigations that need to be done. Assume that the general physical examination and neurological examination are normal.

SUGGESTED APPROACH

This is another common presentation to the emergency department. In the vast majority of people with low back pain, the final diagnosis will be mechanical back pain; however, there are many 'red flags' that should alert you to more sinister causes (Box 25.2) and some features that would suggest a nerve root problem (Box 25.3). The focus of the assessment should be on excluding specific pathologies and nerve root pain.

Box 25.2 Back pain 'red flags'

Box 25.3 Indicators of nerve root problems

Age
- Onset at age <20 or >55 years
- Acute onset in an elderly person

Character and site of pain
- Bilateral or alternating symptoms
- Constant or progressive pain
- Nocturnal pain
- Thoracic pain
- Morning stiffness

Systemic symptoms
- Fever
- Night sweats
- Weight loss

Neurological abnormalities
- Neurological symptoms
- Bladder/bowel dysfunction

Medical history
- History of malignancy
- Immunosuppression
- Current or recent infection
- Tuberculosis

- Unilateral leg pain > back pain
- Radiates to foot or toes
- Numbness or paraesthesia in the same distribution
- Straight leg raising test induces more leg pain
- Localized neurology (limited to one nerve root)

Most patients who do not have any 'red flags' or symptoms to suggest a nerve root problem and who have a normal neurological examination do not require any further investigations.

If there are any 'red flags' elicited in the history then FBC, CRP, urea and electrolytes (U&E), alkaline phosphatase (ALP – for Paget's disease), prostate-specific antigen (PSA – if male >55 years) and urinalysis should be done. A plain X-ray should also be done, although it will be normal in a large number of cases and is not sensitive for early malignancy or infection. CT and MRI of the lumbar spine are indicated for patients with a strong suspicion of underlying infection, cancer or persistent neurological deficit.

The examiner will be looking for you to do the following:

- Introduce yourself.
- Enquire whether the patient is comfortable and offer analgesia if needed.
- Establish character, duration, radiation, etc. of pain, looking specifically for nerve root problems.
- Ask about aggravating and relieving factors and use of analgesia.
- Ask about previous episodes of back pain or previous injury.
- Take a past medical history
- Ask about medications and allergies.
- Ask specifically about 'red flags':
  - systemic symptoms
  - morning stiffness
  - neurological disturbance
  - medical: malignancy, infection and immunosuppression
- Take a social history: employment and home circumstances.
- Discuss initial investigations: bloods (for U&E, WCC, ALP, CRP, ESR and PSA) and X-rays of the lumbar spine.
- Discuss the possible need for further imaging: CT/MRI lumbar spine.

The need for investigation and management will depend upon the answers obtained from the patient in the history taking, and, just as in clinical practice, your discussion of these should be tailored to the individual patient.

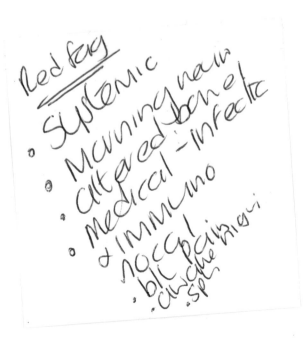

Scoring Scenario 25.2: Back pain and 'red flags'

	Inadequate/ not done	Adequate	Good
Appropriate introduction			—
Ensures comfort and offers analgesia			—
History of back pain, including: • character • duration • radiation			2
Asks about and recognizes symptoms problems: • unilateral versus bilateral leg pai • radiation to foot • numbness and paraesthesias in r • straight leg raise exacerbates pa			2
Exacerbating and relieving factors			—
Asks about previous back problems			—
Asks about past medical history			—
Medications and allergies			—
Asks specifically about 'red flags': • bilateral leg pain • constant/progressive pain • nocturnal pain • thoracic pain • systemic symptoms: fever, sweats, weight loss • previous malignancy • neurological abnormalities • sphincter disturbance	0	1	2
Indicates that would perform additional investigations where appropriate – suggests X-ray and bloods for U&E, ALP, CRP, PSA and ESR	0	1	2
Discusses broader management, including CT/MRI back	0	1	—
Score from patient	/5		
Score from examiner	/5		
Total score	/25		

Handwritten note overlaid on table:
- Radiation to foot
- numbness & pain
- ALR hurts pain

SCENARIO 25.3: EXAMINATION OF THE SPINE

A 42-year-old builder presents to the emergency department with a 2-week history of back pain radiating to his left leg. He reports some numbness in the leg, mainly of the big toe. The pain started when he was lifting a heavy object and is getting progressively worse.

Perform an appropriate neurological assessment.

SUGGESTED APPROACH

Examination of the spine is a common OSCE and one that is surprisingly difficult to do well unless practised beforehand. Examination of a patient with lower back pain should include the range of motion of the lumbar spine, neurological examination, nerve stretch tests and examination of gait. Your neurological examination must systematically test the nerve roots, reflex arcs and dermatomes of the lower limbs, and therefore a sound understanding of these is required. Often, time constraints will not allow all of this to be carried out in the OSCE; the examiner will therefore be looking for a focused examination, and so you should always read the question carefully and do exactly as it requests.

Introduce yourself to the patient. Ensure that they are comfortable and offer analgesia if needed.

Without taking a history, briefly acknowledge that the patient has back pain and the key features of the pain.

Explain that you are going to examine the patient's back and legs.

To determine the range of movement of the lumbar spine, ask the patient to stand, and then check the extent and smoothness of lumbar flexion, extension and lateral flexion.

Perform a neurological examination, testing power, sensation and reflexes and looking for dermatomal patterns (Table 25.1). State that you would wish to perform a rectal examination, looking for perianal tone and sensation.

Table 25.1 Neurological examination of lower limbs

Nerve root	Motor examination	Pinprick sensation	Reflex
L1, L2	Hip flexion	Groin and anterior thigh	
L3	Quadriceps extension	Lateral thigh and medial femoral condyle	Patellar tendon reflex
L4	Ankle dorsiflexion	Medial leg and medial ankle	Patellar tendon reflex
L5	Big toe dorsiflexion	Lateral leg and dorsum of foot	Medial hamstring
S1	Ankle plantar flexion	Sole of foot and lateral ankle	Achilles tendon reflex

Perform nerve root tests:

- Examine for nerve root pain, which is distributed in the relevant dermatomes and worsened by coughing or bending forward.
- Perform a straight leg test for irritation of the sciatic nerve (L4/L5/S1): the test is positive if there is pain below the knee that increases on foot dorsiflexion.
- The femoral nerve (L2/L3/L4) stretch test is positive if there is pain in the groin or anterior thigh when the knee is flexed with the patient lying prone.

Essential background information

Mechanical back pain

This will account for over 80% of all patients with back pain seen in the emergency department. There are a number of structures implicated in the causation of the pain (ligaments, muscles and tendons). The patient often generally attributes onset to an acute traumatic event, but cumulative trauma may also have an important aetiological role. The focus of the assessment is to exclude other causes of the pain. These can be broadly divided into three categories:

Mechanical spinal conditions

- herniated intervertebral disc
- spinal stenosis
- osteoporotic fracture
- spondylolisthesis
- traumatic fracture
- congenital disease: kyphosis and scoliosis

Non-mechanical spinal conditions

- neoplasia: myeloma, metastases, lymphoma and spinal cord tumours
- infection: osteomyelitis, discitis and paraspinous/epidural abscess
- inflammatory arthritis: ankylosing spondylitis and psoriatic spondylitis
- Scheuermann's disease
- diffuse idiopathic skeletal hyperplasia (DISH)
- Paget's disease

Non-spinal causes

- renal disease: calculi, pyelonephritis and perinephric abscess
- aortic aneurysm
- disease of pelvic organs: prostatitis, endometriosis and pelvic inflammatory disease
- gastrointestinal disease: pancreatitis, cholecystitis and peptic ulcer

Usually, no investigations are required unless there are any 'red flags' (see Scenario 25.2). Conservative therapy is the mainstay of treatment in mechanical back pain, and the prognosis is good (97% of cases will settle within 6 weeks):

- regular analgesia (NSAIDs if possible)
- early return to normal activities (avoiding twisting or heavy lifting)

Other modalities have little evidence of benefit in acute back pain (chiropractic, heat packs, acupuncture, etc).

Nerve root compression due to a herniated intervertebral disc

This also generally responds well to non-operative management. Only 2% of patients with sciatica and 4–6% of patients with true disc herniation require surgery. In the absence of cauda equina syndrome or progressive neurological deficit, patients can be managed conservatively for a period of 4 weeks. Opioid analgesia may be required for severe pain. Indications for orthopaedic referral and further investigation are:

- cauda equina syndrome (immediate referral)
- progressive or severe neurological deficit
- persistent motor deficit after 4–6 weeks of non-operative therapy
- persistent sciatica for 4–6 weeks

Cauda equina syndrome

This is a true emergency, requiring urgent referral for decompression to prevent permanent neurological dysfunction. Features are a sudden onset of bilateral leg weakness with urinary or faecal incontinence or urinary retention and saddle anaesthesia.

Scoring Scenario 25.3: Examination of the spine

	Inadequate/ not done	Adequate	Good
Appropriate introduction	0	1	—
Ensures comfort and offers analgesia	0	1	—
Briefly confirms history and symptoms	0	1	—
Explains is going to examine the back and legs	0	1	—
Appropriate examination of lumbar spine: • patient standing • observes for normal lumbar lordosis and for any scoliosis • examines movements of lumbar spine	0	1	2
Performs competent neurological examination of lower limbs: • Examines tone and compares both sides • Tests for power in major muscle groups • Tests reflexes, comparing both sides • Examines for sensation in all dermatomes • Tests plantar reflexes • Indicates would examine for anal tone	0	1	2
Examines for nerve root tests with straight leg raise performed correctly and compared on both sides	0	1	2
Able to interpret the examination of the patient into an appropriate diagnosis, including location of nerve root involved	0	1	2
Score from patient	/5		
Global score from examiner	/5		
Total score	/22		

OTHER TOPICS

These are much less likely to feature in the OSCE and are therefore only discussed briefly here. For each presentation, you need to have a systematic approach to investigation and management.

Acute polyarthropathy

Acute polyarthropathy has a large number of causes:

- polyarticular crystal arthropathy
- viral arthritis: hepatitis B and C viruses, parvovirus and rubella
- bacterial endocarditis
- rheumatic fever
- rheumatoid arthritis
- Still's disease
- seronegative arthritides
- systemic lupus erythematosus
- reactive arthritis
- familial Mediterranean fever
- enteropathic arthropathies

Crystal arthropathies

See the discussion in Scenario 25.1.

Osteoarthritis

Osteoarthritis (OA) is a common incidental X-ray finding. Most patients over the age of 60 will have some evidence of OA on X-ray. Although it is important to include OA in the differential diagnosis of patients presenting with regional pain or an acute monoarthropathy, the presence of X-ray changes of OA does not make the diagnosis nor does it rule out other causes of the pain.

Rheumatoid arthritis

Rheumatoid arthritis (RA) is a chronic inflammatory arthropathy. Presentations to the emergency department may result from acute exacerbations of the joint inflammation process, non-articular complications of the disease (Box 25.4) or complications secondary to drug therapy (Box 25.5). It is important to remember that septic arthritis is more likely in patients with RA, and an acute monoarthropathy should be managed as possible septic arthritis until it is ruled out. Other potential presentations relate to the disease process, and include tendon rupture, atlanto-axial subluxation of the cervical spine and spinal cord compression (often following minimal trauma).

Box 25.4 Non-articular complications of RA

Cardiac
- Pericarditis

Respiratory
- Pleural effusion
- Cricoarytenoid involvement (causing hoarseness and rarely airway obstruction)
- Pulmonary fibrosis

Kidneys
- Amyloidosis

Eye
- Episcleritis
- Scleritis
- Sicca (Sjögren's) syndrome

Blood
- Normochromic, normocytic anaemia

Nervous system
- Peripheral neuropathy
- Carpal tunnel syndrome

Box 25.5 Complications due to drug therapy of rheumatoid arthritis

NSAIDs
- Gastrointestinal ulcer/haemorrhage
- Renal impairment or failure
- Hypersensitivity

Steroids
- Adrenal insufficiency
- Peptic ulcer disease
- Osteoporosis
- Immunosuppression

Disease-modifying drugs (methotrexate and penicillamine)
- Agranulocytosis
- Immunosuppression
- Pneumonitis or fibrosis
- Liver cirrhosis

Tendonitis and tenosynovitis

Tendonitis and tenosynovitis are common presentations to the emergency department. The majority are the result of repetitive action or overuse, and will respond to rest, splintage (where appropriate), NSAIDs and localized steroid injections. The following are common clinical presentations:

Shoulder

- Rotator cuff tendonitis
- Bicipital tendonitis

Elbow

- Tennis elbow (lateral epicondylitis)
- Golfer's elbow (medial epicondylitis)

Wrist and hand

- De Quervain's tenosynovitis (inflammation of the adductor pollicus longus and extensor pollicus brevis tendons)
- Trigger finger (stenosing tenosynovitis of the flexor tendons)

Lower limb

- Adductor tendonitis
- Patellar tendonitis
- Achilles' tendonitis

Bursitis

Bursitis can be due to repetitive injury, but may also result from gout or infection. Similar to acute monoarthropathy, it is not possible to make a definitive diagnosis by history, examination and blood tests, and aspiration of the bursa will be required. Common presentations are:

- prepatellar bursitis – housemaid's knee
- olecranon bursitis
- trochanteric bursitis

Management of non-infective bursitis consists of rest and NSAIDs.

Peripheral nerve syndromes

Reflex sympathetic dystrophy, now referred to as complex regional pain syndrome (CRPS), is a syndrome of pain, swelling, sensory disorder (hyperaesthesia) and autonomic vasomotor dysfunction in a limb. Its onset is usually following trauma, but it can occur after a stroke, or have no obvious cause. It is potentially difficult to diagnose in the early phase, but if missed can lead to skin and muscle atrophy and joint stiffness. A triple-phase bone scan may be of use in diagnosis. Treat with NSAIDs and steroids; refer to orthopaedics or rheumatology for follow-up.

26
Paediatric Emergencies
CHETAN R TRIVEDY

CORE TOPICS

- Paediatric resuscitation (APLS/ATLS)
- The fitting child
- Urinary tract infections
- Meningococcal septicaemia
- The febrile child
- The pulled elbow
- The limping child
- Asthma
- Non-accidental injures
- Ear, nose and throat examination

Paediatric emergencies make up a significant component of the CEM syllabus and are a major topic for the examinations. Paediatric emergency medicine has become a subspeciality in its own right; the syllabus is fairly extensive and can be found on the CEM website.

The following OSCE scenarios give a flavour of the breadth of topics that can be encountered in the CEM examinations, but are by no means exhaustive. It is essential that you be familiar with the advanced paediatric life support (APLS) protocols, as well as the management of common paediatric emergencies.

SCENARIO 26.1: FEBRILE CONVULSION

You are asked to see a 2-year-old boy who has presented to the emergency department after having a witnessed seizure at home lasting approximately 2 minutes. He is accompanied by his mother, who is very worried.

He is alert and his initial observations at triage are:

Temperature 39.4 °C
Pulse 110 bpm
Oxygen saturation 97% on air
RR 24 breaths min^{-1}

Take a focused history and outline your management.

SUGGESTED APPROACH

Febrile convulsions are commonly observed paediatric emergencies, affecting 3% of the population in the age range 6 months–5 years. The seizures are usually of short duration and self-limiting. As the name suggests, they are usually associated with a high temperature, with an underlying source of infection.

The patient's observations suggest that he is stable and not fitting. As he is pyrexial and at risk of further seizures, you must initiate measures to cool him in the first instance. This can be achieved by stripping the child down to their underwear and giving them paracetamol (20 mg per kg body weight) and ibuprofen (5 mg kg^{-1}) as appropriate. You should also ask for an urgent blood sugar to exclude hypoglycaemia.

You should proceed to take a focused paediatric history. Unlike taking histories from adult patients, in a paediatric history you must engage the parent as well as the child. Your approach will vary according to the age of the child and it is important not to exclude the child from the interview. Divide your history into a history of the presenting complaint and a general paediatric history.

History of the presenting complaint

- Ensure that yo_ _____ of the person they are with (parent, guardian, carer_ _____.
- Was the seizure _____.
- Was it generali_ _____.
- Was it simple (_ _____ (a prolonged seizure with a focal component).
- How was the ch_ _____ ack to normal?
- How was the chi_ _____.
- Did they have a _ _____.
- Ask specifically a_out _____ phobia, since these may be indicative of intracerebral i_____.
- Has there been an_ _____ (_____ ed meningitis)?
- Has the child suff_ _____.
- Is there any previ_ _____ en with febrile seizures will have more than one).
- Ask the parents if _____ _____y of febrile convulsions, since 8–20% of cases have a first-degree relative who has had febrile convulsions.

General paediatric history

- Ask about the recent general health of the child. How is feeding going and, if appropriate, are nappies as wet as usual?
- Has the child got any medical history?
- Ask about regular medications, both prescribed and over-the-counter. Does the child have any allergies?
- Ask the mother if the pregnancy went to full term (40 weeks).
- As with all paediatric histories, it is important to know if there were any complications during the pregnancy or delivery.
- Is the child up to date with all of their vaccinations?
- Ask about the health of any siblings as well as the parents.
- Do the parents have any concerns about the child's development (i.e. with speech, behaviour or motor skills)?
- It is useful to take a brief social history and find out what the family structure is and whether there are any social concerns.
- Ask for the 'red book' and plot the weight on the growth chart.

Management

The management of febrile convulsions is dependent upon the following factors:

- Is there a focus of infection?
- How unwell is the child?
- Is this the child's first febrile seizure?
- Is there parental anxiety or social concerns by the healthcare worker?

It is essential that you look for the focus of infection and treat it appropriately. If the focus is clear after a detailed history and examination, the child can discharged with appropriate treatment and follow-up after they have been observed for a minimum of 2–3 hours. In these circumstances, blood tests are not usually necessary, although a urinary tract infection (UTI) should be excluded by performing a bedside urinary dipstick. Where a UTI is suspected, urine may be sent for urgent microscopy and Gram stain. Examination of the ears and throat is essential to look for an upper respiratory tract infection (URTI) as a possible cause.

If the child is unwell or the focus is not clear, they should be investigated to exclude meningitis and/or encephalitis. Such a child should undergo a full septic screen:

- full blood count (FBC) and urea and electrolytes (U&E)
- C-reactive protein (CRP)
- coagulation screen
- lumbar puncture (cerebrospinal fluid analysis for glucose, microscopy and culture, and white and red cells)
- blood culture

In many centres, children who have had their first febrile seizure are admitted overnight for observation. A child who has a prolonged seizure or who has multiple seizures in a short space of time should also be admitted and investigated as above.

Febrile convulsions may be very frightening for some parents, and children are often admitted for observation on the grounds of parental anxiety or other social concerns.

It is important that parents be told that their child is not epileptic and that they do not need a EEG or neurology follow-up. However, a third of patients (especially those under the age of 2 years with a positive family history) will have another febrile convulsion and 3% may go on to have a non-febrile seizure

All patients should have a written fever advice sheet on discharge.

Scoring Scenario 26.1: Febrile convulsion

	Inadequate/ not done	Adequate	Good
Appropriate introduction	0	1	—
Engages parent and child	0	1	—
Elicits history: • recent illness • high fever • type of seizure • length of seizure • family history of febrile convulsions • previous history of febrile convulsions • identifies a focus (URTI) • excludes meningitis, encephalitis and UTI	0	1	2
Takes a general paediatric history and asks for 'red book'	0	1	2
Makes a diagnosis of febrile convulsion	0	1	—
Suggests a full examination of the child: ENT and respiratory	0	1	—
Suggests urine dipstick/MSU to exclude UTI	0	1	—
Management: • Provides reassurance if this is a simple febrile convulsion • Explains that the child is not epileptic • Explains that there is no need for neurological follow-up • Explains that the child may have a further febrile convulsion • Explains that there is a small chance of the child having a non-febrile seizure • Manages fever	0	1	2
Admits and investigates if this is a complicated seizure or is prolonged, if there is focal neurology, or if there is parental anxiety	0	1	—
Suggests appropriate investigations: • bloods: FBC, CRP and blood culture • lumbar puncture (only if complicated seizure) • urine dip and culture	0	1	2
Score from parent		/5	
Global score from examiner		/5	
Total score		/24	

SCENARIO 26.2: NON-ACCIDENTAL INJURY

You are asked to see a 7-month-old boy who has been referred by his GP for an X-ray because his mother noticed that he has been dragging his right leg when crawling for the last week and has been refusing to weight-bear. The X-ray demonstrates a spiral fracture of the shaft of the right femur.

Take a history from the mother and outline your management.

SUGGESTED APPROACH

This OSCE will test your ability to m   **NAI**   ;o test your
communication skills in dealing wit

When dealing with a suspected NAI   **Pc/**   **Hx**   ssible. Taking social
history in suspected cases is often   — **When occurred**   upset when questioned
about their child's injuries. It is im   — **Who noticed.**   gation, and you should
explain that the questions below a   )f injury.

However, safeguarding the child's :   — **delay in presentatn.**   ins be asked and that you
do not avoid asking them because   — **home @ hme.**   you feel that the parents
do not look the type that would d   — **What mob.**   rtant that you remain
objective and do not stereotype c   — **prev. attend**   **eg**

Your history of the presenting con   — **concerns** — **who @ hcm.**
                                      HPC   **Minder**   cy
- Obtain a detailed account of   **social servic**
- When did it occur or was first   **domestc voi...**
- Who noticed the problem and   • **VCC.**   cy
  department?
- If there was a delay betweer   rawling, first
- Who was at home at the time of the ir   **Red book**   ry?
- It is important to establish the level c   rawling, first
  steps, etc.)
- Has the child attended the emergency
- Ask the parents about their concerns r

When taking any history of paediatric traur   ed mechanism of
injury is consistent with the actual injury s   o check to make
sure that the history is consistent with tha   nt between family
members and does not change over time.

Next enquire about the family background

- Establish the structure of the family. Which adults are at home? Ask about siblings and their ages.
- Does the child has a minder or do they attend a nursery or playgroup?
- Have the family had contact with social services before about this or any other child?
- Is there a history of domestic violence?
- Are there any inconsistencies with the history given to the GP or at triage?

In addition, you should take a comprehensive medical history to exclude any causes of a pathological fracture (e.g. brittle bone disease or vitamin D deficiency). It is important to consider possible medical causes of a presentation arousing suspicion of NAI. As with any paediatric history, also ask about:

- length and complications of pregnancy (prematurity is a risk factor for NAI)
- whether the mother suffered postnatal depression
- vaccination status
- medications and allergies

Ask to look at the 'red book' and plot the child's current weight and height. Is there any evidence of failure to thrive?

You should offer to carry out a physical examination. However, where sexual abuse is suspected, the examination should be deferred to a senior paediatrician. Carefully document your findings, making note of the following:

- the child's general appearance
- the child's social behaviour: withdrawn, poor eye contact or tearful
- child–parent interaction: clingy or distant
- bruises of varying ages and in unusual places
- burn marks or scars
- poor dentition (dental neglect)
- finger marks
- retinal haemorrhages (shaken baby syndrome)

MANAGEMENT

The immediate management should involve ensuring that the child is pain-free and treating the fracture appropriately. You should keep the parents informed of what is going on and should explain to them that you will need to contact social services and that the child will be reviewed by the paediatric team.

- Obtain a formal X-ray report
- The fracture should be immobilized appropriately and the child referred for orthopaedic input.
- The child should be referred to the paediatric team and reviewed by a senior paediatrician.
- Contact the duty social worker, who will check to see if the child or other siblings at that address are on the child protection register or known to social services
- If the injury itself does not require admission, any decision to admit the child should be made after liaising with a senior paediatrician and social services.
- Where NAI is seriously suspected, the paediatrician may request a full X-ray skeletal survey and blood tests to exclude medical causes of unexplained injury.

If there is significant concern that the child or other children are at risk of harm, social services will instigate Section 47 of the Children's Act 1989 and contact the police, and will formulate a joint strategy plan with the police and paediatricians to decide if the child needs to be taken into care or can be discharged home. If it is felt that the child needs to be placed in a place of safety, the parents can voluntarily allow the child to be taken into care, which can be the hospital or a with a close relative (Section 20 of the Children's Act). If the parents insist on taking the child out of hospital when there is concern for the child's welfare, the police should be informed. Under Section 46 of the Children's Act, the police have the power to enforce a police protection order that can keep the child in a designated place of safety for up to 72 hours, after which the social worker can apply for an extension in the form of an emergency protection order (Section 44 of the Children's Act).

Scoring Scenario 26.2: NAI

	Inadequate/ not done	Adequate	Good
Appropriate introduction	0	1	—
Engages parent and child	0	1	—
Detailed history of presenting complaint: • How? • Where? • When? • Witnessed? • Who was in the house? • Who noticed the injury? • Why was the presentation delayed? • Establishes normal mobility	0	1	2
Considers inconsistencies in mechanism of injury for mobility of child and notes unexplained delay in presentation.	0	1	—
Takes a focused paediatric history, asking specifically about risk factors for NAI: • prematurity • postnatal depression • significant medical problems or developmental delay	0	1	2
Takes detailed social history: • family structure • siblings • known to social services • history of domestic violence	0	1	2
Asks to see 'red book'	0	1	—
Suggests physical examination for other signs of physical abuse	0	1	—
Management • Manages fracture appropriately • Involves senior paediatrician • Involves social services • Keeps parents informed honestly	0	1	2
Makes decision to admit after liaison with social services	0	1	—
Deals with parents in non-judgemental manner	0	1	—
Score from parent	/5		
Global score from examiner	/5		
Global score	/25		

Circulation

After ensuring that the airway and breathing are stable, assess the circulation by examining for the following:

- heart rate
- pulse volume
- central capillary refill time
- peripheral skin temperature
- cyanosis or mottling
- blood pressure in the older child

Secure intravenous access. This is difficult in the shocked child, and after three failed attempts you should turn to intraosseous access (the technique for intraosseous needle insertion is described in Chapter 31). Once access has been obtained, draw blood for a bedside blood glucose estimation, and then send further blood samples to the laboratory for FBC, U&E, CRP, coagulation screen and culture.

Evidence of circulatory shock should be treated with a fluid bolus of 20 mL kg^{-1} of 0.9% saline, repeated up to three times if required.

Disability

This can be assessed by looking at the following parameters:

- alertness – the AVPU scale ('alert, voice, pain, unresponsive') can be used to gauge alertness in the young child
- neck stiffness
- the pupils
- focal neurological deficits
- abnormal posturing
- evidence of raised intracranial pressure (bulging fontanelle)

Exposure

Remove clothing and quickly examine for signs of acute illness:

- Take the temperature.
- Look for skin rashes. The presence of a non-blanching purpuric rash in this case suggests meningococcal septicaemia.
- Briefly examine the chest, abdomen and joints for a focus of sepsis.

Management

If the blood glucose is low, give 0.5 mL kg^{-1} of 10% glucose and repeat as necessary until corrected.

Manage ongoing seizures with lorazepam 0.1 mg kg^{-1} via the intravenous or intraosseus route. If you do not have intravenous or intraosseus access then 0.5 mg kg^{-1} of buccal midazolam or 0.5 mg kg^{-1} of rectal diazepam are alternatives. The child can be given a second equivalent dose of lorazepam if needed, up to a maximum of 4 mg.

The majority of convulsions in children are controlled with benzodiazepines. However, if seizures continue, the next step in the APLS treatment algorithm is paraldehyde 0.4 mL kg^{-1} diluted with an equal volume of olive oil or saline and administered rectally with a syringe.

An intravenous infusion of phenytoin 18 μg kg^{-1} over 30 minutes should be given if fitting continues despite paraldehyde. If the child is known to be taking phenytoin already for epilepsy then phenobarbital (20 mg kg^{-1} over 20 minutes) should be used instead of phenytoin.

Children whose seizures are resistant to these measures require rapid sequence induction of general anaesthesia, and senior paediatric and anaesthetic help should be summoned.

In the present case:

- This patient has a temperature of 39.6 °C. Remove clothing and give paracetamol 20 mg kg^{-1}.
- In addition to the resuscitation process, treat the suspected cause of seizure and shock. in this case meningococcal septicaemia, with ce͟ ͟   ͟   ͟   ͟   kg^{-1} intravenously.
- The patient should be referred to th͟

Prophylaxis for contacts

There is often concern that contacts of ɛ͟   ͟   ͟   ͟   ͟   iven prophylactic
antibiotics. Close family members and m͟   ͟   ͟   ͟   ͟   ᴨ airway (suctioning,
intubating, etc.) should be offered propɦ

Scoring Scenario 26.3: Meningocc

Neck Stiffness

	Poor	Adequate	Good
Prepares for priority call ('WET FLAGS') Correctly calculates doses			2
Takes handover from ambulance			—
Asks for: • high-flow oxygen through a reservo • cardiac monitoring • saturation monitoring • requests blood glucose and asks for result			2
Rapid assessment of airway and uses adjuncts appropriately	0	1	2
Rapid assessment of breathing	0	1	—
Rapid assessment of circulation: assesses BP, pulse and capillary refill Secures IV access Suggests IO access if IV fails twice Sends appropriate blood samples, including blood cultures Gives fluid bolus for shock and assesses effect (correct dose)	0	1	2
Rapid assessment of disability: • Uses AVPU • Looks for neck stiffness	0	1	—
Treats seizures appropriately: Knows lorazepam dose: 0.1 mg kg^{-1} (IV) Conversant with steps of APLS treatment algorithm	0	1	2
Examines child for non-blanching petechial rash and suggests treating with appropriate antibiotic	0	1	—
Diagnosis of meningococcal septicaemia with shock	0	1	—
Admits to PICU	0	1	—
Discusses prophylactic antibiotics for close contacts	0	1	—
Keeps parent involved and uses assistant appropriately	0	1	—
Score from assistant	/5		
Global score from examiner	/5		
Total score	/28		

SCENARIO 26.4: THE LIMPING CHILD

A 5-year-old girl with learning difficulties presents to the emergency department with her mother. She has had a 2-day history of a painful limp and today the mother noted a temperature of 38.8 °C. She is now refusing to weight-bear.

Take a focused history from the mother and give a differential diagnosis and management plan for this patient.

SUGGESTED APPROACH

The management of the limping child is a topic that often crops up in the written and OSCE components of the CEM examinations. It is useful to start with the identity and relationship of the adult accompanying the child, and then assess, using a paediatric pain score, the level of discomfort of the child and offer appropriate analgesia.

Next take a history of the presenting problem:

- When were symptoms first noticed?
- Confirm the site of pain.
- Is the child able to weight-bear?
- Is there any history of a preceding injury?
- What is the nature of the pain?
- Is there pain at rest?
- What analgesia has been given?
- Have the parents noticed any swelling?
- Is the limb tender to touch?
- Has the child been unwell recently?
- Has the child had any problems with the limb before?
- Has there been any recent use of antibiotics?

[handwritten annotation:] limping Child — Sickle Cell — Salmonella (Om) — Mumps)

As with all paediatric cases, take a general paediatric history as outlined in Scenario 26.1, but with additional questions specific to this presentation:

- Ask about previous orthopaedic problems and operations.
- Consider if sickle cell disease is a possibility.
- Ask about any family history of rheumatological disorders.
- Ascertain the age at which child began walking.
- Ask to see the 'red book'.

Differential diagnosis of a limping child

The mnemonic 'NICE TODI' (Box 26.2) may help to remember the differential diagnosis for a limping child of any age.

Box 26.2 Differential diagnosis of a limping child: 'NICE TODI'

N	Neurological	• Cerebral palsy • Guillain–Barré syndrome
I	Infective/inflammatory	• Transient synovitis (irritable hip) • Septic arthritis • Osteomyelitis • Psoas abscess • Cellulitis • Tuberculosis
C	Congenital	• Congenital dysplasia of the hip (from birth onwards) • Sickle cell disease
E	Environmental	• Lack of sunlight/vitamin D deficiency • Malnutrition
T	Trauma	• Sprains • Fractures • NAI
O	Oncological	• Lymphoma/leukaemia • Primary (osteosarcoma) or secondary bone tumours
D	Developmental	• Perthes' disease (common between ages 4 and 9 years) • Slipped upper femoral epiphysis (SUFE) (common in early adolescence: 10–15 years of age)
I	Immunological	• Juvenile idiopathic arthritis • Henoch–Schönlein purpura (HSP)

Physical examination

You should state that you would carry out a thorough physical examination of the child as well as the joints involved. In addition, you should examine below the joints as well as the joints on the other side for comparison.

Observe the child walking.

You should suggest a detailed neurological examination of the lower limbs.

Examine the spine and back.

Look for bruising and features to suggest NAI.

Investigation and management

Investigations should include:

- FBC (raised white cell count, WCC)
- CRP (which is increased in osteomyelitis)
- erythrocyte sedimentation rate (ESR) (see Kocher's criteria below)
- sickle screen if appropriate
- blood cultures
- X-ray (anteroposterior and lateral with or without frog leg views of the hip if SUFE is suspected)
- screening X-ray of lower limb in younger children (hip to feet) for fractures
- ultrasound scan to look for effusions
- urine dipstick for haematuria

Most important in the management of this patient who is febrile and non-weight-bearing is exclusion of septic arthritis. You should be familiar with Kocher's criteria for differentiating between transient synovitis and septic arthritis (Box 26.3).

Box 26.3 Kocher's criteria

- History of a fever > 38.5°C
- The child is not weight-bearing
- ESR > 40 mm h^{-1}
- Serum wcc > 12 × 10^9

Handwritten annotation overlaid:

Kocher's Criteria
(1) Temp >38°5.
(2) NWB
(4) WBC >12.
(5) ESR >40mml⁻
=1 40-90% septic
arthritis.
2 =

Children with two or more of these criteria are at high risk of having septic arthritis (Table 26.2) and should be admitted (may require IV antibiotics and orthopaedic referral for joint aspiration). The child in this scenario has a Kocher score of at least 2 and warrants admission and further management.

Patients with one or none of the criteria have less than 3% chance of having septic arthritis and an alternative diagnosis should be considered.

Table 26.2 Risk stratification of septic arthritis using Kocher's criteria

Number of Kocher's criteria present	Risk of septic arthritis (%)
0	0.2
1	3
2	40
3	93
4	99

Scoring Scenario 26.4: The limping child

On re "red" book (handwritten note)

	0	1	2
Introduces self to adult and confirms their identity relationship to child			
Engages child appropriately to age group			
Calculates pain score and offers analgesia			
Takes history of presenting complaint: • onset of pain • location of pain • characteristics of pain • history of recent trauma • weight-bearing or not			
Takes an appropriate paediatric history: • previous orthopaedic problems • rheumatologic conditions in the family • recent illnesses, coughs and colds • asks to see 'red book'			
Asks about analgesia use, drug history and allergies	0	1	2
Offers to perform detailed examination of affected limb	0	1	—
Offers an appropriate differential diagnosis, including: • septic arthritis • transient synovitis • osteomyelitis • cellulitis • trauma	0	1	2
Investigations: • inflammatory markers • blood cultures • X-rays: AP and lateral hip • ultrasound scan of hip	0	1	2
Knows Kocher's criteria • Temperature > 38.5 °C • WCC > 2×10^9 L^{-1} • unable to weight-bear • ESR > 40 mm h^{-1}	0	1	2
Calculates Kocher's score for this patient as 2 Decides to admit for further investigations for septic arthritis	0	1	—
Summarizes findings	0	1	2
Score from parent	/5		
Global score from examiner	/5		
Global score	/29		

SCENARIO 26.5: UTI IN A CHILD

An 18-month-old boy is bought to the emergency department by his elder sister. The child has had a 2-day history of intermittent vomiting and has been crying whenever he wets his nappy.

He is crying and unhappy but fully alert, and his initial observations at triage are:

Temperature 38.4 °C
RR 26 breaths min^{-1}
Pulse 130 bpm

Take a focused history from the sister and suggest appropriate investigations. Outline your management plan.

SUGGESTED APPROACH

Paediatric fever is a very common problem presenting to the emergency department. It is important to find the focus of fever, and urinary tract infection (UTI) should always be on the list of possibilities, especially when vomiting is also a feature. Your initial history should probe for the specific symptoms of UTI, ask more generally about symptoms of infection elsewhere and also gain information on how unwell the child might be. As always, start with the identity and relationship of the person accompanying the child; in this case, it is an elder sister and it would be pertinent to ensure that she is not a minor herself.

Then ask about:

- duration of fever
- associated symptoms: cough, runny nose, difficulty breathing, diarrhoea
- dysuria
- abdominal pain
- loin pain or tenderness
- offensive-smelling urine
- rigors
- number of episodes of vomiting
- poor feeding
- constipation

Ask whether the child is tolerating fluids and whether they have been alert or more sleepy.

Enquire whether anybody else (e.g. siblings) has been unwell.

Then take a general paediatric history as outlined in Scenario 26.1, but also ask specifically about:

- previous UTI
- previous recurrent undiagnosed fevers
- family history of vesicoureteric reflux or renal disease

Plot the child's weight in the 'red book' and check for poor growth.

The child has been brought to the emergency department by an elder sister, and it would be pertinent to enquire about the family circumstances and why the parents were not with the child. Who looks after the child most of the time?

You should suggest that you would carry out a thorough examination, looking for the focus of infection. In the case of suspected UTI, examining for loin tenderness is of particular importance.

Investigation

Children under the age of 3 years should have a clean-catch urine specimen sent for urgent microscopy and culture, since dipstick testing alone is unreliable. If the child is over the age of 3 years, a negative urine dipstick is adequate for excluding a UTI.

This child is 18 months old and so you should indicate that a clean-catch urine be sent for urgent microscopy. The examiner tells you at this point that the urine you send is positive for bacteriuria but negative for pyuria.

Management

Deliver symptomatic treatment first. Remove clothes and consider antipyretics and analgesia to make the child more comfortable.

The 2007 NICE guidelines on UTI in children set out clear advice on its management in all age groups. A positive microscopy result for bacteriuria with or without pyuria (white cells) indicates the presence of a UTI; the next step is to decide whether it is an upper or lower UTI (Table 26.3).

Table 26.3 Classification of UTI in children

Upper UTI/ pyelonephritis	Lower UTI/ cystitis	Atypical UTI	Recurrent UTI
• Bacteriuria with fever >38 °C or • Bacteriuria with loin pain/tenderness	• Bacteriuria ± pyuria but no systemic features	• Acutely unwell • Septic • Raised creatinine • Not responding to antibiotics after 48 h • Atypical organism (non-*Escherichia coli*)	• Two or more upper UTI pyelonephritis • One upper UTI and one or more lower UTIs • Three or more lower UTIs

Treatment of proven UTI should be along the lines shown in Table 26.4.

Table 26.4 Treatment of UTI in children

Type of UTI	Treatment
Any UTI where the child is <3 months old	Paediatric admission for IV antibiotics
A child >3 months old with an upper UTI	Oral antibiotics for 7–10 days Where oral antibiotics are not possible (i.e. vomiting), admit for IV antibiotics until oral therapy is possible
A child >3 months old with a lower UTI	Oral antibiotics for 3 days and reassess response in 48 h

In the present case, it will be necessary to admit the child for intravenous antibiotics until their vomiting settles and appropriate oral therapy can be instituted. All children placed on antibiotics for UTI should be reassessed at 48 hours. Children over 6 months old who respond rapidly to treatment and in whom symptoms resolve at 48 hours do not need follow-up or further investigation. Failure to respond to treatment after 48 hours should prompt referral to a paediatrician for ultrasound of the renal tract during the acute illness and follow-up.

The NICE recommendations for imaging in children with UTI are summarized in Table 26.5.

Useful resource

National Collaborating Centre for Women's and Children's Health. *Urinary Tract Infection in Children: Diagnosis, Treatment and Long-Term Management* (NICE Clinical Guideline 54). London: RCOG Press, 2007. Available at: http://guidance.nice.org.uk/CG54.

Table 26.5 Recommended imaging in children aged 6 months to 3 years with a UTI

Imaging	Patient responds well to treatment within 48 hours	Atypical UTI	Recurrent UTI
Ultrasound scan during the acute infection	No	Yes [a]	No
Ultrasound scan in 6 weeks	No	No	Yes
DMSA in 4–6 months	No	Yes	Yes
MCUG	No	No [b]	No [b]

DMSA, dimercaptosuccinic acid scintigraphy; MCUG, micturating cystourethrogram.

[a]If the infection is not due to *Escherichia coli* and is responding well, the scan can be performed in 6 weeks.

[b]This is not routinely performed unless dilation on ultrasound, poor urine flow, non-*Escherichia coli* or family history vesico-ureteric reflux.

Scoring Scenario 26.5: UTI in a child

	Inadequate/ not done	Adequate	Good
Introduces self to carer, confirms her identity and checks that she is not a minor	0	1	—
Engages child appropriately to age group	0	1	—
Delivers symptomatic treatment	0	1	—
Takes history of presenting complaint: • duration of fever • dysuria/frequency • abdominal pain • loin pain or tenderness • offensive-smelling urine • severity of vomiting/toleration of fluids • symptoms of infection at other sites • poor feeding	0	1	2
Asks about: • previous UTI • previous undiagnosed fever • family history of vesico-ureteric reflux or renal disease	0	1	—
Takes competent general paediatric history and asks for 'red book'	0	1	2
Enquires about family background and why parents have not brought child to emergency department	0	1	—
Suggests MSU for urgent microscopy to confirm UTI and is aware that dipstick is not reliable in this age group	0	1	2
Confirms upper UTI and suggests antibiotic treatment	0	1	2
Admits child because of vomiting and unsuitability for oral therapy	0	1	—
If the child does not respond in 48 hours, suggests ultrasound scan during acute infection and DMSA scan in 4–6 months	0	1	2
Score from child's sister	/5		
Global score from examiner	/5		
Total score	/26		

27
Psychiatric Emergencies
NICOLA DRAKE AND CHETAN R TRIVEDY

CORE TOPICS

Deliberate self-harm

- NICE guidelines on deliberate self-harm
- Risk factors for suicide
- Liaison with psychiatric services

Acute psychosis

- Causes, including organic
- Initial management options, including drug indications/contraindications

Alcohol and drug abuse

- Intoxication
- Dependence
- Withdrawal
- Patients warranting admission

Violent behaviour

- NICE guidelines on violent behaviour
- Domestic violence
- Sexual assault
- Staff safety
- Restraint

Dementia

- Assessment and causes

Mental health law

- Capacity
- Consent
- Mental Health Act

Psychiatric emergencies can be very complex, and usually need a multidisciplinary approach, sometimes involving external agencies. Calm, logical assessment of all medical, psychiatric, social and legal aspects is essential.

SCENARIO 27.1: ALCOHOL HISTORY

You are the registrar on duty in your clinical decision unit and are asked to see a 48-year-old man who has been admitted to recover from acute alcohol intoxication. A CT of his brain prior to admission was normal and he has no injuries.

Carry out an assessment of his alcohol use and outline your management. You are not expected to take a medical history or examine the patient.

SUGGESTED APPROACH

A high proportion of emergency department attendances are alcohol-related. The ability to assess if the patient has a problem with the level of alcohol he is drinking is an important skill. Many presentations may be related to alcohol, including falls, head injury, burns, fits and other collapses, gastrointestinal symptoms, repeat attendance, and depression and other psychiatric presentations. A formal assessment of drinking (and drug) habits should be made in patients who present in this way.

It is very important that if a patient is admitted with what is thought to be alcohol intoxication then other causes for their clinical state have been sought and excluded before admitting them to an observation or clinical decision unit to 'sober up'. There should be a full clinical assessment to look for injuries as well as any medical consequences of hazardous drinking. A blood glucose level should always be obtained for intoxicated patients.

Alcoholics frequently neglect themselves and may have malnutrition. If there is evidence of chronic alcohol misuse, Wernicke's syndrome or Korsakoff's syndrome (Box 27.1) then thiamine (Pabrinex) should be given intravenously – one pair of ampoules in 200 mL 0.9% saline over 20 minutes. Two pairs of Pabrinex ampoules should be given three times a day for Wernicke's and Korsakoff's syndromes, and once a day otherwise.

Box 27.1 Clinical features of Wernicke's and Korsakoff's syndromes

Wernicke's syndrome
- Ataxia
- Confusion
- Nystagmus
- Ophthalmoplegia

Korsakoff's syndrome
- Selective memory impairment
- Confabulation
- Disorientation in time
- No clouding of consciousness

You should start by introducing yourself and explaining the purpose of your interview with the patient. You should ensure that the patient's main reason for attending has been dealt with. This way, you gain rapport and the patient is more likely to be receptive to pertinent alcohol questions. You should assume an empathetic and non-judgemental approach, using open-ended questions where possible. Bold accusatory statements such as 'You are an alcoholic aren't you!' and a moralistic attitude will damage the therapeutic relationship and are counterproductive. Express interest and concern. Show reflective listening so that the patient can see ... trying to understand their point of view. Do not interrupt ...

Establish how much the patient ... its are:

- for a man: 21 units per wee...
- for a woman: 14 units per w...

Some alcoholics can be vague an... you exactly what they drank the previous day. Ask them ... vy intake to one type of drink may indicate dependent... nk and how much they are spending on alcohol, so this ... quite an eye opener. Remember that some beers and w... dard.

You should ask about the pattern... with whom? Drinking alone and early in the morning ar... particular pattern or situation. Find out if they belong ... lism, for example barmen, publicans, members of the armed ... they took their last drink, since this may be useful for estima...

You will now be able to assess if th... aviour. The CAGE questionnaire (Box 27.2) may be u... ...pendence. If the patient answers 'yes' to 3 out of 4 of the CAGE questions, they are likely to be dependent on alcohol. The Paddington Alcohol Test (PAT) combines assessment of drinking habits with questions that form the start of a brief intervention. Patients are offered an appointment with an alcohol worker if deemed 'PAT-positive', and/or offered written information.

[Handwritten annotation: CAGE — C = cut down — A - angry — G - guilty — E + eye opener. If 3/4 = 1 dep.]

Box 27.2 The CAGE questionnaire

- Have you ever tried to **C**ut down your drinking?
- Do you ever get **A**ngry when people talk to you about your drinking?
- Do you ever feel **G**uilty about your drinking?
- Do you ever take an '**E**ye opener'?

'Yes' to 3 out of 4 questions indicates likely dependence.

Paddington Alcohol Test (PAT)

The PAT questionnaire is a relatively quick and easy screening tool. Essentially, it asks three questions:

1. **Quite a number of people have times when they drink more than usual – what is the most (in total number of units per day) you will drink in any one day?**

Table 27.1 shows the average number of units (pub measures) for a variety of alcoholic beverages. It is important to note that the units consumed when people drink at home are likely to be higher, and a single shot of vodka may be up to 3 units in volume.

2. **If you drink more than 8 units a day (for men), or 6 units a day (for women), is this at least once a week?**

If the patient answers 'yes' then they are PAT-positive and should receive alcohol advice. If they answer 'no' then move onto Question 3:

3. **Do you feel your current attendance at the emergency department is related to alcohol?**

If the patient answers 'yes' then they are PAT-positive; if they answer 'no' then they are PAT-negative. However, this should be interpreted carefully, since many patients presenting to the emergency department will deny alcohol as a cause for their attendance, despite being obviously intoxicated.

Table 27.1 Units of alcohol per volume in a variety of alcoholic beverages

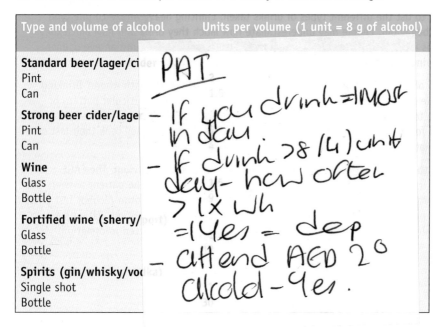

Type and volume of alcohol	Units per volume (1 unit = 8 g of alcohol)
Standard beer/lager/ci[der] Pint Can	
Strong beer cider/lage[r] Pint Can	
Wine Glass Bottle	
Fortified wine (sherry/...) Glass Bottle	
Spirits (gin/whisky/vo[dka]) Single shot Bottle	

Handwritten note:

PAT
- If you drink = most in day
- If drink >8 (4) unit day - how often
  > 1x wk
  = Yes = dep
- attend AED 2°
  alcohol - Yes.

Hazardous drinking

This is defined as drinking more than twice the recommended daily limit – i.e. more than 8 units for a man and 6 units for a woman. This group can benefit from a brief intervention involving advice and information about reducing alcohol intake.

Dependent drinking

This is defined as drinking more than twice the recommended daily limit every day, or demonstration of other signs of dependence. This group do not benefit from brief intervention and need more complex management form specialist alcohol workers. You must ask the patient about signs of dependence:

- Do they feel a compulsion to drink?
- Do they show signs of tolerance – i.e. can they have a heavy intake without becoming intoxicated or feeling drunk?

You should ask the patient if they get any of the symptoms of withdrawal listed in Box 27.3 and whether they have had to take a drink to relieve symptoms. Have they had repeated failed attempts to stop drinking? Any of these points indicate likely dependence. You should suggest scoring any potential withdrawal using the CIWA scale and treat with benzodiazepines such as chlordiazepoxide as indicated. It is likely that if you are asked to perform this assessment, you will be given the CIWA proforma as a template (it is scored out of 67).

Box 27.3 Signs of acute alcohol withdrawal, forming the basis of the Clinical Institute Withdrawal Assessment for Alcohol (CIWA) scoring system

- Nausea and vomiting
- Tactile disturbances
- Tremor
- Auditory disturbances
- Paroxysmal sweats
- Visual disturbances
- Anxiety
- Headache, fullness in head
- Agitation
- Reduced orientation and clouding of senses

If you have established the presence of hazardous or dependent drinking, find out the effect that this has had on the patient in terms both of his health and of his social circumstances. Comorbid psychiatric illness is common in alcohol-dependent people (up to one-third of cases), and specific questions should be directed at detecting this. The most common are the mood disorders: depression and anxiety. Antisocial personality disorder is also common. Always remember that alcohol abuse is a risk factor for suicide, and you must enquire about ideas of self-harm.

Throughout the interview, you should encourage the patient to make the connection between the problem drinking and the negative consequences of that behaviour: 'Do you think your attendance is related to alcohol?' Letting the patient come to this conclusion will be more helpful to them than pointing it out. If there are denials in the face of likely alcohol issues, the previous question could be followed up with 'Would you be in hospital if you had not been drinking?' You should help the patient see any gaps between their own goals/values and where they are or are likely to be with continued problem drinking. Encourage the patient to weigh up the pros and cons of changing or not changing their behaviour.

Also encourage belief in the possibility of change and reinforce statements of intention to change. You should also reinforce any statements that the patient might make that indicate alcohol has had a negative effect. Do the same if they express concern about their drinking levels. These reinforcement techniques are part of 'motivational interviewing'.

Finally, offer help to the patient while allowing them to choose between options – for example counselling, Alcoholics Anonymous or help from their GP. It is valuable for the patient to be offered an appointment and to be given a time there and then. Striking while the iron is hot increases the chances that the patient takes up the appointment offer. It is also preferable if the appointment is scheduled very soon. The longer the patient has to wait, the less likely they are to attend. They should also be offered written information to take away, consisting of advice about safe levels of drinking, health issues, and sources of help for drinking and social problems. If there is a coincident mental illness, a referral should be made to the local mental health team.

Scoring Scenario 27.1: Alcohol history

	Inadequate/ not done	Adequate	Good
Appropriate introduction	0	1	—
Explains purpose of interview	0	1	—
Uses open-ended questions to commence interview: • How are you feeling today? • What are the circumstances related to emergency department presentation?	0	1	—
Asks specifically about alcohol intake and assesses PAT status: • pattern of drinking • units per day: >8 units male, 6 units female • type of alcohol • was admission related to alcohol?	0	1	2
Performs CAGE questionnaire: • Cutdown • Anger • Guilt • Eye opener	0	1	2
Asks about symptoms of acute withdrawal: • anxiety • tremor • headaches • nausea/vomiting • sweating • hallucinations (visual/auditory) • agitation • tactile disturbances • confusion Needs 4 (to score 4 marks)	0	1	2
Enquires about previous attempts at detox	0	1	—
Asks about: • depression/medications/recreational drugs • Previous psychiatric history	0	1	—
Takes social history (employment) Social status	0	1	—
Empathetic approach and does not interrupt	0	1	—
Non-judgemental	0	1	—
Engages patient and involves them in treatment plan	0	1	2
Suggests scoring according CIWA scale and prescribes chlordiazepoxide as appropriate	0	1	—

Continued

Scoring Scenario 27.1 *Continued*

	Inadequate/ not done	Adequate	Good
Gives written alcohol advice sheet	0	1	—
Refers to community and drug and alcohol team	0	1	—
Score from patient	/5		
Global score from examiner	/5		
Total score	/29		

SCENARIO 27.2: DELIBERATE SELF-HARM HISTORY

You are on duty in the emergency department and are asked to see a 24-year-old woman. She has tried to hang herself in her bedroom following an argument with her boyfriend. She is alert and orientated with normal vital signs and a normal clinical examination. She is refusing treatment and wishes to leave.

Take a history and perform a risk assessment. Briefly outline your management. You are not expected to examine the patient.

SUGGESTED APPROACH

It is important to remember that there are two aspects to management of the patient who self-harms: physical health and mental health. Your assessment should cover both. You must also include an assessment of risk of further acts of self-harm. The key to management decisions is to assess whether a patient has the capacity to refuse treatment. In this particular OSCE, the phrasing of the question indicates that the emphasis is on risk and mental capacity issues.

Introduce yourself and ensure that the interview is carried out in an environment that offers privacy. Explain the purpose of your interview and that you wish to help.

Establish the circumstances of the act of self-harm and confirm if she is still suicidal.

The patient must be given an opportunity to express the motivation for the act of self-harm. Do not make assumptions about this. Reasons may include a cry for help, to escape worries, to change another person's behaviour, to punish someone, etc.

Your risk assessment should cover three main areas:

- characteristics of the act of self-harm
- characteristics of the person
- social circumstances and provoking events

Characteristics of the act that are associated with increased risk of repetition include:

- violent means (e.g. attempted hanging or jumping off a bridge)
- evidence of planning:
    - Were there any arrangements to prevent being found (telephones off, doors locked, etc.)
    - Was the patient discovered by accident or did they know that another person was due to visit?
    - Was there any evidence of sorting of affairs (writing of a will, cancelling deliveries, calling work to say they would not be in, arranging care for pets, etc.)
    - Was there a suicide note?

Characteristics of the person indicating a higher risk of repetition include:

- stated intention to die
- previous episode of self-harm
- presence of a mental illness or personality disorder (particularly depression)
- substance misuse

A person who states suicidal intent must be believed. An indication of great intent means that there is a need for close care and observation of the person concerned. A person who very calmly states their intention to die should not be thought of as less at risk because of their incongruent affect. It is known that patients can become very calm once they have firmly come to a decision to kill themselves. Previous self-harm episodes are a common risk factor for completed suicide.

Current and previous psychiatric history (particularly as an inpatient) indicates increased risk, Between 30% and 40% of general hospital attendees who self-harm are given a psychiatric diagnosis, and one-third have prior contact with psychiatric services. The most common diagnosis is depressive disorder, so you should enquire about depressive symptoms (Box 27.4). Alcohol dependence is diagnosed in 10% of people with depression and in a similar percentage of people with schizophrenic and bipolar disorders. Hopelessness is a psychiatric trait particularly associated with self-harm and has been found to be a better predictor of suicide than depression. Therefore, your assessment should include questions that ask how the patient feels about the future. Older age, male sex and poor health are also risk factors for completed suicide.

You should also use the SAD PERSONS score to assess the patient's risk for future suicide attempts. (Box 27.5)

Box 27.4 DSM-IV criteria for major depression (need 5 or more to diagnose major depressive episode)

- Low mood for most of the day every day
- Fatigue
- Recurrent suicidal ideation
- Lack of concentration
- Weight loss > 5%
- Low self-esteem
- Disturbed sleep
- Weight loss
- Loss of interest
- Agitation

Box 27.5 SAD PERSONS scale for risk of suicide

		Score
S	Sex: female	1
A	Age: 15–24, 45–54, >75	1
D	Depression/hopelessness	1
P	Prior history	1
E	Ethanol (alcohol use)	1
R	Rational thinking loss	1
S	Support system lacking/isolation	1
O	Organized plan	1
N	No significant other half	1
S	Sickness (terminal illness/cancer/HIV)	1

Score	Action
0–2	Discharge with follow-up
3–4	Discharge with close monitoring
5–6	Consider admission
7–10	Definite admission

It is also important that you screen for any organic (biological) causes of the patient's depression (Box 27.6) and investigate and manage these conditions appropriately.

Social circumstances and trigger events are also important. Ask about recent crises, such as relationship break-up, divorce, loss of job and deaths. Social isolation due to difficult living arrangements or to lack of friends and relatives can increase risk. Are there any other factors that may cause vulnerability, such as unemployment, debt, homelessness or domestic violence? In the majority of cases, self-harm is reported to have occurred because of social factors. If problems are perceived to be unsolvable, patients tend to a greater level of feelings of hopelessness.

Having performed a risk assessment, you should then turn your attention to the question of capacity. This is often a difficult decision, and different members of staff can reach different conclusions depending on their interpretation of the law. It is good practice to obtain another opinion (usually from a psychiatrist) if possible and to record this in the notes. If a competent patient is refusing treatment, particularly if the treatment is lifesaving, they should repeatedly be given the opportunity to change their mind. In cases where there is some doubt about capacity, advice from a defence organisation is wise, and even an application to the courts may be required if time allows.

In order for a patient to have capacity, you must be satisfied that they demonstrate all of the criteria in Box 27.7. The treatment being proposed must be explained in language and terms appropriate for the patient. You must take steps to overcome communication issues, for example in a patient who is deaf or who cannot speak. The consequences of treatment and of non-treatment must be explained. You should be happy that the patient is able to weigh up the pros and cons and come to a reasoned decision, free from coercion (including from you!).

Box 27.6 Medical causes of depression (not exhaustive)

- Hypothyroidism
- Diabetes
- Addison's disease
- Systemic lupus erythematosus
- Addison's disease

Box 27.7 Assessment of a patient's capacity

The patient should be able to:

- Understand in broad terms what is proposed
- Retain the information
- Weigh up the risks and benefits, including the consequences of no treatment
- Come to a reasoned decision

The decision should be free from coercion

Remember that different treatments require different levels of understanding, so a patient may have capacity to decide about some things but not others. Also remember that a patient may be temporarily incapable of making a decision owing, for example, to distress, anger, pain or intoxication.

If it is decided that the patient does not have capacity then the common law 'doctrine of necessity' applies – usually known colloquially as 'common law' – and you must treat the patient according to their best interests. This involves giving treatment only to save life or to prevent a serious deterioration in health, and nothing more. The use of force or restraint is a matter of last resort, and these should only be used to the minimum possible degree. With the advent of the Mental Capacity Act 2005, common law has been placed on a statutory footing. The act also allows for an independent mental capacity advocate to be appointed to make health decisions on behalf of an incapacitated adult should there be no close relative or person with lasting power of attorney. In an emergency situation where there is no time for such an appointment, you should proceed with treatment in the patient's best interests.

If the patient does have capacity then their decision to refuse treatment should be respected, no matter how irrational that decision might seem. You must remember that you still have a duty of care towards this patient despite their refusal, and they should be offered other treatments as necessary, plus appropriate observation and follow-up. The only exception to acceptance of the refusal is if the patient is mentally disordered and can be treated under the Mental Health Act 1983 (Box 27.8). If a patient satisfies the relevant criteria and is detained under Section 2 or 3 of the act, they can be compulsorily treated for their mental disorder. Under Section 2, they may also be treated for the conditions arising directly as a consequence of that disorder, such as treatment for a suicide attempt. For other sections and for other conditions not directly arising as a consequence of the mental disorder, treatment is by consent or under common law.

Box 27.8 The use of The Mental Health Act 1983 for the compulsory detention of patients with psychiatric disorders

---

Criteria for detention under the Mental Health Act 1983

A person suffering from a mental disorder may be detained under the act if they are considered to be a risk to themselves or to others. Mental disorder is defined as:
- mental illness
- mental impairment (arrested or incomplete development of mind)
- psychopathic disorder

(These are legal, not medical, definitions.)

Section 2
- Compulsory admission for up to 28 days
- Requires two practitioners (one must be approved)
- Application made by social worker or nearest relative

Section 3
- As above
- Compulsory admission for up to 6 months

Section 4
- Emergency section when an urgent admission is required
- To be used when the patient poses a significant risk to others or themselves
- Can be used when there is not enough time to get a second medical practitioner

Section 5(2)
- Emergency section – 'doctor's holding powers'
- Only applicable to inpatients; cannot be used in the emergency department
- Can be used to detain patient for 72 hours
- Cannot be renewed

Section 5(4)
- Emergency section – 'nurse's holding powers'
- Trained mental health nurse can detain a high-risk patient following an informal assessment for up to 6 hours
- Only applicable to inpatients

Section 135
- This section allows an approved social worker to remove an 'at risk' patient to a place of safety
- Requires a magistrate's warrant

Section 136
- This section allows the police to remove a patient to a place of safety
- Hospital or police station (not all emergency departments are places of safety)
- Cannot extend section by using Section 5(2) or 5(4)
- Convert to Section 2 or 3 if admission is required

Scoring Scenario 27.2: Deliberate self-harm history

Handwritten note overlaid on table:

Depression
- DM
- hypothyroidism
- addison
- ALE

			Good
Appropriate introduction			—
Finds private area to take history			—
Establishes circumstances surrounding attempt: • mechanism: overdose, hanging, etc. • triggers • planning: suicide note, financial affairs • impulsive act • previous attempts at self-harm • remorse after attempt • continuation of suicidal ideation			
Previous psychiatric history and treatment			
Recent medical history to exclude organic cause • hypothyroidism • diabetes • Addison's disease • systemic lupus erythematosus			
Ascertains features of major depression (needs 6 out of 9): • low mood • agitation • sleep disturbance • fatigue • low self-esteem • thoughts of self-harm • weight loss • loss of libido • poor concentration	0	1	2
Performs a risk assessment using SAD PERSONS score	0	1	2
Assesses patient's capacity to refuse treatment	0	1	—
Explains to the patient that they will need to be assessed by the on-call psychiatric liaison team	0	1	—
Suggests making arrangements to detain the patient under Section 2 of the Mental Health Act: • Informs social services • Two independent medical practitioners (one is approved practitioner with a background in psychiatry)	0	1	2
Demonstrates non-confrontational approach • Is non-judgemental • Explores patient's concerns	0	1	—
Score from patient		/5	
Global score from examiner		/5	
Total score		/26	

SCENARIO 27.3: MENTAL STATE EXAMINATION IN MANIA

You are asked to review a patient who has been brought in by the police after he was found wandering on the dual carriageway. Perform a mental state examination and outline your management plan. You are not required to perform a detailed assessment of the patient's cognitive state.

SUGGESTED APPROACH

This scenario tests your ability to make a rapid assessment of a patient's mental state and formulate a management plan.

Taking a psychiatric history in less than 7 minutes in a patient who is acutely disturbed is a major challenge for candidates taking the CEM examination. The key to this type of OSCE is to have a structured approach to your interview and to keep engaging the patient throughout the scenario. From the outset, you should have a good idea whether the patient is:

- manic
- psychotic
- depressed
- acutely confused

One approach to this OSCE is to remember the mnemonic 'All Brides Should Make Tea Cakes In Summer' – this is not only useful in your assessment but also provides a model for a structured way to present your findings to the examiner:

- **A**ppearance
- **B**ehaviour
- **S**peech
- **M**ood
- **T**hought
- **C**ognition
- **I**nsight
- **S**ummary

Appearance

From the moment that you enter the room, make a mental note of the patient's appearance and whether it is normal or abnormal. You should consider their cultural beliefs and the circumstances of their presentation to the emergency department. For example, a patient in cricket whites wearing batting gloves, cricket pads and a helmet may be appropriate in a cricket ground but not in a supermarket.

Is the patient kempt and what is their personal hygiene like? Patients who are manic may present with a bizarre sense of dress, wearing bright colours, which often match and reflect their extreme euphoric mood. In contrast, a schizophrenic patient may present with silver foil on the frames of their glasses to distract penetrating X-rays from space.

It is essential that you do not mock the patient's appearance, since not only will this make them more defensive, but you also risk losing rapport (and global marks in the OSCE). However, it is important to enquire about any incongruities in appearance in a non-threatening way, since these will be important clues to the underlying condition. For example, a patient sitting in the room under an umbrella may divulge that the umbrella is preventing other people from reading their thoughts.

Behaviour

Once you enter the room, you should introduce yourself and outline the purpose of the interview. Take time to observe the patient's behaviour and do not fall into the trap of trying to make them do what you want. A manic patient may refuse to sit down and may wander around the room. Attempts to get the patient to sit down may waste valuable time and not help your rapport. Instead, you should try to observe their behaviour and explore why they are pacing. Make a note of any unusual behaviour and explore it without trying to control it.

Assess the patient's ability to make eye contact and whether this is appropriate for the circumstances. A depressed patient may make little eye contact and be withdrawn, whereas a patient who is in a manic phase is likely to be hyperactive and loud.

You should remember that, in the examination, everything the actor does is deliberate and a potential clue for you to interpret. It is important that you are not thrown by the actor, since they are very realistic, and you should remain calm and composed throughout the scenario.

You should ask the patient about the circumstances that led them to be brought to hospital:

- What were they doing at the time? (Swimming in the fountains in Trafalgar Square.)
- Did the act have any significance? (Washing the devils away, since the water is blessed.)
- Do they believe that their behaviour is unusual or strange in any way?

Speech

Listening to the patient often provides important clues to the underlying condition. A depressed patient may say a few words in a low quiet tone. In contrast, you may not get a word in edgeways when faced with a manic patient in the examination (**pressure of speech**).

Patients with schizophrenia also present with speech changes where the patient will often move onto talk about unrelated topics abruptly (**knight's move thinking**). They may also make up words that make no sense (**neologisms**) and use words that rhyme but are not in context (**clang associations**). The content of the speech may deteriorate to the point that the patient makes no sense at all (**word salad**).

Mood

By observing the patient's appearance, behaviour and speech, you should get a fairly good idea of their mood. The use of open-ended questions such as 'How are you feeling today?' should be used to directly assess the patients mood. Manic patients will often be euphoric and tell you that they feel great despite having been hit by a car only an hour ago. They will appear to be full of energy and highly excitable in nature. In contrast, the acutely depressed patient is likely to be withdrawn and may become very tearful during the consultation.

Thought

Until this stage, your assessment will have been largely observational and should have taken less than a minute or two, and it will not necessarily have required you to engage the patient. To assess the patient's 'thought' process is often difficult, especially when the patient is exhibiting extreme behaviour. The key is to develop a rapport and keep the patient engaged.

Patients who are depressed may have thoughts of worthlessness, guilt and low self-esteem and generally feel miserable. They may be slow to respond to your questions, and you should ensure that you ask about any thoughts of self-harm and if they have ever had any suicidal ideations. These should be explored further, since they will impact significantly on your management plan.

In striking contrast, a manic patient will have their thoughts rushing at a hundred miles an hour and they will change the topic of discussion rapidly (**flight of ideas**). They may suggest that they have special powers or that they have been sent by god to save mankind, as well as other **delusions of grandeur**. Although some of these ideas may be very far-fetched, you should avoid mocking the patient or being confrontational and should try to explore the thoughts behind their thoughts.

In schizophrenia, the thought process is delusional; the patient may hold beliefs that are not consistent with rational thinking and cannot be explained by their cultural, religious or educational background. The patient may feel that they are being persecuted and that their neighbours are spying on them through their television or that they are being followed. They may also have primary delusions that are out of the blue or where they attach a delusional belief to a normal perception – for example 'I looked out of the window and saw a red car and I knew it meant that the aliens were coming.' In addition, patients with schizophrenia may also display the following:

- thought insertion
- thought withdrawal
- thought broadcasting
- echo de la pensée (a belief that thoughts can be read or spoken out loud)
- passivity phenomenon (mood, actions and bodily functions are controlled by an external force)
- auditory hallucinations – often the person may hear several voices that talk about the patient among themselves (third person) or refer to the patient directly (second person); visual and other sensory hallucinations are possible but less likely

Cognition

Cognition is often disturbed in patients who present with acute psychiatric emergencies. You may not be able to perform a detailed assessment of the patient's cognitive function in the time available in the OSCE, but you should try to gauge their cognitive state by testing their:

- orientation
- memory
- concentration
- calculation skills

If the patient is in a manic phase or acutely psychotic, you may find that they have poor cognition and may not be able to concentrate on the tasks that you set them. If the patient is uncooperative or does not respond to your calls to spell the word 'world' backwards, do not get bogged down – move on to the next task quickly. You will not have the time to perform a full mini-mental state examination (MMSE).

Insight

You should make an assessment of the patient's insight into their illness by asking them if they are ill and how they feel about it. Patients with schizophrenia or who are manic will refuse to accept that they are ill. They may also feel that any medical intervention is a conspiracy against them. Patients who are depressed often have some insight into their illness in that they accept that they are unwell, but may attribute their symptoms of depression to an underlying medical condition.

Focused medical history

Before you present to the examiner, tell them that ideally you would like to take a detailed medical and social history.

It is important to know if the patient has any previous medical or psychiatric illnesses and if they are on any medications. You should enquire about any previous formal detentions under the Mental Health Act. Ideally, you should take a formal developmental and social history, but for the purpose of the OSCE this is not required and you should focus on assessing the patient's current mental state

Summary

You should allow a minute or so at the end of your time to summarize your findings to the examiner and offer a differential diagnosis. It may be helpful to use the structured 'All Brides Should Make Tea Cakes In Summer' approach to your answer, as well giving a differential diagnosis and management plan for your patient.

Differential diagnosis

The three main psychiatric conditions that come up in the CEM examinations are depression, mania and the psychoses; they are summarized in Table 27.2.

Table 27.2 Acute features of common psychiatric OSCE scenarios

Characteristic	Mania	Schizophrenia	Depression
Appearance	• Bright garish clothes that may clash	• Inappropriate attire • May use everyday objects inappropriately	• Withdrawn • Poor eye contact
Behaviour	• Hyperactive • Fidgety • Over-familiar	• May experience hallucinations • Agitation • Bizzare postures • Violent/aggressive	• Poor eye contact • Withdrawn • Mute • Tearful
Speech	• Pressure of speech • Loud	• Neologisms • Clang associations • Word salad	• Quiet
Mood	• Euphoria out of context of situation	• Variable • May not show any emotion (flattened affect)	• Low mood • Tearful
Thought	• Flight of ideas • Thoughts of grandeur	• Delusions (primary/secondary) • Thought broadcasting • Thought insertion • Thought removal • Auditory hallucinations (third person)	• Poor self-esteem • Guilt • Worthlessness
Cognition	• Poor in acute phase	• Poor in acute phase	• Limited
Insight	• Poor	• Poor	• Limited

Management

The management of an acute psychiatric emergency in the emergency department will vary according to the nature of the emergency and whether the patient is a risk to themselves and/or to others. It is highly likely that the patients in examination scenarios may need to be sectioned, and you should suggest involving relevant bodies to organize an urgent section.

Remember that many patients brought in with psychiatric emergencies may also have other problems or injuries as a result of their psychiatric behaviour, and these should be addressed. For example, a manic patient struck by a car may have significant injuries, which they may underplay because they feel invincible.

As a part of your management, you should perform at least basic investigations to exclude any organic cause, although this may be complex since the patient is often reluctant to have any investigation. If the patient is under the influence of recreational drugs or alcohol, they may have to be observed in the emergency department under close supervision until the effects of the intoxicants have worn off and the patient can be formally assessed.

The basic investigations include:

- low/high blood sugar
- bloods, to exclude sepsis
- urine, to exclude infection in the elderly
- chest X-ray, to exclude sepsis
- CT head, to exclude tumour or head injury

If the patient is acutely psychotic, violent or exhibiting aggressive behaviour, an emergency sedation may be considered, but this is usually the last resort and should be performed after discussing with a senior experienced clinician.

Scoring Scenario 27.3: Mental state examination in mania

	Inadequate/ not done	Adequate	Good
Introduces self and explains purpose of interview	0	1	—
Observes: • appearance • behaviour • speech	0	1	2
Uses open-ended questions to engage patient	0	1	—
Ask about the events leading up to the presentation to the hospital	0	1	—
Assesses mood using open-ended questions	0	1	—
Enquires about thought disturbances: • flight of ideas • knight's move thinking • delusions • thought insertion • thought withdrawal • thought broadcasting	0	1	2
Elicits any thoughts of grandeur: • 'special powers' • special role in the world • fantastical achievements	0	1	—
Asks about hallucinations: • Second-person auditory: Are the voices talking to you? • Third-person auditory: Are the voices talking about you?	0	1	—
Makes attempt to test cognition (patient has poor cognition)	0	1	—
Addresses patient's insight and understanding of their illness	0	1	—
States intention to take a focused medical and social history: • previous medical history • sleep/appetite loss/mood • use of alcohol and recreational drugs • previous psychiatric history • previous sections • family history • social history	0	1	2

Continued

Scoring Scenario 27.3 *Continued*

	Inadequate/ not done	Adequate	Good
Summarizes effectively	0	1	2
Offers diagnosis of acute mania	0	1	—
Maintains good rapport with patient	0	1	—
Non-confrontational			—
Non-judgemental approach to patient'			—
Performs a psychiatric risk assessment			—
Makes a recommendation that the pat ⎯ detained under Section 2 of the Menta and two medical practitioners, one of ⎯ perform a section)			2
Suggests investigations to exclude orga head. Treats any additional problems/inj			2
Score from patient			
Global score from examiner			
Total global score			

(handwritten note) Are their voices talking to you or about you. – test cognition. & insight.

SCENARIO 27.4: ACUTE CONFUSION

You have been asked to see a 74-year-old r ....rgency department after his carer found him to be acutely confused .... self. The carer is present at the time of your assessment.

Take a focused history and perform a mini-mental state examination (MMSE). Outline any investigations and your management of this patient. You are not expected to examine the patient.

SUGGESTED APPROACH

This is a common clinical scenario in everyday emergency department practice and therefore a potential OSCE. The key approaches to this type of OSCE include:

- obtaining a detailed history of the presenting complaint
- previous medical history
- previous psychiatric history (depression)
- assessing premorbid activities of daily living (ADL)
- performing an MMSE and appropriate investigations
- looking for predisposing factors: infection, trauma, cerebral event or medication-induced
- formulating an agreed management plan, involving the patient, next of kin and carers

After introducing yourself to the patient and the carer, ask about the events preceding presentation to the hospital:

- Over what time period did the patient become confused: minutes, hours, days or months?
- What are the carers and patient's main concerns?
- Has there been any episode of loss of consciousness?
- Is there any history of falls or trauma?
- Have there been any previous episodes of confusion?
- Is there a risk of accidental or deliberate drug overdose?

- Because of this omission, the plaintiff suffered a legally recognized harm. This constitutes the causation: the defendant caused the plaintiff's harm. This is established on a balance of probability, i.e. it was more likely that the defendant caused the harm.

Should all three elements be proven, the plaintiff is entitled to monetary compensation. Thirty percent of medical cases are proven in this way – considerably less than the 86% in other negligence cases.

Vicarious liability involves delegation of tasks to juniors by seniors, who must be confident that the juniors are capable of these tasks. Likewise, a junior must actively seek the advice of a senior – and therefore ignorance cannot be used as a defence. It is also important to realize that if you exercise reasonable skill, caution and care in establishing a course of treatment then you cannot be held to be negligent even if the decision was wrong.

The Bolam test is the test used to establish that a professional breaches their duty of care if they fail to achieve the level of competence of their peers. It constitutes practising in accordance with a competent responsible body of opinion. This responsible body of opinion must be judged as sensible, and is established by the court.

MENTAL CAPACITY ACT 2005

This is a framework to protect vulnerable people who are unable to make appropriate decisions for themselves. The act makes clear who can make the decisions, and has five key principles:

- Presumption of capacity assumes capacity unless proved otherwise.
- People have the right to be supported to make their own decisions – all appropriate help must be given before it is assumed that they cannot make decisions.
- People retain the right to make eccentric, unwise decisions.
- Anything done on behalf of people must be in their best interests.
- Anything done without capacity should be least restrictive of rights and freedoms.

30
Communication Skills
CHETAN R TRIVEDY AND ANDREW PARFITT

CORE TOPICS

- The angry patient
- Breaking bad news
- Making a difficult referral
- Dealing with a complaint

Within the acute medical setting, clear and effective communication with patients and colleagues is a fundamental skill for all emergency medicine trainees. Communication skills are therefore tested extensively in Part C of the MCEM and FCEM examinations and it is an area that many candidates find particularly difficult to master. Many try to prepare specifically for the communication skill stations of the OSCE without addressing any shortcomings in their underlying ability to communicate in everyday practice. It is here where the real preparation is. Every candidate will have their own style of communicating with others. Some are natural communicators, others struggle. The important point is that we all have our own style, and it is essential to preserve this in the examination to avoid seeming artificial or false. In this chapter, we will attempt to introduce some key concepts in communication skills and look at some methods that may be incorporated into the everyday practice of these skills. We will also look at some typical communications skills stations that are old favorites in the MCEM and FCEM examinations.

It may seem obvious, but the first and perhaps most important goal in the communication skills test is to completely understand what you are asked to do by the examiners. This corresponds in clinical practice to understanding clearly the issue or problem that requires effective communication as the solution. There is no point in making a cake, however grand it may be, when your examiner – or the patient – has asked for a loaf of bread! Obvious, yes, but many candidates will steer the consultation away from the original problem and consequently fail the station. In this type of test, you will often have the opportunity to study a pie chart indicating the distribution of the marks between practical skills, knowledge and communication skills for that station. As an example, you may be asked to see a 7-year-old asthmatic child who has presented with his mother. Your task may be to demonstrate and explain how to use an inhaler. Most marks will be awarded for the actual communication element of the scenario. Remember also that a significant number of marks will be given to the actor to score you on how well they thought you communicated!

In any communication with patients, it is important to use language that they will understand and to explain medical matters to them in terms that they will be familiar with. You will have been told this many times, but it is a point that is easily forgotten. For example, having patiently explained to a patient that they have fractured their wrist and described in detail what you are going to do about it, you will be familiar with the frequent response 'So it isn't broken then?' The term 'fracture' is meaningless to most people. The examiner will be watching for technical

Scoring Scenario 30.1: The angry patient

	Inadequate/ not done	Adequate	Good
Reads relevant notes to confirm facts	0	1	—
Appropriate introduction	0	1	—
Takes patient to private area to discuss problem	0	1	—
Listens to patient's complaints without interrupting	0	1	2
Apologizes for long wait	0	1	—
Ascertains patient's concerns: • long wait in emergency department • not seen by a doctor • missed meeting • cancellation of skiing trip • litigation against bus company	0	1	2
Offers to examine patient's ankle	0	1	—
Explains to patient why X-ray is not necessary	0	1	—
Explain role of emergency nurse practitioner and their significant experience and skills in managing minor injuries	0	1	—
Suggests an agreed treatment plan: • rest/elevation/analgesia • crutches • GP to review • physiotherapy • letter to travel company	0	1	2
Responds to patient's concerns effectively	0	1	—
Does not appear to collude with emergency nurse practitioner	0	1	—
Does not arrange X-ray to keep patient happy	0	1	—
Remains calm and professional throughout consultation	0	1	2
Avoids use of technical jargon	0	1	—
Effective use of silence as well as verbal and non-verbal communication skills	0	1	2
Ends interview effectively	0	1	—
Score from actor	/5		
Global score from examiner	/5		
Total score	/32		

SCENARIO 30.2 BREAKING BAD NEWS

You are the emergency department registrar and have just attended a trauma call involving a 32-year-old man who was severely injured in a motor vehicle collision. He suffered severe head injuries and arrived in the emergency department in cardiac arrest. After 45 minutes of CPR, the trauma team agreed that further attempts to resuscitate the patient would be futile, and he was pronounced dead.

You have been asked to speak to his wife, who has rushed to the emergency department after learning that her husband has been involved in an accident. You have 7 minutes to break the news.

SUGGESTED APPROACH

This is a difficult scenario that we face all too often in the emergency department, and one that, with a few variations, often crops up in OSCEs. The following is a suggested approach.

First, establish the facts before you speak to the relatives. Make sure that you know the patient's name. Obtain information on the accident and pre-hospital care from the police and ambulance crew. Review the details of resuscitation and the findings of the primary survey. Relatives will often ask for a lot of information – be prepared.

Find an appropriate place to talk to the relatives. The waiting room or the resuscitation bay is inappropriate. Most emergency departments have a dedicated relative's room. Failing that, use any room that is comfortable and where there is adequate privacy and seating facilities. Ask for a member of the nursing staff who was involved in the resuscitation to accompany you. Turn off your pager, as well your mobile. There should be no interruptions.

Introduce yourself and your colleague to the relatives, clearly stating your involvement with the patient. Take care to find out who they are and to establish their relationship to the patient:

'Hello, my name is Dr_____. I am the emergency department registrar looking after Mr_____.' 'Can I ask, you are Mrs_____, his wife?'

After establishing the relationship and identity of the relatives, you can prepare them and yourself for the difficult process of breaking the news.

Ask the relatives to take a seat. If there is just one person on their own, ask if there is anyone else they would like to be present. You can also ask if they would like a glass of water or a cup of tea.

Ask the relatives how much they know about the situation and what they have been told so far. Do not interrupt. Wait until they have finished, and then say:

'I have some very bad news, I am afraid. Mr_____ has died.'

You have to use the words 'died', 'dead' or 'death' explicitly. Avoid terms such as 'passed on', 'gone to heaven' or 'is no longer with us'. These phrases may sound more comforting, but they are not explicit enough. The relative has to get the clear message that their loved one has died.

Once you have imparted the bad news, the best approach is to remain silent and expect anything. Responses may range from anger or hysteria to complete denial, or even silence. Shock is a common response and it essential that you give the relatives time to accept the situation. You may have to repeat the fact that the patient has died. At an appropriate moment, offer your apologies. Be prepared to answer any questions from the relatives, but give only the facts that you have. Do not speculate on a cause of death if it is not clear.

Touch is a contentious issue. Put simply, only consider touching the relatives to show sympathy if this is something you do naturally and with success when dealing with such situations in everyday practice. If you do not use touch normally, do not use it in the OSCE, since it will look forced and make both you and the relative uncomfortable. There are never marks awarded for touching the relative, so not doing so is always safest.

Once the relatives are more collected, you should attempt to engage them. Explain to them in simple terms the circumstances surrounding the admission to hospital and what medical treatment was provided. Occasionally, relatives arrive while CPR is ongoing. It is acceptable for them to be present, especially when children are being resuscitated. A dedicated team member should stand with them and explain what is taking place.

The relatives should be given the opportunity to see the patient, but this should be done once the body has been prepared and cleaned. It is important to pre-warn the relatives that there may be tubes (endotracheal, central lines or cannulae) present and that these may have to remain in case there is a coroner's inquest.

This may also be the opportunity to ask the relatives if they would like a representative from their religious community to be contacted. Most hospitals have dedicated staff available on-call.

You should allow the relatives the opportunity to grieve in private and encourage them to hold the patient's hand if they want to. Do not feel pressurized to give them too much information at this stage. It may be appropriate to leave them and return in half an hour or so and then ask if they are OK or if they have any questions. It is always appropriate to ask if there is anything you can do to help.

It is often surprising how quickly relatives focus on the practical issues now facing them. Common questions include:

- What will happen to the body once it leaves the emergency department?
- When can the funeral be organized?
- How is the paperwork organized?
- Will they be able to visit the deceased?

The relatives should be given the appropriate leaflets on bereavement and also the telephone number of the bereavement office. There are also several national organizations that deal with bereavement counselling, such as Cruse Bereavement Care, which provide free advice and a helpline for those who are bereaved.

It is also vital that you consider and approach the sensitive issue of organ transplantation. This is a difficult area, but, if organ donation is a viable option, it should not be avoided. The issue can be raised by asking the relatives if the deceased carried an organ donor card. The transplant coordinator may also be contacted where organ donation is a possibility.

As with all OSCEs, you should end with a management plan or follow-up. In this case, you should ensure that the relatives have been referred to the bereavement office and that you have answered any relevant questions.

Scoring Scenario 30.2: Breaking bad news

	Inadequate/ not done	Adequate	Good
Read relevant notes to confirm facts	0	1	—
Appropriate introduction and confirmation of relative's identity and relationship to patient	0	1	—
Explains own role in looking after patient	0	1	—
Takes relative to private area to break news. Asks for nurse to be present	0	1	—
Asks relative if she wants anyone to be present	0	1	—
Enquires how much she knows about what ʰ	0	1	—
Explains facts and implicitˡʸ Avoids use of tᵉ	0	1	2
Makes good useᵉ	0	1	—
Checks understaⁿ	0	1	—
Does not give relᵉ	)	1	—
Explores relative's • Can she see thᵉ • coroner's inqueˢ • funeral arrangenᵗ • request for Islamⁱ		1	2
Explains need for post		1	—
Demonstrates good useᵉ		1	2
Demonstrates empathy		1	2
Avoids use of technical jₐ	0	1	—
Raises issue of organ donₐ	0	1	—
Offers details of bereavemeⁿ ᵃⁿᵈ relevant literature	0	1	—
Ends interview effectively	0	1	—
Score from actor		**/5**	
Global score from examiner		**/5**	
Total score		**/32**	

[handwritten note: organ donation / No PCME]

SCENARIO 30.3 THE DIFFICULT REFERRAL

As the emergency department registrar, you are asked to see a 50-year-old roofer who has fallen off some scaffolding. His C-spine is immobilized and plain radiography demonstrates a fracture at C5. Your F2 has unsuccessfully attempted to refer this patient to the orthopaedic registrar on call. You examine the patient and find the patient fully orientated with a GCS of 15 and no neurology apart from tingling in his right hand.

You call the orthopaedic registrar with a view to making a referral. You have 7 minutes to make the referral. You have access to the patient's notes and X-ray for your information.

SUGGESTED APPROACH

Negotiating a referral with a difficult colleague is a common practice in the emergency department. The ability to turn a diagnosis and treatment plan into action often requires specialist input, and it is crucial that the emergency department trainee can make appropriate referrals, even in the face of adversity. Further, the smooth handover of responsibility for patients is essential for safe management across specialties.

There are several factors that may contribute to a difficult referral:

- The referring doctor has insufficient knowledge about the patient to adequately refer.
- The receiving doctor is under pressure themselves and does not want additional work.
- There are personality clashes from either party, which result in 'referral meltdown'.
- The receiving doctor feels that the referral is inappropriate.
- The referring doctor believes that the accepting doctor is being lazy by not wanting to accept the patient.

Ensure that you know the facts before you make the call. This means that you should take a focused history, and at least perform a brief examination yourself. In addition, you should personally review the relevant tests that have been carried out (ECGs, blood results, X-rays and observations). The results should be at hand at the time of the referral. It is important that you explain why you are referring the patient and that the other party understands the need for the referral – you should clarify this to make sure that there is no misunderstanding.

As with all professional communication, a good introduction is a key step in achieving good rapport. The following phrase is a good opener, since it demonstrates that you appreciate that the person may be extremely busy and that you would like some of their time:

'Hello. My name is Dr _____. I am the emergency department registrar. I would like to refer a patient to you. Do you have a moment to discuss?'

In the OSCE, and occasionally in real life, you may get a torrent of abuse about how you or emergency department clinicians are making inappropriate referrals and wasting time. It is imperative that you do not take the bait and become embroiled in a slanging match. In real life, this will certainly result in referral meltdown; in the OSCE, it will not look good on your global score. Retaliation to aggression from a colleague is not an option, and you should ride out the storm. Once you have an appropriate platform, you should defuse the situation by the use of one of the following phrases:

'I am sorry you feel that way, but I feel that this patient needs admission because ...'

'I understand that you are really busy, but I have seen this patient and I think that they need to be seen because ...'

'I am quite concerned about this patient and really value your opinion because ...'

You should not agree to any management plan that you think might compromise patient safety, or back out of a referral because of friction. If you cannot refer, you should at least insist that the patient be reviewed by the specialist team for an opinion.

Another strategy to use when making a difficult referral is to compromise or negotiate an agreed treatment plan, provided that this does not compromise patient safety. In this scenario, for example, it may involve the emergency department registrar organizing a CT scan of the neck prior to the requested orthopaedic opinion. Admitting the patient to a clinical observation unit or sending them to the orthopaedic ward without being seen is not a safe outcome of compromise. In the OSCE, the actor playing the difficult colleague will propose numerous inappropriate, and some unsafe, management options, and may even try to bully you into accepting one of them. The examiners are looking for you to put the patient's safety first in any agreed plan that you do make with the difficult colleague.

If you continue to meet with implacable obstruction and things are getting heated then you can acknowledge this and suggest ways out for both of you. For example:

'I feel that we are not getting anywhere. Maybe we should both think about the situation, and can I call you back in five minutes. Is that OK?'

'I feel that we are not getting anywhere and that I do have concerns about this patient. I think I will have to discuss this with my consultant. Is that OK?'

Whatever the outcome, remember to remain courteous and polite at all times

Ultimately, you will have to talk to your consultant if an appropriate management plan cannot be negotiated. It is important to realize that asking for senior help is not a sign of failure or 'snitching'. Often, a fresh approach is required once you have exhausted your diplomatic attempts to refer a patient. It is important that you carefully document the outcome of your discussion. It is possible that your consultant may not even be on site, and so they will be relying not only on your history and examination, but also on your synopsis of the discussion that you have had with the orthopaedic registrar. It is vital that you record the salient points of your discussion accurately.

Once the patient has been referred, it is useful to make a transcript of the referral in your notes, or at least document the time of referral, the accepting doctor's details and contact number, as well the agreed outcome.

Scoring Scenario 30.3: The difficult referral

	Inadequate/ not done	Adequate	Good
Reads patient's notes and states intention to review patient (does not actually have to do so). Looks at X-ray and confirms fracture	0	1	2
Appropriate introduction, stating his/her role and ascertaining name, grade and bleep number of orthopaedic registrar	0	1	2
Asks if it is a good time to discuss patient	0	1	—
Gives details of referral: • significant mechanism of injury • fracture at C5 on plain film • neurology (tingling in fingers)	0	1	2
Listens to orthopaedic registrar: • Avoids interrupting or talking over colleague • Refrains from entering into an argument • Remains calm and professional at all times	0	1	2
Explores and deals with orthopaedic registrar's concerns: • F2 who referred earlier not knowledgeable about facts • Short-staffed and under pressure • Previous poor referrals from emergency department • About to start a case in theatre	0	1	2
Does not give into unsafe management options: • Review on fracture clinic tomorrow • Refer to neurologists for opinion • Admit to clinical decision unit under emergency department	0	1	2
Politely but firmly insists that patient is reviewed by orthopaedic registrar	0	1	—
Checks understanding on need for referral	0	1	—
Agrees on safe plan of action: • Emergency department to organize further imaging (CT) • Patient to be reviewed by orthopaedic registrar after emergency case	0	1	—
Remains calm and professional at all times	0	1	2
Deals with aggression and is non-judgemental	0	1	—
Avoids blaming F2 or criticizing registrar for their behaviour	0	1	—
Agrees time for further discussion to ensure resolution to conflict	0	1	—
Clearly documents conversation, with times and outcome	0	1	—
Effective use of silence as well as verbal and non-verbal communication skills	0	1	2
Ends interview effectively and suggests consultant input if there is no resolution	0	1	—
Score from actor	/5		
Global score from examiner	/5		
Total score	/35		

SCENARIO 30.4 DEALING WITH A COMPLAINT

A 60-year-old woman presented with a 1-week history of dysuria and increased urinary frequency. She was diagnosed with a urinary tract infection (UTI). Despite having a documented allergy to penicillin, she was prescribed a course of co-amoxiclav. The pharmacist picked up the potential drug error and another doctor prescribed the patient an alternative antibiotic. The patient has returned from the pharmacy and is unhappy with her treatment. She has spoken to the nurse in charge of the department and is planning to write to the chief executive about the incompetence of the junior doctor as well as his manner and lack of professionalism.

You have 7 minutes to discuss her concerns.

SUGGESTED APPROACH

As an emergency department trainee, you will be expected to deal with complaints made against your junior colleagues and take the appropriate action. The Citizens Charter Complaints Taskforce defined a complaint as 'an expression of dissatisfaction requiring a response'. Dealing with complaints requires tact, diplomacy and, above all, integrity and transparency. It is important not only to resolve the complaint, but also to look critically at how such complaints can be prevented in the future. All complaints from patients should be taken seriously, since there is still a public perception that doctors work in collusion and that complaints are never dealt with. Furthermore, it is important not alienate or negate the member of staff against whom the complaint was made. Most emergency department have complaints procedures in place, and it is advisable that you familiarize yourself with the policies of your department to use both in practice and as an example for examination purposes.

The patient in this case has raised an important concern about a drug error that could have had serious implications for her. She has also raised concerns regarding the junior doctor's manner and level of professionalism, which should also be addressed. We recommend the following approach when dealing with this particular complaint.

Start with the patient. As with all of the communication skill stations, you should find an appropriate room where you are not likely to be disturbed. Turn off your bleep and telephone and introduce yourself to the patient, stating your name and position. Explain that you are the most senior person in the department at night and that you consider it important to hear what she has to say.

You can start off with a statement such as:

> 'I'm sorry that you feel that you have not had good treatment in our department. Can you tell me more about what you are worried about so that we can do something about it.'

You are not apologizing for what happened, but are sorry that the patient has not been satisfied with her treatment.

You should allow the patient the opportunity to speak without interruption. Many patients who make a complaint want to be heard, and listening to their concerns goes a long way in resolving the complaint in the emergency department and preventing it going further. You should ask the patient to give specific examples of behaviour from the doctor that she felt was unprofessional or rude. With regard to the drug error, assure her that this is a serious concern and will not be ignored. Describe the procedures that you will undertake to flag this up – filling out an incident form and alerting the consultant of the error – and explain that, where necessary, a review of policy will result.

Once you have heard the patient's side of things, you need to gain further information from the junior doctor, the emergency department record and other staff who may have been involved. Use this to respond to questions that the patient may have about her treatment, but not to judge whether mismanagement has occurred or to make what might be taken as a formal response to the complaint yourself.

If the patient indicates that she wishes to make a written complaint, do not try to dissuade her from doing so. Instead, outline the procedure for written complaints and to whom she must write – give her details of the trust's Patient Advice and Liaison Services (PALS). Assure her that all complaints are taken seriously and let her know how long after her compliant she can expect to receive a response from the Trust.

Finally, it is likely that the patient will not have confidence in her diagnosis and treatment so far. Review with her the history and offer to re-examine her to ensure that a UTI is the correct diagnosis. Arrange follow-up. Ensure detailed documentation in the notes.

Scoring Scenario 30.4: Dealing with a complaint

	Inadequate/ not done	Adequate	Good
Reviews relevant notes to confirm facts	0	1	—
Takes patient to private area to discuss complaint	0	1	—
Listens to patient's complaints without interrupting	0	1	2
Apologizes for error and checks that patient has correct medications	0	1	—
Ascertains and addresses patient's concerns: • drug error • rude/unprofessional junior doctor • death of husband in emergency department after missed aneurysm • concerns over hospital cover-up • wish to make formal complaint	0	1	2
Agrees to speak to junior doctor regarding patient's concerns	0	1	—
Gives patient details of the PALS and offers information on departmental complaints procedure	0	1	—
Avoids blaming or colluding with junior doctor	0	1	—
Suggests filling an adverse incident form and looking at departmental drug policies	0	1	—
Remains calm and professional throughout consultation	0	1	2
Demonstrates empathy	0	1	—
Avoids use of technical jargon	0	1	—
Effective use of silence as well as verbal and non-verbal communication skills	0	1	2
Ends interview effectively	0	1	—
Score from actor	/5		
Global score from examiner	/5		
Total score	/28		

31
Practical Skills for the Emergency Department
NATALIE S SHENKER AND CHETAN R TRIVEDY

Procedures form an important part of emergency medicine practice and are often tested in the MCEM and FCEM OSCEs. Some procedures that we must be able to perform are rarely encountered in working practice but are lifesaving when applied, such as pericardiocentesis. Others are the 'bread and butter' of the daily job, such as male urethral catheterization. Regardless, the examiners want to see that you know how to perform the procedure safely with an accepted methodology. This chapter suggests approaches to those procedures most commonly examined in the OSCE stations. It is not an exhaustive list, and you are referred to the CEM curriculum for detail of all the procedures you are required to know. Many commonly performed procedures, for example applying a backslab plaster of Paris or application of a splint, are much more readily learned from an experienced plaster technician or nurse in the emergency department, and written instructions, being of limited value, are not included here. Other procedures, such as procedural sedation, vary considerably between departments and practitioners alike, and we recommend that you consult local policy as an example of good practice to use if asked in an examination.

When encountering an OSCE scenario requiring demonstration of a practical skill, it would be a mistake, however, to focus solely on the procedure itself. You must also know and be able to describe to the examiner the following in relation to any procedure that you might perform:

- indications
- contraindications (absolute and relative)
- complications (early and late) and how to deal with them

To avoid repetition, there is a generic approach to practical procedures that should be followed in clinical practice as well as in examination situations:

1. Review the need for the procedure with the patient and how it will benefit them.
2. Ask about and minimize the influence of anything that would increase the risk of the procedure (e.g. warfarin therapy). Check for any absolute contraindication.
3. Describe the procedure and what the patient can expect to feel. Answer any questions as appropriate.
4. Obtain consent (verbal or written). This requires openly discussing the complications that the patient needs to know about.
5. Before you begin, ensure that all equipment is to hand and that you have any assistance you require.
6. Wash your hands.
7. Set up a sterile field where you can work.
8. Put on sterile gloves for all procedures – surgical gowns for the more invasive procedures.
9. Prepare the patient with drapes and clean the skin with saline or antiseptic (povidone–iodine or chlorhexidine).

The needle should be angled to 'hit' the clavicle. It can then be worked downwards to enter the vessel. This minimizes the risk of a pneumothorax and injury to the subclavian artery, which also lies posteriorly to the vein.

The central line is placed using the Seldinger technique as described above. The line should be inserted to 17 cm on the right and 19 cm on the left, but its position should always be checked with radiography before use to minimize the risk of arrhythmias.

Complications

- Haemorrhage int
- Misplacement
- Air embolus
- Arrhythmia
- Carotid artery (
- Pneumothorax
- Late complica   , followed by sepsis), erosion of the
  containing ve

IJ- blk 2
heads sterno
-clomastoid
Muscle △

Useful resour

McGee DC, Gould   ral venous catheterization. *N Engl J Med* 2003; **348**: 112

National Instit   *e of Ultrasound Locating Devices for Placing Central Venous Catheters (.lable at: http://guidance.nice.org.uk/TA49.*

SCENARIO 31.6: ARTERIAL LINE PLACEMENT

Indications

- Invasive monitoring of arterial blood pressure
- Frequent arterial blood sampling

Equipment

- Local anaesthetic (1% lidocaine)
- Arterial cannulae
- Heparinized syringe
- Three-way tap with extension, flushed
- Gauze and adhesive clear bandage
- Flushed infusion set, attached to pressure transducer and monitor

Procedure

Usually the left radial artery is used at the wrist.

Check for collateral circulation by occluding both the radial and ulnar arteries and ask the patient to repeatedly clench their fist. With the palm open and pale, release pressure on the ulnar. In the presence of good collateral flow, the palm should become pink (Allen's test).

Avoid areas of infection and skin damage. Other potential sites include the brachial, posterior tibial, dorsalis pedis, ulnar and femoral arteries.

Extend the patient's wrist. This can be done in an obtunded patient with an assistant holding the hand or, if you are alone, by using a sandbag beneath the wrist, with tape attaching the patient's thumb to the bed.

Prep the skin and infiltrate over the artery with local anaesthetic.

Insert the arterial cannula attached to a syringe at a 30–45° angle over the artery. Advance slowly – the artery is often more peripheral than you think.

Once the cannula is inside the artery, blood will pulsate into the syringe. Holding the needle steady at this point, advance the cannula over the needle into the artery.

Remove the needle and prevent blood flowing freely by compressing the artery proximally. Connect the three-way tap or T-connector, ensuring that these are flushed in advance with 0.9% saline.

Secure the cannula with tape or sutures (tape is usually adequate) and cover with a transparent dressing.

Connect the infusion set and calibrate the monitoring system before use.

Complications

- Arteriospasm
- Haematoma
- Bacterial colonization and sepsis
- Damage to surrounding structures (e.g. the radial nerve)
- Pseudoaneurysm

Useful resource

Tegtmeyer K, Brady G, Lai S et al. Videos in Clinical Medicine: Placement of an arterial line. *N Engl J Med* 2006; **354**: e13.

SCENARIO 31.7: INTRAOSSEOUS CANNULATION

Indications

- Where urgent venous access is required in children and three attempts at venous cannulation have failed
- Paediatric cardiac arrest

Equipment

- Cleaning solution
- Intraosseous needle
- Syringe and flush
- 0.9% saline infusion set

Procedure

Explain to the parent(s) why such an apparently brutal procedure is required, stressing the importance and necessity of timely access in this emergency.

Position the child's leg slightly flexed at the knee. The landmarks are the anteromedial surface of the tibia 2–3 cm below the tibial tuberosity (other locations are possible, but this is the most accessible). Avoid the site of any lower limb trauma.

Clean the site with antiseptic. Draping is not required.

Insert the intraosseous needle at 90° to the skin and advance by twisting it into the cortex until there is a give. The inner needle is removed and the cannula first aspirated for blood samples and then flushed with saline.

It is important to remember that you may not be able to aspirate blood from the marrow space, but, if you can, remember that the same range of tests can be performed on blood aspirated from the marrow space as on venous blood. You should, however, inform the laboratory if you send any marrow blood for analysis.

Any medications or fluid infusions should be given by hand or run via a syringe driver to overcome the resistance of the bone marrow.

Complications

- Fracture of the bone
- Misplacement and extravasation of infusion fluid into soft tissue
- Late complication: osteomyelitis

SCENARIO 31.8: INSERTION OF A MALE URETHRAL CATHETER

Indications

- Relief of urinary obstruction, either acute or chronic
- Monitoring of urine output in a shocked patient
- Part of general care in an obtunded patient

Equipment

- Sterile gloves
- Topical analgesic gel (e.g. Instillagel)
- Catheter pack with sterile drape and forc...
- Urethral catheter, usually Foley; size 12– ... be used for bladder irrigation in retention caused by ...
- Bladder bag, ideally with hourly volume m...

Procedure

Inform the patient what you are going to do an...

Always check for blood at the meatus in a traum... ...xclude urethral injury before passing a catheter.

Put on two pairs of sterile gloves. Use your left h... ...right hand sterile to handle the catheter.

Using the left hand, elevate the penis and clean and retract the foreskin using gauze soaked in sterile skin prep.

Place the sterile drape, and then remove the first pair of gloves.

Using the same technique, infiltrate topical analgesic gel (e.g. Instillagel) into the meatus. In a conscious patient, allow at least 2 minutes for this to work. It also provides vital lubrication.

Pass the catheter, initially with the penis held upright; then, to help passage through the narrow prostatic urethra, point the penis towards the feet of the patient. If you encounter difficulty, try a larger catheter (which, because it is stiffer, may more easily negotiate the bends in the urethra where a smaller catheter would simply coil up, particularly when passing through the prostate).

Pass the catheter to the hilt and wait for urine to appear. Attach the urine bag. Inflate the balloon, watching the patient's face for discomfort in case the tip is still in the urethra.

Pull back the catheter and replace the foreskin.

Measure the residual volume in the catheter bag after half an hour if the catheter has been placed for retention.

Complications

- Trauma through creation of a false passage
- Failure of the procedure (e.g. due to prostatic obstruction of the urethra)
- Post-obstruction diuresis – the catheter may need to be clamped to slow this

SCENARIO 31.9: INSERTION OF A SUPRAPUBIC CATHETER

Indication

- Where bladder catheterization is required but it is impossible or unsafe to pass a urethral catheter

Equipment

- Skin preparation
- Local anaesthetic
- Suprapubic catheter pack, including sterile drape, filled 10 mL syringe, gauze, trocar and sheath
- Suprapubic catheter

Procedure

Lay the patient supine.

Palpate and percuss the lower abdomen to assess bladder size. This can also be determined by bladder ultrasound. Identify the point of catheter insertion as roughly three fingerbreadths above the pubic symphysis in the midline.

Prep the lower abdomen and apply sterile drapes.

Infiltrate local anaesthetic into the skin and underlying tissues. Often, as you infiltrate deeper, urine is aspirated.

Nick the skin at this point with a scalpel blade.

Push the trocar and sheath gently through the tissues, using a straight, down-pointing index finger to prevent injury when the bladder is breached.

At this point, a rush of urine occurs. Remove the trocar, pass the catheter through the sheath and either inflate the balloon or remove the catheter stylet, which allows some suprapubic catheters to curl within the bladder as an alternative to a balloon for anchorage.

Attach the catheter to a urine bag.

Remove the sheath and apply a dressing.

Measure the residual volume of urine after half an hour if the catheter has been placed for urinary retention.

Complications

- Bowel perforation where bowel was present between the bladder and abdominal wall
- Bleeding, although this is usually insignificant
- Infection

SCENARIO 31.10: NEEDLE CRICOTHYROIDOTOMY

Indications

- If a patent airway cannot be achieved by other means
- In an emergency, as a last resort
- Needle cricothyroidotomy is preferred in children under the age of 12 years
- Surgical cricothyroidotomy (Scenario 31.11) allows better protection of the airway for adults and children over 12

Equipment

- Antiseptic swabs
- Cricothyroidotomy needle (or, if this is not available, a large-bore intravenous cannula) attached to a 5 mL syringe containing a little water
- Oxygen delivery tubing and Y-connector

Procedure

Position the patient lying supine with neck extended (unless there is significant concern about a C-spine injury).

Locate the cricothyroid ligament between the prominent thyroid cartilage and the cricoid cartilage below it.

Clean the neck quickly with antiseptic swabs.

Stabilize the cricothyroid membrane between the fingers and thumb and insert the needle and cannula through the cricothyroid membrane at a 45° angle into the trachea. Gradually aspirate the attached syringe constantly during insertion.

When air is aspirated, advance the cannula over the needle.

Withdraw the needle and recheck that air can be aspirated through the cannula.

Attach the oxygen delivery tubing to the Y-connector and the cannula, and set the flow rate to the rate in litres per minute equivalent to the child's age.

Occlude the Y-connector with your thumb to inflate the child's lungs and allow passive exhalation for 4 seconds by removing your thumb. If the chest does not rise, check the cannula position and do not inflate for longer than 1 second.

Auscultate to check for bilateral breath sounds.

Examine the neck to check for crepitus in case the cannula has become dislodged into the soft tissues.

Secure the cannula.

Arrange for an urgent definitive airway such as a tracheostomy. Needle cricothyroidotomy can only maintain oxygenation for 20–40 minutes at best.

Complications

- Failure of the procedure and death
- Pneumomediastinum and surgical emphysema from tracheal trauma
- Haemorrhage: venous and arterial
- Aspiration of blood or secretions
- Pulmonary barotrauma

SCENARIO 31.11: SURGICAL CRICOTHYROIDOTOMY

Indications

- As for needle cricothyroidotomy, but oxygenation can be maintained for longer
- Only suitable for adults and for children older than 12 years

Equipment

- Skin preparation
- Scalpel and blade
- Tracheal spreader
- Range of endotracheal tubes or a tracheostomy tube
- Oxygen delivery set
- Suture set and appropriate non-absorbable suture
- Gauze bandage

Procedure

Prepare the patient and locate the cricothyroid membrane as for a needle cricothyroidotomy.

Holding the trachea stable between the fingers of your left hand, make a 2–3 cm transverse incision over the cricothyroid cartilage in the midline.

Incise carefully downwards until the cricothyroid membrane itself is divided.

Insert the tracheal spreader. If one is not available then place the handle of the scalpel into the hole and rotate it sideways to enlarge the hole.

Insert the largest-diameter endotracheal or tracheostomy tube possible through the incision.

Connect the oxygen delivery set and ventilate the patient.

Suture the skin around the tube on either side to ensure that the tube is secured and apply a gauze bandage.

Complications

- As for needle cricothyroidotomy, although the risk of causing bleeding is much greater

Useful resource

Henderson JJ, Popat MT, Latto IP, Pearce AC. Difficult Airway Society guidelines for management of the unanticipated difficult intubation. *Anaesthesia*. 2004; **59**: 675–94.

SCENARIO 31.12: LUMBAR PUNCTURE

Indications

- Suspected subarachnoid haemorrhage (remember, however, that xanthochromia is present only after 12 hours following the bleed)
- Suspected central nervous system infection
- Other, non-acute, indications: diagnosis of demyelination or benign intracranial hypertension

Equipment

- Skin preparation
- Sterile drapes, gown, gloves
- Local anaesthetic
- Lumbar puncture needles
- Manometer
- Three specimen-collecting pots
- Adhesive bandage

Procedure

Perform fundoscopy, looking for papilloedema, or review any prior CT scans to ensure that there is no possibility of raised intracranial pressure before lumbar puncture. Where there is any doubt, the procedure should not be performed.

Explain to the patient what you are about to do and why.

Position the patient on their left side, rolled in a ball such that their knees are tucked into their chest as far as possible. This opens up the intervertebral spaces.

Identify and mark the entry site. This is typically at L3–L4, below the termination of the spinal cord at L1. The L4 intervertebral space is always located at the level of a line drawn between the two iliac crests.

Ensuring sterile technique, prepare the overlying skin and apply drapes. Ensure that you are comfortable by using a chair next to the bed.

Infiltrate 1% lidocaine into the overlying skin and paravertebral muscles.

Insert a spinal needle, aiming approximately towards the umbilicus. Slowly advance the needle into the intervertebral space. A distinct 'pop' is felt as you breach the tough ligamentum flavum between the vertebral lamina. A further 'give' is felt as you enter the spinal canal by passing through the dura and arachnoid meninges.

The stylet should then be withdrawn, and, after a moment, cerebrospinal fluid (CSF) should drip from the end of the spinal needle. The colour and turbidity of the fluid should be noted. First attach the manometer and measure the opening pressure (typically 10–15 mmHg).

CSF can then be dripped into three separate specimen pots, and sent for culture, microscopy, cytology, and protein and glucose analysis, depending on the indication.

At the end of the procedure, withdraw the needle and apply an adhesive bandage.

Some recommend that the patient lie flat for 1 hour to minimize post-lumbar-puncture headache.

Complications

- Post-lumbar-puncture headache – very common
- 'Coning', i.e. herniation of the brainstem through the foramen magnum due to raised intracranial pressure
- Introduction of infection

SCENARIO 31.13: REDUCTION OF A COLLES' FRACTURE WITH HAEMATOMA BLOCK

Indication

- Colles' fracture requiring manipulation

Equipment

- Analgesia as appropriate (intravenous morphine or midazolam; nitrous oxide)
- Syringe, needle and local anaesthetic (1% lidocaine or bupivacaine) for haematoma block
- An assistant to apply counter-traction
- Plaster trolley

Procedure

Clean the skin overlying the fracture site on the dorsum of the arm.

Infiltrate local anaesthetic into the skin 1–2 cm proximal to the wrist joint. Infiltrate deeper, aiming towards the fracture deformity while aspirating until a small flashback of blood into the barrel of the needle indicates that the fracture haematoma has been reached. Infiltrate 10 mL of 1% lidocaine into the haematoma.

Allow 5 minutes for the anaesthetic to become effective. Use this time to prepare the plastercast material.

An assistant applies counter-traction by grasping the arm above a flexed elbow.

Apply traction by positioning your thumbs over the distal fracture fragment of the radius, encircling the wrist with your fingers.

First apply traction until spasm of the surrounding muscle relaxes, and then push the fragment ventrally and to the ulnar side. This aims to reverse the mechanism of injury.

Still applying traction, position the wrist in ulnar deviation with slight palmar flexion and ask the assistant to apply the plaster backslab. Maintain the wrist in the correct position until the cast is solid.

In the case of a Colles' fracture, the cast should not interfere with elbow or metacarpophalangeal flexion.

Arrange for another set of anteroposterior and lateral X-rays to assess the reduction.

Complications

- Inadequate reduction – may need to be done under general anaesthesia
- Slippage of the bone fragments due to inadequate immobilization
- Theoretically, there is a danger of introducing infection into the fracture site with the haematoma block, but this is extremely rare in practice

SAMPLE SCORE SHEET FOR PRACTICAL SKILLS

Scoring Scenario 11.2: Chest drain insertion

[Handwritten note overlaying table: "Chest drain 2cm – over inferior rib to avoid NV bundle."]

	Inadequate/ not done	Adequate	Good
Explains need for procedure	0	1	—
Appropriate	0	1	—
Asks about	0	1	—
Selects app	0	1	—
Identifies c	0	1	—
Gives appro	0	1	—
Adopts appr	0	1	—
Inserts drain safely	0	1	2
Makes 2–3 c			
Blunt dissec			
Inserts drain without trocar			
Connects tubing to underwater seal			
Is able to describe suture placement	0	1	—
Bandages drain appropriately	0	1	—
Checks drain for bubbling and fluid. Is aware of guidelines for management of massive haemothorax	0	1	—
Asks for post-insertion chest X-ray	0	1	—
Arranges appropriate referral	0	1	—
Documents procedure accurately in notes	0	1	—
Conducts procedure in a fluent and logical manner. Talks to patient and reassures them throughout procedure	0	1	—
Can list major complications of procedure	0	1	2
Score from patient/role player	/5		
Global score from examiner	/5		
Total score	/28		

32
Management Skills
DAVID ROE

SCOPE OF THIS CHAPTER

At present, the management elements of the FCEM curriculum are assessed only through the viva examination. This chapter explores some of the material required for the management viva and suggests approaches to the kind of scenario that may be encountered in the form of either an 'in-tray' exercise or a long-case 'management scenario'. A number of examples are given, grouped according to in-tray priority. The differentiation into in-tray and long-case is somewhat artificial, since the examples are equally applicable to the long-case element. The latter part of this chapter contains a variety of useful information about some aspects of management, and some further examples are embedded in the text to illustrate these.

Both the FCEM examination and the underlying curriculum continue to be developed and refined, and the most current information on the curriculum, the structure of the examination and marking schemes is always available online via the College of Emergency Medicine gateway at www.collemergencymed.ac.uk or at the emergency medicine Trainees Association (EMTA) micro-site. At the time of writing, one of the interactive in-tray exercises, with accompanying long case from a previous examination diet and suggestions for answers and scoring, is available for download, and a generic marking scheme is also highlighted within the examination regulations.

THE MANAGEMENT VIVA

Familiarize yourself with the latest information from the CEM about structure and marking. For recent diets of the examination, there has been fairly equal weighting across questions, but this may not always be the case. The viva currently consists of a 15-minute interactive in-tray exercise followed by a 15-minute management scenario ('long case'). The long case is merely an extension of the in-tray, with an opportunity to explore a scenario or particular issues in more depth. The domains of assessment include a selection from the following areas:

- analytical skills
- prioritization
- time management
- clinical governance
- medicolegal awareness
- human resources issues
- communication skills
- handling the media
- lateral thinking

- team building
- education
- medical ethics

STRATEGIES FOR SUCCESS AT THE IN-TRAY EXERCISE

TIME MANAGEMENT

You must look at all of the in-tray material that you are given, so use your 5 minutes' reading time to consider *everything*. You cannot score well if you miss material out, particularly where the neglected material is the most important. As a consultant, you have a secretary: use this resource.

MANAGE YOUR DIARY FOR THE DAY

Time management includes your management of the 'schedule' in the diary that you are given as part of the exercise. Below are some examples of how you might manage your schedule for the day:

- Departmental and patient safety comes first, so serious clinical or immediate staffing matters need your attention.
- A registrar can probably do your review clinic if there is an over-riding need for you to do something else.
- Look for links to your diary. If your diary has teaching in the afternoon and you have a critical incident in the pile then link these via immediate feedback. The same is true if there is a governance meeting in your diary and a governance issue in the pile
- Meetings can be rescheduled if risk/benefits dictate. If the Chief Executive wants to see you now, acknowledge the importance of that, but not above clinical need – use your secretary.

PRIORITIZATION

Try to prioritize the in-tray material that you are given – for example priority 1, 2 and 3 or today/tomorrow/never. There may be a couple of priority 1 things, so look for these. Be aware of what you can delegate, and use other departments within the Trust, as you cannot/should not do everything yourself.

Priority 1

These include:

- staffing for today (departmental safety)
- under-performing doctors: for example, the sister from nights is waiting to speak to you because the night doctor could not cope, made poor decisions, could not read an ECG, etc.
- personal behaviour issues: for example intoxication or sexual advances to a staff member
- adverse clinical events
- alerts from the National Patient Safety Agency that relate to your equipment: for example, the pregnancy testing kits or ventilators that you use are faulty
- threats to your service: for example, some of your observation beds are going to be used for day surgery to meet surgical waiting targets, or the fracture clinic is going to expand into minors
- theft of controlled drugs

Priority 2

This is a somewhat indeterminate group, generally being defined as neither priority 1 nor priority 3:

- complaint letters – *but make sure that they do not contain a priority 1 issue*. The Trust has 25 working days to respond, so you have some latitude with time
- letters from patients – *but make sure that they do not contain a priority 1 issue*

Priority 3

These include:

- flyers for courses and meetings
- requests to see drug company representatives
- leaflets promoting new equipment

USE OF OTHER PROFESSIONAL GROUPS AND DELEGATION

Delegation is necessary, since you are a finite resource, and other groups may have more appropriate skills. Many candidates in mock examinations approach the management viva from a theoretical perspective that reflects the difficulties of getting management experience within their training scheme. A reflection of this is the candidate who tries earnestly to sort out all difficulties personally, rather than either delegating or using the resources that the Trust makes available.

If the issue is primarily a nursing issue then liaise with your directorate nurse manager.

If the issue is a Human Resources (HR) issue then involve the HR team.

If you have a review clinic but there are urgent issues to address then delegate the clinic to a middle-grade colleague.

Poorly performing trainees require local support through their educational supervisor, Director of Medical Education (DME) and Clinical Tutors, with Deanery involvement if the problem is more serious.

Poorly performing career-grade doctors need local support through mentoring. Involve the Clinical Director and/or the Medical Director. Persistent failure should involve the National Clinical Assessment Service (NCAS).

PRIORITY 1 SCENARIOS

SCENARIO 32.1: THE UNDER-PERFORMING DOCTOR

The sister from nights is waiting to meet you at 8.30 a.m. The doctor who just started nights has been a challenge for the whole team. He was very slow and struggled to make decisions. He did not recognize an ST-elevation myocardial infarction (STEMI) on ECG but referred to the medical team, who recognized and treated it.

SUGGESTED APPROACH

First thoughts

This is clearly important. The night sister's comments are likely to be fair and accurate. It would be unsafe to let this continue without decisive action being taken.

FACT FIND

Get all the details from the night team to corroborate the night sister's report. Pull the emergency department records of all the patients seen that night. Look in detail at the missed STEMI and get feedback from the admitting team. Look for errors in other patients.

Enlist the help of a couple of senior colleagues and act on what is found.

Contact HR. Ask them to look at the references. Have any previous problems been identified?

You need to interview the doctor concerned – ideally straight away if he has not gone home yet. If he has left and does not live on site then it is probably better to telephone in the afternoon for an interview that afternoon.

Do not interview alone, since complaints of bullying or harassment may result. Have a senior colleague, an educational supervisor or an HR representative present. *Keep detailed records.*

If the evidence supports a case of serious underperformance then you must protect the department and patient safety:

- Take the doctor concerned off nights.
- Ensure that the nights are covered with an appropriate person. Swap shifts or arrange a locum.
- Report the clinical incident.

Educational/regulator response

This depends on the severity of the issues, but the following are some possible strategies:

- Allow the doctor concerned to do supervised daytime work with supporting CEX/DOP/CBD evidence
- Involve the Educational Supervisor for mentoring.
- Involve the DME and/or Clinical Tutor for doctors in training posts, and probably for non-training SHO equivalents.
- Inform the Deanery if a trainee is in difficulty.

If local remedial action is not effective then the NCAS can be approached – through the Deanery for trainees and through the Medical Director for other grades.

SCENARIO 32.2: ADVERSE CLINICAL EVENT

You have received a telephone call from a consultant in the paediatric intensive care unit (PICU) at your regional centre. A child was transferred from your Trust last night after treatment for status epilepticus. The child was accidentally given a large overdose of lorazepam on two occasions by your team. The child is now doing well, and the parents have been informed of the error by the PICU consultant.

SUGGESTED APPROACH

First thoughts

This is a significant error. You need to find out urgently how this came to happen, and make sure that there can be no repetition of it. You are going to need to involve stakeholders such as the paediatric department and PICU, and communicate with the family. There are reporting matters to be addressed.

Fact find

Get the notes. Speak to the doctors and nurses involved. Written statements will be needed at some point, but you need to rapidly identify the personal or system error that allowed this to happen.

Initial findings

The doctors concerned are a CT1 in emergency medicine, an emergency medicine staff grade and a general emergency medicine nurse. The staff grade ordered the drugs, but the CT1 colleague worked out the dose from a list of emergency drug doses that had been written with a marker pen on a white board in the paediatric resuscitation area. Unfortunately, the lorazepam dose was transcribed wrongly on the board, which led to the drug calculation error. The doctor felt under pressure to act quickly, and but did not confirm it with an authoritative source. The generally trained nurse was not aware that the dose was too high.

You must act to protect the department and its patients:

- The white board is not an authoritative source – it can be altered, and this has led to the error. Remove it – immediately.
- Ensure that colleagues have access to emergency protocols (APLS etc.), and that these are accurate and authoritative.
- Is prescribing for children immediately available?
- Does the Trust have guidance documentation for the management of children? Is this available?

Do you have the right skills mix?

- A nurse with paediatric training or skills should be available for sick children in the emergency department.
- Do all your senior colleagues have an appropriate minimum standard of competence for seeing sick children (e.g. APLS)?
- Was a member of the paediatric team involved? They should have been.

Reporting and clinical governance issues

- Reporting is mandatory (IR1).
- Ensure that there is a formal critical incident review.
- Do you have a critical event forum in the emergency department to allow feedback and implement change?
- New doctor induction – they cannot be provided with teaching on everything that they need to know at the start of the job, but they can be told where to get help and what information sources to use.

Communication

Keep the paediatric department apprised of your investigation and action. They will be supportive with necessary system changes.

It would be a courtesy to inform the reporting PICU consultant.

Make yourself available to speak to the family as soon as possible. Keep records of telephone discussions, provide a follow-up letter and offer to meet with them personally.

Inform the Trust's complaints department. Any meeting with the family needs a representative present to keep records.

You may choose to inform the Medical Director about the event and your actions. There is often a Trust-level committee to look at errors, and the Medical Director is often the executive representative.

Clinical performance

This is a system error, not one of a failing trainee, but be aware of the ways of addressing the failing trainee.

SCENARIO 32.3: ISSUES WITH PERSONAL BEHAVIOUR

The matron has left a confidential note with your secretary. One of her staff nurses has complained that one of your juniors made an unwanted sexual advance during the night shift. This allegedly took the form of grabbing her bottom and making sexually suggestive comments when she was alone with him in the one of the equipment store rooms. The staff nurse is in tears in the matron's office and is formulating a statement.

SUGGESTED APPROACH

Fact find

The nurse appears to be going on record by formulating a statement.

Is there corroborating or supporting testimony from other staff on the shift? This needs to be approached with some sensitivity, to avoid undermining either party.

You will need to interview the doctor and get his statement – today. Do not interview him on your own. Ideally, have an HR manager present.

Service

The doctor concerned is on nights. Whether he is guilty or not, his effectiveness may be compromised. Consider taking him off service and getting locum cover.

The nurse's shifts are a matter for the nurse manager, although it would be sensible for her to do the same. Avoid making one party look guilty until the facts are known.

Stakeholders

Human Resources

This is an HR issue, and so an HR manager must be involved. They should sit in on any interview.

Does either party have 'form', i.e. evidence of previous behaviour issues in this or previous employment. HR are well placed to investigate this.

Deanery and their representatives

Is the doctor a trainee? If so, notify the DME and/or Clinical Tutor. If there is clear evidence of wrongdoing then this will escalate to the Deanery.

Senior management

Notifying the Medical Director is a judgement call, but it is probably a courtesy, and is required if there is supporting evidence.

Disciplinary actions if there is evidence of wrongdoing

There will be a local framework to be followed. The action is unlikely to be less than a final written warning, to be kept on file.

The nurse may choose to involve the police, who will investigate separately.

Deanery escalation is required.

With regard to referral to the General Medical Council (GMC), they can give telephone advice.

DEALING WITH DEPARTMENTAL THREATS

Threats to your department come in many forms: from management, other departments competing for space and resources, budgetary issues, and access to essential services. We explore a selection of these below, but remember that if such a threat is presented as part of the viva in-tray exercise, you can be fairly sure that the action date is today or tomorrow and you need to make it priority 1.

SCENARIO 32.4: LOSS OF DEPARTMENTAL BEDS

Ten of your observation ward beds are to be converted to surgical day-case beds to reach 18-week surgical wait targets.

SUGGESTED APPROACH

Be firm (say no!), but acknowledge that as an emergency medicine consultant you need to be a good corporate citizen, and there is a balance between Trust objectives and departmental needs.

The emergency department is not your personal empire – it is a Trust resource, and the Executive Board can reassign your workspace. However, you have compelling clinical need and risk management issues why that should not be done.

Flows and targets

- The 18-week targets are important to the executive, but the consequence of losing observation beds is at the expense of 4-hour targets.

Safety and expertise

- If you cannot admit to your own beds then there will be pressure on acute medical and surgical beds.
- Emergency medicine physicians are the experts in emergency medicine, and patients are not well served by being forced onto other teams. Do not 'shroud-wave', but make your point.
- Does the Trust want poisoning cases to go to the physicians? Do they have the expertise?
- Does the Trust want head injuries looked after by general surgeons who have not done so for a decade, and to be nursed by a team more interested in flatus and urine output than neurological observation?
- It does not seem appropriate for postoperative surgical patients to be nursed by emergency department nurses, and there are some serious risk management issues.

SCENARIO 32.5: LOSS OF WORKSPACE TO ANOTHER DEPARTMENT

The orthopaedic department is going to expand fracture clinic provision by taking a chunk of your 'minors' facility.

SUGGESTED APPROACH

No other directorate or division has a call on your workspace, so say no to a fracture clinic invasion decided by the surgical division.

As in Scenario 32.4, the Executive Board can reassign your workspace, but again you have compelling clinical need and risk management issues why that cannot be done.

Flows and targets

- Your 'minors' always hits the 4-hour target because of 'see and treat', so losing 'minors' facilities is potentially going to impair your performance
- Crowding and access to cubicle space will adversely affect targets.
- Patient flows will be impaired.

Safety

- There will be overcrowding.
- There will be reduced access to assessment spaces.
- The risk of critical events and adverse outcomes will be increased.

Human Resources

- There are likely to be consequences in terms of staff retention, stress and absenteeism.

SCENARIO 32.6: REDIRECTION OF GP ADMISSIONS TO THE EMERGENCY DEPARTMENT

Direct GP admission to the acute medicine unit is struggling from lack of capacity, slow turnover and egress block. From tomorrow, all GP referrals to medicine will be seen in the emergency department, be triaged, and have initial investigation and treatment. You have expertise in triage and your medical support workers can front-load the investigations.

SUGGESTED APPROACH

This touches lots of nerves – inadequate capacity, not enough clinician and patient safety – and needs urgent action.

You raise the following issues.

Capacity

- It is likely that your emergency department is already used to capacity.
- There are limited trolley spaces.
- There is limited clinical space.
- The waiting room is likely to be at capacity
- There will be an unacceptable burden on phlebotomy and cardiology technicians as you are resourced for your patients – not yours and someone else's – assuming that no new resources come with this.

Safety

- Triaging someone else's patients delays emergency department triage and assessment.
- Self-presenting serious illness (myocardial infarction etc.) is already a problem before adding new delays. There will likely be an effect on MINAP figures.
- Your expertise is emergency medicine, not general medicine.
- Capacity and resource inadequacy will compromise care.
- The change is unacceptable from a risk management perspective.

Action

The emergency department team need to have a single view, and have that relayed coherently via the Clinical Director for Emergency Medicine.

Communicate with:

- the Clinical Director for Medicine
- the Divisional Manager for Medicine
- the Medical Director and Chief Executive

- the Operational Services Team
- local GPs via the Primary Care Trust's Professional Executive Committee – do they know that patients that they refer in for specialist opinion and treatment, and pay for via PBR, are being diverted into a crowded environment to be triaged?

FURTHER EXAMPLES

A few more examples of threats to the department are:

- Children's inpatient facilities are being moved to a neighbouring Trust, along with several of your emergency department F2s.
- Your CT scanner is unreliable. If it fails again then it will not be replaced until your department moves into the new Private Finance Initiative (PFI) build in 18 months. You can still use general CT, which is at the other end of the site.

PRIORITY 2 SCENARIOS

Priority 2 issues are somewhat indeterminate, and will not raise any priority 1 issues, but will be more important, for example, than flyers for conferences of little relevance. There may be important issues involved, but the time frame may make them priority 2. Complaints can fall into this category, since the Trust has 25 working days to respond.

COMPLAINTS

The structure varies from Trust to Trust, and it is something that you should familiarize yourself with locally. The usual complaint letter flow is from the complainant to the Complaints Office or to the Executive (who routes them to the Complaints Office). The Complaints Office has to acknowledge written complaints within 2 working days, and needs to respond to them within 25 working days, i.e. 5 weeks. It is at this point that the emergency medicine consultant gets the complaint letter, with a deadline to allow a reply within the 25-working-day time frame. This means that most complaint letters do not need your immediate attention unless the issue is a very important clinical issue or safety matter, and so can be temporarily redirected to your 'pending' tray. Issues around serious clinical incidents, near-misses and patient safety will generally be flagged up in an alternative way, either by medical or nursing colleagues, in person, the next day.

PRIORITY 3 SCENARIOS

Some of this will be of little relevance, and be immediately consigned to the waste bin.

COURSES AND CONFERENCES

Many departments have a weekly consultants meeting, when everyone is together with their diaries. Assuming that the course or conference has some merit, this is often a good time to decide, since you can see who is available, deserving or most interested.

MEDICAL EQUIPMENT

In terms of the in-tray, the equipment-related issues that should most concern you are notices about faults in crucial equipment, such as ventilators (priority 1).

Adverts for new equipment are never going to be a time priority unless the closure date for the annual round of capital bids is imminent! This means that you can put them aside for another time. Equipment that you aspire to must be requested via capital bids, accompanied by a business case, which contains clinical need, risk management aspects and capital cost, as well as revenue implications (service contract, consumables, etc.)

NOTES

Inexpensive equipment (<£1000) usually does not need a capital bid. PFI Trusts are increasingly common, and may have a managed equipment service, with equipment provided and cycled for replacement as part of the contract.

REQUESTS TO SEE COMPANY REPRESENTATIVES

These are up to you. Either you do not see the rep, and so consign to the waste bin, or you are interested, and so get your secretary to organize a convenient date and time.

ADDITIONAL MATERIAL

This final section contains miscellaneous useful information, with a couple of examples of in-tray or long-case management viva scenarios.

HUMAN RESOURCES (HR) DEPARTMENT

All Trusts have HR departments and they an incredibly important resource. Most emergency medicine consultants have a strong relationship with colleagues in HR management and call on their expertise frequently. If the problem that you are confronted with is one the following issues then you should pick up the telephone to your HR contact – usually the Medical Staffing Manager:

- sickness
- timekeeping
- absence
- probity
- personal behaviour at work
- recruitment and selection

They have access to references and previous employment records, and can link to HR colleagues in previous Trusts. This can be a useful way of establishing previous behaviour, or if someone has 'form'. Sometimes, it is necessary to interview a colleague over an HR matter, and it usually makes sense to have someone from HR present.

SCENARIO 32.7: DISCIPLINARY PROCEDURES

You have received a letter from the HR department of a local factory. It has attached a copy of a sick note (Med3) giving 3 months off work, including Christmas and New Year, with the reason given as 'back pain'. It has been signed by one of your current doctors and bears your departmental stamp. You have asked your secretary for the patient's notes, but there is no record of such a patient on that day.

SUGGESTED APPROACH

Issues

- Preserve confidentiality.
- Is this a fraudulent note on a factitious patient?
- Did the doctor sign it or is it a forgery?

- Is this a police or GMC issue?
- Do you have an issue with Med3 security?

Fact find

Maybe the patient is real but the date is wrong.

If the note is not fraudulent:

- Arrange an informal interview with the doctor concerned for feedback and education.
- Do you have guidance (handbook or emergency department education programme)?
- There must be no dialogue with the employing HR department without the patient's consent.
- Write to the patient and GP suggesting that the GP is more appropriate to assess the need for long-term sickness absence.

If the note is potentially fraudulent:

- Meet with the doctor concerned, but make sure that you have a neutral party present (ideally from HR) and keep detailed records. Get the doctor's version of events.
- Involve HR, both for the interview and to check on the doctor's background – they may have 'form'.

Are there grounds for professional misconduct (e.g. a fraudulent Med3 done for a friend)?

- The GMC can give advice over the telephone.
- The Medical Director can offer useful advice – and ought to know anyway.
- Is the doctor concerned a trainee (Deanery property)? Involve the Deanery through the DME or Clinical Tutor.

If the note is a likely third-party forgery from a genuine note:

- Refer back to the referring HR department and leave them to take action.
- With regard to Med 3 security:
  - Are they left lying around?
  - Control access.
  - Log use against patient attendance.

RECRUITMENT AND SELECTION (R&S)

Curriculum knowledge for this area involves:

- recruitment
- job descriptions
- employment law
- interviewing

If you are going to interview at a Deanery level then it is mandatory to have had formal recruitment and selection training, along with diversity training. This is usually done as a 1- to 2-day Deanery-backed short course. Local recruitment can be more informal, but the same standards should apply.

The recruitment sequence for an appointment at Trust level is as follows:

- Identify funding and obtain manpower approval, usually through a manpower committee.
- Draw up a job description, person specification and advertisement.
- Advertise on BMJ Careers or, increasingly, NHS Jobs.
- Shortlist against the person specification.
- Interview.

The person specification is important and states mandatory and desirable qualities. Shortlisting is done against the person specification, which allows you interview the right candidates, as well as defend a decision not to shortlist.

For example, for an SHO-equivalent Trust-grade job, you want clinicians with the right skills. You do not particularly want a candidate with 5 years of orthopaedics and no medicine. Address this by making foundation competencies mandatory; for overseas candidates, you might require 4 months' medicine at foundation level or a previous emergency medicine post.

If the interview is to appoint a consultant or associate specialist colleague then there is a defined structure of how the Advisory Appointments Committee (AAC) should be constituted:

- lay chair (non-executive director, Trust Chair or external Chief Executive)
- Chief Executive or board-level representative (e.g. HR Director, Director of Nursing or Finance Director)
- College representative
- at least one local emergency medicine consultant
- university representative if the post has research or teaching responsibilities

For local posts, such as Trust grade or clinical fellow, two consultants, or a consultant and specialist registrar, together with an HR representative are adequate.

The following are the key points:

- Ask every candidate broadly the same questions.
- Keep records.
- Use a quasi-numerical scoring system, such as 0 = poor, 1 = average, 2 = above average, for each domain of questioning. This helps to identify outliers in either direction and supports your final decision.
- You cannot use references to choose candidates, unless there is no other way to separate them.

SCENARIO 32.8: THE AGGRIEVED CANDIDATE

You have a letter from a doctor who has not been shortlisted for a Trust-grade job in your emergency department. He feels that he is highly qualified and is aggrieved at not being selected for interview. His letter contains threats of legal action or involvement of the Equality and Human Rights Commission.

SUGGESTED APPROACH

Although this is important, it is unlikely to be the most pressing thing in your in-tray (priority 2).

You should delegate – this is largely an HR matter, so telephone them and get them to make the initial response. If you did not shortlist this doctor, it was because he did not meet the person specification – and that should be the basis of the HR response.

Make yourself available to HR to clarify issues with the candidate if they have issues after HR have responded.

Reasonable candidates can be dealt with verbally, otherwise respond (if needed) by letter.

Have you have had R&S and diversity training?

Deaneries, Schools, Colleges and their representatives: Who does what?

If the doctor concerned is in foundation or specialty training then you will need to have dialogue with some of the above. Bear in mind that your post-foundation CT1/2 (SHO equivalents) may belong to schools of general practice, medicine or surgery, as well as Acute Care Common Stem (ACCS)/emergency medicine.

Director of Medical Education (DME) and Clinical Tutors

These posts have dual lines of accountability to both the local Deanery, and the Trust's Chief Executive. They oversee the foundation trainees, so persistent problems with doctors in these grades needs to involve them. As they link to the Deanery, they are better placed to refer on to the appropriate structure. Issues with specialty trainees historically involved them in the same way, although the inception of specialty schools may replace some of their functions, since the schools may have directors for CT1/2 and ST3 onwards. The release of trainees to regional training, the provision of local education and study leave are all within their remit. At present, the situation concerning medical education is in a state of flux, in view of Modernising Medical Careers, the Tooke Report and the Department of Health response.

Undergraduate Sub-Dean and Tutors

These are analogous to the DME and Clinical Tutors, but for issues that involve medical students.

Medical director

The Medical Director is a permanent member of the Trust's Executive Board, and thus is the link between the consultant body and the Board. The Medical Director is of great value as an 'honest broker' if there are relationship breakdowns between consultant colleagues either within emergency medicine or between the emergency department and other departments. The Medical Director should become involved in the following situations:

- serious concerns about colleagues
- interspecialty conflict
- threats to departmental safety caused by egress block or medical team unavailability
- for a general 'wise' opinion
- serious performance problems
- probity issues

33
Evidence-Based Medicine
CHARLES YOUNG

It is important that you know the principles of evidence-based medicine, which evidence to use and what to do if the ideal evidence is not available.

Evidence-based medicine as a term has been interpreted in a variety of different ways. Many people assume that it means to base clinical practice on the results of published randomized controlled trials (RCTs). Although true in part, this is a very limited definition. Biomedical evidence takes many forms, and these include not only RCTs, but also observational studies (prospective or retrospective cohort studies, case series, case reports, etc.), opinion-based publications and secondary research (systematic reviews of randomized or observational evidence, or meta-analyses of numerical data from more than one trial, often based on the reults of a systematic review). All of these types of evidence may be published or unpublished, and all form part of the ever-accumulating mass of biomedical evidence.

Evidence-based medicine therefore may be seen to mean basing clinical practice on any form of biomedical evidence. To complicate this already tricky area further, different sorts of evidence are more or less suited to answering different types of clinical questions. For example:

- If the question is 'Are beta-blockers effective in reducing mortality in people aged 50– 70 years with mild to moderate biventricular heart failure?' then the best sort of evidence would probably come from a systematic review and associated meta-analysis of placebo-controlled RCTs in this population.
- If the question is 'Is beta-blocker 1 better than beta-blocker 2 in reducing mortality in people aged 50–70 years with mild to moderate biventricular heart failure?' then the best sort of evidence would probably come from a systematic review and associated meta-analysis of RCTs comparing beta-blockers 1 and 2 in this population.
- If the question was 'Does beta-blocker 1 cause important side-effects in people aged 50–70 years with mild to moderate biventricular heart failure?' then the best type of evidence would probably be one or more large, long-term, prospective cohort studies in this population.

As these examples illustrate, a key principle in evidence-based medicine is that the best/level 1/gold standard evidence is defined not only by what sort of evidence it is (randomized or observational), but more importantly by the type of question being addressed.

In spite of the very varied nature of evidence-based medicine, there are four fundamental principles that can be applied to any sort of evidence and that underlie any sort of evidence-based medicine.

First, the clinical question must be clearly defined. This is best done using the PICOT approach:

Population
Intervention in question
Comparator intervention
Outcome
Time frame

So, an example of a good evidence-based question would be the following:

'In people taking the MCEM examination [Population], does reading this chapter on critical appraisal [Intervention in question], compared with not reading the chapter [Comparator intervention], increase the risk of their passing the MCEM examination [Outcome], after 6 months [Time frame]?'

Second, the type of evidence most suited to answering the question needs to be identified. If the best type of evidence is not available then alternative forms will be required, bearing in mind their limitations. Expanding this point further, it may not be possible to collect the ideal form of evidence for practical or ethical reasons. For example, it would be neither practical nor ethical to conduct an RCT of a new thrombolytic medicine versus placebo in a group of patients with myocardial infarction, however useful the information from such an RCT might be, as it has already been established that thrombolytics in general reduce mortality in these patients. In situations like this, it may be necessary to use more pragmatic evidence that, although not ideal, helps answer the question in some way. In using more pragmatic evidence, however, it is crucial to identify and consider carefully its limitations before drawing any firm conclusions.

Third, any evidence identified needs to be contextualized, i.e. a thorough literature search must be carried out to find all the available relevant evidence – published and unpublished – not just one or two pieces seen in isolation. In considering the importance of contextualizing individual pieces of biomedical evidence, it should be borne in mind that some trial results occur by chance and some occur as a result of methodological errors. In other words, a trial may indicate that an intervention works, whereas many previous or subsequent trials show that the same intervention in the same population does not work. If the trial showing that the intervention works is considered in isolation, a potentially erroneous view of the intervention's effectiveness may be formed. Evidence must also be contextualized in terms of individual clinical experience and ability, as well as patients' views and preferences. In this way, evidence-based medicine involves not only research but also clinical abilities and patient priorities.

Finally, the evidence must be scrutinized and evaluated to identify any possible methodological shortcomings before summary conclusions are drawn. Clearly, these principles will be limited by time, resources and experience, but nonetheless they form the basis of any evidence-based approach to medical practice.

GUIDELINES, NSFs AND NICE GUIDANCE

Guidelines are another sort of evidence that may influence clinical practice. They are usually created by groups of experts and contain more or less didactic advice on how to manage specific groups of patients. The purpose of guidelines is broadly to standardize care to ensure that patients in a certain group all receive the best care possible and that resources are used in the most effective way. In this capacity, guidelines are very helpful for clincans (who may require guidance in unfamiliar areas), resource controllers (who need to make sure that limited resources are rationed appropriately) and patients (who should reasonably expect to receive good-quality standardized care). All guidelines, however, come with three key considerations:

- Their basis is very likely to be a mix of evidence (any sort) and expert opinion. This basis is often not apparent to the user, and so caution is required when applying their recommendations to any clinical situation. In other words, guidelines should not be followed blindly when situations are not going acording to plan. Clinicians should be prepared to use guidelines in a flexible way, since no single guideline will cover every eventuality.
- Guidelines may reflect practice at a variety of levels (international, national, local, departmental, etc.). On this basis, it can be seen that, for many reasons (resources, technological, legal, etc.), it may not be possible to

strictly apply an international guideline for example at a departmental level. Again, flexibility is required and the guidelines' overall aims should be considered.

- Guidelines should not be seen as a replacement for medical training and expert experience, and need to be interpreted carefully in the context of an individual patient.

Two key sources of national UK guidelines are National Service Frameworks (NSFs) and National Institute for Health and Clinical Excellence (NICE) guidance:

- NSFs are long-term strategies for improving specific areas of care. They set national standards, identify key interventions and put in place agreed time scales for implementation. As such, they represent a type of contextualized national-level guideline for treatment of a key disease area.
- In comparison, NICE is an independent organization responsible for providing national guidance on promoting good health and preventing and treating ill health. NICE guidance comes in a variety of forms, key among which are guidelines.

KNOW HOW TO SEARCH FOR EVIDENCE

Conducting a literature search is a difficult challenge, and is far more complex than typing 'beta-blockers AND mortality' into PubMed. It is also a very skilled task, which is best done by, or with explicit guidance from, an expert in this area – usually an information specialist or librarian. The key issue about literature searching is that an incomplete search may miss determinant articles. The summary derived from such an incomplete search may then be lacking key pieces of information (e.g. all the trials that show that the intervention in question does not work) and so present a misleading conclusion (continuing the example, that the intervention in question has a positive effect when in reality it does not).

If the first requirement for literature searching is that it is guided by experience in searching, the second requirement is that the question being addressed is clearly defined. The requirements for any question of this type are, as before, Population, Intervention, Comparator, Time frame. Other key considerations for searching are that all appropriate databases are included (PubMed, EMBASE, Cochrane Library, *Clinical Evidence*, etc.), that a consistent and appropriate approach is taken to publications in different languages, and that a consistent and appropriate approach is also taken to unpublished data.

Unpublished data is worthy of a particular note in this context. The main concerns about unpublished data are that a single important piece of information that could affect the overall search conclusions may be missed or that a systematic loss of all of one type of data may occur (e.g. all of the negative trial results relating to an intervention may be unpublished, whereas all the positive results are published).

It is unlikely that any search will discover every piece of data on a given intervention, but tactics such as searching the reference lists of identified publications for other publications not found by the search, and contacting key researchers directly, are important to maximize literature search effectiveness.

The final part of any literature search is the initial appraisal of the search results. No literature search will be 100% accurate, and so every search is likely to identify some data that are not relevant to the question being investigated. The appraisal process then sorts which search results are relevant and should be evaluated further, and which are not and so can be disregarded. The initial appraisal process should be based on very clear principles derived from the research question (disregarding, for example, any publication with the wrong population group), should be done in a consistent way, and ideally should be done by more than one person, with an a priori plan of how to deal with disagreements between appraisers.

EVALUATION OF BIOMEDICAL EVIDENCE, AND LIMITATIONS OF EMERGENCY MEDICINE RESEARCH

Biomedical evidence is not of homogenous quality. Published evidence may be intentionally misleading, with, for example, one or more research studies being designed and run specifically to show a predetermined result, with this result actually being incorrect. Such intentionally misleading research is, however, fortunately quite rare. Unintentionally misleading research is usually caused by poor presentation of the research findings, bias (a systematic error caused by the research design or interpretation), confounding (where an additional variable confuses an observed association) or statistical uncertainty.

Any evaluation of biomedical evidence needs to consider all of the possible intentional and unintentional shortcomings in a systematic and thorough way. Many systems exist for this type of research evaluation, and usually the best approach is to stick to one that you are familiar with and that you know works. Having said that, any good evaluation system should consider biomedical evidence in terms of its internal and external validity (truthfulness).

In this context, external validity really means 'Does this information tell us what we need to know to make a decision?' and can be considered in terms of whether the information in question is practical (Can it be done by those who need to do it?), important (Does the patient or clinician think that the result is important enough to bother using the intervention?) and generalizable (Does the information relate to the group of patients in question).

In contrast, internal validity means 'Has the research been done appropriately, and is it presented in a way that allows us to understand it properly?' Internal validity is assessed by considering each part of the publication in turn (usually introduction, methods, results and conclusions), and deciding whether they are appropriate in themselves and whether they relate correctly to all the other parts of the publication. For example, do the methods clearly explain the results and do the results support the all of the categorical conclusions that are not supported by other references.

An important principle of biomedical research evaluation is not to be too critical, and to look for useful parts of the publication as well as identifying any flaws. It is all too easy to dismiss every publication because of often relatively minor flaws, where a more time-efficient and useful approach is to think 'There may be problems with this, but do they really affect the result I am interested in, and, even if they do, can I take anything away from this publication, even accepting that it has problems?'.

Considering emergency medicine in particular, there are some specific issues that may affect research quality or generalizability of research findings:

- Emergency medicine research is often conducted in environments that are hard to standardize, with inconsistent staffing, very varied patient presentations and high patient volumes.
- Ethical problems are frequently encountered, including the ability to gain informed consent for research.
- The subjects of investigation are interventions or outcomes that are hard to capture using standard trial designs.
- Taken together, these issues mean that emergency medicine research, although very valuable, is often skewed towards the more pragmatic end of the research spectrum.

BIOMEDICAL STATISTICS

It is beyond the scope of this chapter to provide a detailed description of the entirety of biomedical statistics and statistical interpretation. However, there are some important statistical principles that will facilitate a general understanding of this area, and guide further reading. Broadly speaking, the important statistical concepts that relate to practical research evaluation include:

- deciding whether a trial had sufficient statistical power to observe an effect if one exists
- assessing the statistical significance of a trial result
- assessing the size of an observed effect
- assessing statistical confidence in the observed effect size

Power calculations are a fundamental part of any trial statistics plan, and are necessarily based on an assumption of what the trial effect size is likely to be. This effect size assumption should be supported by previously published research, where possible, and it is important for the reader to assess this assumption when considering if the power calculation was appropriate. Remember that although an underpowered trial will not observe an effect that does not exist, it may miss a real effect when one does exist.

Statistical significance is conventionally assessed using probability (p) values, with $p < 0.05$ being the arbitrary cut-off for statistical significance, at which point the null hypothesis (e.g. that there is no difference between intervention and placebo) is rejected. This significance level is often described by using the Greek letter alpha (α). Considerations here are that statistical significance at the 0.05 (i.e. 5%) level means that there is still a 1 in 20 chance that the observed result occurred by chance, that clinical significance and statistical significance are not the same (a result may have statistical significance but be of only very limited clinical significance because of the small effect size) and that a trial should not be dismissed as useless simply because the p-value is marginally above the 0.05 level.

Typical effect size measurements include relative risks and odds ratios.

* Risk in this context is defined as the the number of patients with an outcome divided by the total number of patients in that particular group. The relative risk is the ratio of the risk in the intervention group to the risk in the control group.
* In contrast, odds can be described as the number of patients with the outcome divided by the number without the outcome. The odds ratio is the ratio of the odds in the treatment group to the odds in the control group.

Risk and odds cannot be used interchangeably, and, although they may be numerically similar when their values are low, they are clearly quite different in the ways in which they are calculated and interpreted.

Other key comparative statistics include the number needed to treat (NNT) and the number needed to harm (NNH).

The confidence interval (or confidence limits) is usually reported at the 95% level. This means that we can be 95% certain that the true value for a result lies within that range. For example, if the estimated relative risk from a trial is 2 and the 95% confidence interval is 1.5–3.5, this means that we are 95% confident that the true relative risk for the population will lie somewhere in the range from 1.5 to 3.5. Clearly then, the wider the confidence interval, the less confident we are of exactly what the true value for the result is. Furthermore, if the result to which the confidence interval relates is a ratio (e.g. a relative risk) and the confidence interval includes 1 (e.g. relative risk 2, 95% confidence interval 0.5–3.5) then we can be 95% certain (which equates to the conventional α of 5%) that the trial result is not statistically significant, since a ratio of 1 means that there is no difference in the observed effect between the two groups being investigated.

CONCLUSIONS

Evidence-based medicine is the process by which clinicians and patients interpret and utilize biomedical information. Without the application of evidence-based medicine principles, it is not possible to keep up to date with the almost daily advances in every aspect of clinical care or to appropriately interpret the biomedical research findings that form the basis of the majority of clinical developments. This process of continuing professional development or continuing medical education is appropriately seen by clinical regulatory bodies and patients alike as essential to the safe and effective practice of medicine. It is then the clinician's responsibility to ensure that they are able to use an evidence-based approach to defend their patients from treatments that may not work or may be harmful, while at the same time making full use of those treatments, old and new, that are of benefit.

USEFUL RESOURCES

Bandolier website: www.medicine.ox.ac.uk/bandolier.

Clinical Evidence website: http://clinicalevidence.bmj.com.

Cochrane Library website: http://cochrane.co.uk/en/clib.html.

National Institute for Health and Clinical Excellence website: www.nice.org.uk.

National Service Frameworks are available at the Department of Health website: www.dh.gov.uk/en/Healthcare.

34

Instructions for actors in relevant OSCEs

CHETAN R TRIVEDY

It is useful for actors who are playing the role of patients (or other participants, such as parents or students) in the OSCE scenarios to have a guide on how to approach the scenario. We would encourage the actors to build upon the briefs that we have provided in order to make the OSCEs more challenging and complex. Not all of the OSCE scenarios have patients/actors – we have omitted these from the list of instructions.

CHAPTER 3: ANAESTHETICS AND PAIN RELIEF

SCENARIO 3.1: ANALGESIA AND CONFLICT RESOLUTION

- You are a 39-year-old male patient.
- You have fallen and fractured your ankle.
- You are upset because you have had a long wait and are in pain.
- Your mother had a bad reaction to pethidine once and you are very anxious about analgesia.
- You have are due to go skiing in 2 weeks.
- Your girlfriend is also upset and insists on private treatment.
- You are otherwise well and have no medical problems.

SCENARIO 3.2: TEACHING LOCAL ANAESTHESIA

- You are a fourth-year medical student.
- You have heard of local anaesthesia but have not used it.
- You should ask about safe doses, complications and signs of toxicity.

SCENARIO 3.3: FEMORAL NERVE BLOCK

- You are 34 years old and have broken your right leg.
- You have had morphine but are still in pain.
- You are concerned about the junior doctor performing the procedure.
- You are worried about a football match that you have in 2 weeks.

SCENARIO 3.4: CONSCIOUS SEDATION

- You are a 75-year-old man
- You have fallen in the park and thought that you had sprained your ankle.
- The X-ray shows that you have broken your leg.
- You have high blood pressure and had a heart attack 10 years ago.
- You had an operation to remove your gallbladder, after which you felt sick.
- You are a retired publican who smokes 15 cigarettes a day and used to drink heavily.
- You have problems with snoring and are waiting to see the ENT specialist.
- You are on antihypertensives, statins and aspirin.
- You live alone and are worried about going to the toilet, which is upstairs.

CHAPTER 4: WOUND MANAGEMENT

SCENARIO 4.1: DOG BITE

- You are 35 years old and have been attacked by a dog.
- You are right-handed and work as a graphic designer.
- You are worried about rabies and having a scar.
- You are allergic to penicillin.
- You are not up to date with your tetanus vaccination.

CHAPTER 6: MUSCULOSKELETAL EMERGENCIES

SCENARIO 6.1: EXAMINATION OF THE SHOULDER

- You are 40 years old and fell off your bike 2 days ago.
- The injury has affected your dominant arm.
- You have pain and are unable to put your arm behind your back or lift it to the side.
- You are concerned about going back to work and about playing golf.
- You friend had a similar injury and needed an operation.

SCENARIO 6.2: EXAMINATION OF THE WRIST AND HAND – BONY INJURY

- You are a 30-year-old painter and decorator.
- You fell last night after having a few drinks.
- You have pain and deformity in your right (dominant) wrist.
- You have some tingling in your fingers.
- You are well, but felt sick after having sedation to reduce a dislocated shoulder.

SCENARIO 6.3: EXAMINATION OF THE WRIST AND HAND – SOFT TISSUE INJURY

- You are a 22-year-old art student who has cut the palm of her right (dominant) hand.
- You have no significant neurovascular deficit.
- You are concerned about whether it will affect your studies.

SCENARIO 6.4: CERVICAL SPINE INJURY

- You are a 36-year-old driving instructor.
- You car was hit from behind at 15 mph when your student braked suddenly. You were wearing a seatbelt.

- You were not knocked out, and managed to walk out of the vehicle.
- The accident happened 2 days ago,
- You now have pain in the back of your neck, which is stiff.
- No have no change in your bowel or bladder habits.
- You had some tingling in your fingers.
- You can move your neck from side to side, but it feels stiff.
- You are worried that you will be off work, and need a letter for your insurance company.

SCENARIO 6.5: EXAMINATION OF THE BACK

- You are 65 years old and have a 2-week history of lower back pain.
- You have had a history of breast cancer and have noticed that you have had some weight loss recently.
- You have not noticed any urinary or bowel incontinence.
- You are unable to straight raise your right leg.
- You have some numbness in your right foot.

SCENARIO 6.6: EXAMINATION OF THE HIP

- You are a 65-year-old man with a 1-month history of a painful right hip.
- You have a history of osteoarthritis and had bilateral knee replacements 5 years ago.
- You walk with a stick.
- You had a fall a week ago when you slipped on some leaves in the garden.

SCENARIO 6.7: EXAMINATION OF THE KNEE

- You are 28 years old and have hurt your right knee, which suddenly gave way when you were jogging.
- You cannot straight-leg raise and are unable to weight-bear.
- You are worried that you have torn something. You were planning to run the London marathon in 8 weeks time.

CHAPTER 7: VASCULAR EMERGENCIES

SCENARIO 7.1: ABDOMINAL AORTIC ANEURYSM ASSESSMENT

- You are a 60-year-old man with central abdominal pain.
- You initially thought that it was food poisoning, but it is getting worse.
- You have high blood pressure and diabetes, for which you take tablets.
- Sometimes you wake up at night with pains and tingling in your legs.
- You have smoked 20 cigarettes a day for over 30 years.
- You work as a banker.
- You are worried that you have appendicitis.

SCENARIO 7.2: DEEP VEIN THROMBOSIS – HISTORY AND EXAMINATION

- You are a 30-year-old woman who has had a 2-day history of pain and swelling in your right calf.
- You noticed that the right calf was bigger than the left and tender to touch.
- You had been to the gym and thought that you had pulled a muscle.
- Your mother had a DVT and died from pulmonary embolism.
- You are on the oral contraceptive pill.
- You flew back from New York 2 weeks ago, but flew business class.
- You do not smoke and are otherwise well.
- You have heard that there is a blood test to tell if you have a clot or not, and would like more information.

CHAPTER 8: ABDOMINAL EMERGENCIES

SCENARIO 8.1: ABDOMINAL PAIN

- You are a 44-year-old editor for a fashion magazine.
- You have an 8-hour history of epigastric pain radiating to your back after going out a work party the night before, where you thought you had a dodgy kebab.
- You have taken paracetamol, which has not helped, and you came to hospital because you felt light-headed.
- You have vomited four times and noticed a little of blood in the vomit.
- You drink about a bottle of wine and smoke 5 cigarettes a day.
- There has been no change in your bowel habit.
- You are otherwise well and have no allergies and are not on any regular medications.
- Your periods are regular and you are not currently sexually active.

SCENARIO 8.3: UPPER GI BLEED

- You are a 65-year-old architect.
- You have been vomiting blood for the last 2 hours. It is dark brown in colour, although there was also some fresh blood.
- You have atrial fibrillation and take warfarin. Your last blood test was last week and your INR was 2.6.
- You are currently on amoxicillin for a dental abscess.
- You have not noticed any change in your bowel habits or weight.
- You do not smoke or drink alcohol.
- Your father died of stomach cancer and you are worried about having cancer.

SCENARIO 8.4: LOWER GI BLEED

- You are a 70-year-old retired shopkeeper.
- You have had a 2-week history of passing fresh blood with your stool.
- There has been no pain or mucus associated with the motions, but you feel constipated and have been taking senna.
- You have dropped 2 inches on your waist over the last 3 months.
- You are otherwise well and gave up smoking 10 years ago.
- You drink socially and have had no foreign travel.
- You have recently been started on iron tablets after your GP found you to be anaemic.

SCENARIO 8.5: GASTROENTERITIS

- You are a 20-year-old medical student.
- You are currently doing a placement on one of the surgical wards.
- You have passed loose watery stools with a little bit of blood but no mucus 4 times a day for the last 2 days.
- You have also felt feverish, but have not had any vomiting.
- You were on holiday in Chile and did not have any medical problems during your travel.
- You are on the oral contraceptive pill but not on any other medications and have no known allergies.
- There has been an outbreak of *Clostridium difficile* on the ward.
- You are worried that if you are taken off the ward, you will not get your rotation signed off.

CHAPTER 9: GENITOURINARY EMERGENCIES

SCENARIO 9.1: TESTICULAR TORSION

- You are a 19-year-old engineering student
- You were masturbating, following which you developed a sudden onset of acute testicular pain.
- The right testicle is exquisitely tender.
- You were too embarrassed to tell anyone, but the pain has got worse and you have vomited twice.
- You are otherwise well and have no medical problems.
- You are extremely embarrassed and do not wish your parents, who are in the waiting room, informed.

SCENARIO 9.2: HAEMATURIA – HISTORY

- You are a 78-year-old retired lawyer.
- You have noticed blood in your urine for the last 2 days.
- There is no pain associated with passing urine.
- The blood appears to be fresh.
- You are otherwise well, but take tablets for high blood pressure and high cholesterol.
- You have no known allergies.

CHAPTER 10: OPHTHALMOLOGICAL EMERGENCIES

SCENARIO 10.1: ACUTE RED EYE

- You are a 25-year-old hairdresser.
- You have had a painful red eye for 2 days.
- You think that some hair got into your eye and that you may have rubbed it.
- It has been watering and very painful, with a little bit of discharge.
- You are otherwise well and have no medical problems or allergies.
- You wear contact lenses.

SCENARIO 10.2: ACUTE LOSS OF VISION

- You are a 70-year-old retired teacher.
- You noticed that the right eye has become painful and that you have pain in your scalp when you comb your hair or when you chew .
- Your have high blood pressure and diabetes.
- You are worried because you have to drive your disabled husband to his dialysis twice a week.

SCENARIO 10.3: TRAUMATIC EYE INJURY

- You are a 20-year-old student.
- You were assaulted the night before.
- You were punched over the left side of your face.
- You have blurred vision when you look up and numbness over your left cheek.

CHAPTER 11: EAR, NOSE AND THROAT CONDITIONS

SCENARIO 11.1: ACUTE OTITIS MEDIA

- You are the parent of Jimmy, who is 6 years old.
- He has had a painful ear for 2 days after he went swimming.
- Jimmy is otherwise well, but gets a lot of ear infections.
- You use cotton buds routinely to keep his ears clean.
- You are concerned that Jimmy has got the infection form the swimming pool after one of the other boys in his class confessed to urinating in the pool on the day Jimmy went swimming.

SCENARIO 11.2: ACUTE EPISTAXIS

- You are a 60-year-old businessman.
- You have had a profuse nose bleed for 2 hours and, despite pinching your nose, you have not managed to stop it.
- It is your third nose bleed in a week.
- You have high blood pressure and your GP has just increased your medication in an attempt to control it.
- You take warfarin for atrial fibrillation and an antihypertensive medication, but cannot remember what it is called.
- You have no known allergies and do not drink alcohol or smoke.
- You are due to fly to Sweden for a meeting tomorrow and are concerned about having another nose bleed on the flight.

CHAPTER 13: OBSTETRICS AND GYNAECOLOGY

SCENARIO 13.2: VAGINAL BLEEDING

- You are a 26-year-old pharmacist.
- You are generally well, with no known allergies.
- You have lower abdominal pain and have noticed that you are passing some blood from the vagina.
- You and your partner have been trying for a baby and you have had two attempts at IVF, both of which have failed.
- You are sexually active and do not have any discharge or pain during intercourse.
- You have had two previous miscarriages and no successful pregnancies.
- Your periods are irregular and your last period was 6 weeks ago.
- You are concerned that you are having a miscarriage and want an ultrasound scan.

SCENARIO 13.3: VAGINAL DISCHARGE (SEXUAL HISTORY)

- You are a 36-year-old sex worker.
- You have had a 3-day history of an offensive vaginal discharge and itchiness.
- You have had seven male partners in the last 4 days.
- You usually use condoms when having sex with clients, but have unprotected sex with your boyfriend.
- You participate in oral and vaginal sex but not anal sex.
- You were tested for HIV, hepatitis B and hepatitis C only 4 months ago and were cleared.
- You have previously received treatment for *Chlamydia* 6 months ago.
- You are concerned that your boyfriend has been unfaithful to you, since your clients are upmarket citizens.

SCENARIO 13.4: EMERGENCY CONTRACEPTION

- You are a 15-year-old girl who has skipped school to come to the emergency department.
- You had unprotected sex with your boyfriend, who is also 15 and in your class.
- You have had sex on four previous occasions and your boyfriend thinks that the withdrawal method is safe.
- You had sex 6 hours ago, when the withdrawal method failed, and you are worried about being pregnant.
- Your parents are very strict and you do not want them to find out.
- You are otherwise well and have no illnesses.
- You understand what emergency contraception is and have been reading about it on the Internet.
- You would like the emergency contraceptive pill.
- You are scared that the doctor will tell your parents or the school.
- You would like to know where you can get confidential advice on safe sex.

CHAPTER 14: RESPIRATORY EMERGENCIES

SCENARIO 14.2: PNEUMOTHORAX

- You are a 27-year-old graphic designer.
- You have had a sudden onset of pain in your chest when you breathe and have found it difficult to breathe.
- There has been no history of trauma and you were perfectly fine yesterday.
- You are otherwise well and have not had any recent travel.
- You enjoy diving.
- You are a non-smoker and drink alcohol occasionally.
- You are worried about a diving trip that you have planned for next month.

SCENARIO 14.3: INTERPRETATION OF THE WELLS SCORE

- You are a 37-year-old banker who has pleuritic chest pain, shortness of breath and a swollen leg.
- You have just returned from a business trip to China.
- You are worried about a clot on the lung and have been told that your D-dimer blood test is negative.
- You are keen to go home, since you have been travelling for 5 days and have come straight to the hospital from the airport
- You are on the oral contraceptive pill.
- You are a non-smoker and drink occasionally.

SCENARIO 14.4: COPD

- You are a 64-year-old woman who has had a 3-day history of a cough and progressive shortness of breath over the last 24 hours.
- You are producing green sputum.
- You are a chronic smoker and have smoked 20 cigarettes a day for over 30 years.
- You live in a third-floor flat and have home oxygen and nebulizers and take a lot of medications.
- You do not think that you can stop smoking.
- You do not always take your medications, because they give you a sore throat.
- You have been admitted several times to the hospital, but never to HDU or ITU.
- You are keen to go home, since you have three cats to look after.

SCENARIO 14.6: ASTHMA IN PREGNANCY

- You are 28 years old and have had asthma for over 13 years.
- Your asthma is normally well controlled, although you have had two previous admissions for acute exacerbations, but have never been admitted to HDU or ITU.

- You are 18 weeks pregnant, and have stopped taking your asthma medications since you feel that they will harm your baby.
- You smoke occasionally, but only have had one or two cigarettes a day since you became pregnant.
- You are not sure about when you should use your inhalers.
- You have poor inhaler technique, but improve when you are shown.

CHAPTER 15: CARDIOLOGICAL EMERGENCIES

SCENARIO 15.1: CHEST PAIN – HISTORY AND MANAGEMENT

- You are a 38-year-old banker who has had a 2-hour history of palpitations and central chest pain, which are associated with sweating and nausea. The pain has been eased with the aspirin that you have received.
- The pain radiated into your left arm and scored 8/10.
- These symptoms were relieved by the medications that the paramedics gave you, but you still feel discomfort in your chest
- You are otherwise well and have no serious illnesses and not currently taking any medications.
- You have never had chest pain before and admit to having taken two lines of cocaine earlier on in the day. You smoke 10 cigarettes a day.
- You father died of a heart attack at the age of 69.
- You are worried that you will be in trouble with the police and do not wish it to be disclosed that you take cocaine.

SCENARIO 15.3: ARRHYTHMIA (I)

- You are a 32-year-old university lecturer who has been unwell with diarrhoea and vomiting for 2 days. You have not been able to eat, but have managed to drink black coffee. You had four cups and then noticed that your heart was racing, about 2 hours ago.
- You have had a similar episode in the past and have got an old ECG for the candidate if they ask you.
- You are generally well, but have a condition known as Wolff–Parkinson–White syndrome and you are due to have ablation surgery.

SCENARIO 15.4: ARRHYTHMIA (II)

- You are a 68-year-old housewife who has a 3-hour history of palpitations and a feeling that your heart is racing.
- You were shopping in the supermarket and felt dizzy and short of breath.
- You have been investigated for an overactive thyroid and are awaiting the results. You are currently on antibiotics for a chest infection.
- You had breakfast this morning, but have not eaten for 4 hours.
- You are worried about being 'shocked' and are concerned about it being painful.

CHAPTER16: NEUROLOGICAL EMERGENCIES

SCENARIO16.1: HEADACHE HISTORY

- You are a 28-year-old postman.
- You have presented with a severe headache that started suddenly after you had sex with your girlfriend a few hours ago.
- It was not resolved with paracetamol and ibuprofen.

- You only occasionally get headaches, which are mild and respond to simple painkillers.
- You have no other medical problems and do not smoke.
- Your father died of a stroke.
- On a couple of occasions, you have had post-coital headaches, but these have been mild.
- You now have nausea and photophobia and feel that your neck is stiff.
- You are concerned that you have meningitis.

SCENARIO 16.5: TRANSIENT ISCHAEMIC ATTACK

- You are a 80-year-old retired policeman.
- You were in the kitchen when you collapsed.
- You cannot remember much about what happened, but feel well now and want to go home.
- You live with your wife and are otherwise independent.
- You suffer from high blood pressure and tablet-controlled diabetes, and had a mild stroke 10 years ago from which you have totally recovered.
- You take tablets for blood pressure and diabetes.
- You gave up smoking 10 years ago.

CHAPTER 18: TOXICOLOGICAL EMERGENCIES

SCENARIO 18.1: PARACETAMOL OVERDOSE

- You are a 17-year-old student
- You took a deliberate overdose of paracetamol about an hour ago.
- You think that you took 30 tablets, but vomited afterwards.
- You wanted to kill yourself and texted your sister to say that you took the overdose. You were planning it for 2 days, and you took the overdose when you knew your sister would be away.
- You have had no previous episodes of self-harming
- You have an eating disorder and are receiving counselling.
- You are currently not on any medications.
- You split up from your boyfriend 2 weeks ago.
- You are currently sharing a flat with your sister.
- You do not smoke or drink.

SCENARIO 18.4: DIGOXIN TOXICITY

- You are a 82-year-old retired builder.
- You have had a recent chest infection, for which you have been started on erythromycin because you are allergic to penicillin.
- You have atrial fibrillation and take digoxin.
- You take quinine for muscle cramps.
- You have noticed that everything looks yellow and that your vision is blurred.
- You feel more tired than usual.
- You have had some vomiting and diarrhoea and thought that you had food poisoning.

CHAPTER 19: RENAL EMERGENCIES

SCENARIO 19.1: ACUTE RENAL FAILURE

- You are a 74-year-old retired orthopaedic surgeon.
- You had a blood test today, which showed that your potassium was too high, and your GP advised that you attend the emergency department to be followed up.
- You have just recovered from an episode of acute diarrhoea, but otherwise feel well.
- You have problems with your kidneys, and your GP sends you for a blood test every 6 months.
- You have high blood pressure and take bendroflumethiazide and lisinopril, and you could not tolerate beta-blockers.
- You have been taking diclofenac for your osteoarthritis.
- You do not smoke or drink.
- You had a heart attack 6 years ago and have diet-controlled diabetes.

SCENARIO 19.2: RENAL COLIC

- You are a 32-year-old lawyer.
- You have had a 3-hour history of severe left-sided flank pain that is radiating to your testicle.
- You have taken some paracetamol and your wife's codeine phosphate, which has helped marginally.
- You have had no fever, but have noticed a little bit of blood in the urine.
- You have diabetes and are currently on metformin.

SCENARIO 19.3: URINARY TRACT INFECTION

- You are a 69-year-old retired window cleaner
- You had an operation on your prostate gland 5 days ago for an enlarged prostate (TURP).
- You have been feeling feverish and today had two episodes of vomiting.
- You are able to pass urine, but it is painful and you have noticed some blood in the urine. You were told by the urology doctor that it is OK to notice some blood in the urine.
- Your wife was worried because you were confused and did not know where you were this morning.
- You are otherwise well and not on any regular medicines.
- You are allergic to penicillin and you got a rash the last time you were given amoxicillin.

CHAPTER 20: ENDOCRINE EMERGENCIES

SCENARIO 20.1: DKA HISTORY AND MANAGEMENT

- You are a trainee bus driver.
- You have been unwell for 2 days with abdominal pain and tiredness, and today you had some shortness of breath and felt faint.
- You are otherwise well, but have noticed some weight loss over the last couple of months and also some blurred vision on occasions, as well as a recurrent urinary tract infection.
- You are not on any medications and do not have any allergies.
- You are worried about being diagnosed with diabetes and concerned that you may not be able to work as a bus driver.

SCENARIO 20.3: ADDISONIAN CRISIS

- You are a 43-year-old shop assistant.
- You woke up this morning feeling very dizzy and light-headed.
- You collapsed at work and have vomited once.
- You have lost weight in the last 2 months.
- You were diagnosed with pulmonary tuberculosis and are on antituberculous medications.

CHAPTER 21: HAEMATOLOGICAL EMERGENCIES

SCENARIO 21.1: SICKLE CELL CRISIS

- You are a 23-year-old Nigerian trainee accountant.
- You have had severe pain in your right knee as well as some chest discomfort after having a flu-like illness last week.
- You do not have any history of trauma or recent travel.
- You have taken dihydrocodeine and diclofenac, which have not helped.
- You have a history of sickle cell disease and are on regular folic acid and penicillin.
- You have not had a sickle cell crisis for over 6 months and you have a haematology appointment next week.
- You have your examinations next week, but cannot revise because of the pain.

SCENARIO 21.2: DIC

- You are an F2 doctor who has just started your emergency department placement.
- You have come from an orthopaedic placement and have not had much exposure to acutely unwell medical patients.
- You had to manage a sick patient yesterday and were too scared to ask for senior support.
- You are worried that you mismanaged a patient with meningococcal septicaemia.
- You need help in interpreting the blood results.
- You are worried about the need for antibiotic prophylaxis, since you treated the patient.

CHAPTER 22: INFECTIOUS DISEASES

SCENARIO 22.1: COMMUNITY-ACQUIRED PNEUMONIA

As the F2, you give the patient's history as follows:

- Mr Jessop is age 63 and presents with fever, productive cough and worsening shortness of breath over 3 days. He has no significant comorbidities, is a non-smoker and lives independently with his wife. On examination, he is fully alert, with mental test score 10/10.
- His vital signs are as follows: pulse 96 bpm, BP 115/55 mmHg, oxygen saturation 94% on room air, respiratory rate 24 breaths min^{-1}. There are coarse crepitations in the right lung.

SCENARIO 22.2: THE FEBRILE TRAVELLER

- You are a 36-year-old Nigerian businessman.
- You travelled to Nigeria for 4 weeks, returning 5 days ago.
- You did not take any antimalarial treatment.
- You were born in Nigeria and moved to the UK when you were 16 years old, and you think that you have had malaria 'a few' times before.

- The fever is coming in waves every day or so, when you shiver uncontrollably.
- You do not have sickle cell disease and are otherwise fit and healthy.
- You have no specific respiratory, gastrointestinal or urinary symptoms.

SCENARIO 22.3: HIV SEROCONVERSION

- You are a 26-year-man.
- You are currently unemployed and have been backpacking in Australia for the last 3 months.
- You have had multiple male and female partners in the last 3 months. Most of them were casual and you did not always use contraception
- You have had a sore throat and generalized aches and pains, as well a rash on your face. You do not have any symptoms to suggest an STI.
- You smoke occasionally, but have never used intravenous drugs.
- You went to a sexual health clinic 2 years ago, where you were tested for HIV as well as hepatitis B and C, and were cleared for all three.
- You currently have a male partner who is not aware of your sexual contacts in Australia. You are worried that you have AIDS, and become upset when the candidate suggests that you may be at risk of HIV.

SCENARIO 22.4: BACTERIAL MENINGITIS

- You are worried about your girlfriend, who is a medical student. She was meant to meet you at the student union bar but had a headache and decided to have an early night. She has had a sore throat and a cough for 2 days.
- She is otherwise well, with no allergies, and has had no recent travel history.
- When you got home, she seemed confused and you thought that she was drunk. She also complained of neck pain and was unable to tolerate bright lights. She has vomited on two occasions.
- You are worried about having caught meningitis from your girlfriend, and want to know if you need antibiotics.

SCENARIO 22.5: NEEDLESTICK INJURY

- You are a 28-year-old nurse on one of the renal wards. You were giving insulin to an elderly patient subcutaneously, and you gave yourself a needlestick injury in your left index finger.
- You made the wound bleed and washed it under the tap.
- You had a full course of the hepatitis B vaccination 3 years ago and you think that your levels are OK.
- You do not know much about the source, but were told that he is an 80-year-old man who was admitted with a UTI and is not known to have any risk factors for having any bloodborne viruses.
- You are worried about getting HIV and request to be given post-exposure prophylaxis (PEP), and you would like a blood test to see if you have got HIV.
- If you are given an adequate explanation of why this is not necessary, you are reassured and do not push for PEP.
- You are up to date with your tetanus vaccination.

CHAPTER 23: DERMATOLOGY

SCENARIO 23.1: ECZEMA HISTORY

- You are a 19-year-old trainee chef.
- You were working in a restaurant and developed a rash on your arm.
- You were recently cleaning dishes using a new concentrated detergent.
- You do not wear gloves when washing the dishes.

- You are otherwise well.
- You suffer from asthma and hay fever.
- You are concerned about the appearance of the rash, and your colleagues are asking if it is contagious.

SCENARIO 23.3: EXAMINATION OF A RASH (IMPETIGO)

- You have come to the emergency department because you are very worried about your 2-year-old son's rash.
- It developed 2 days ago and is getting worse.
- Your son is eating and drinking.
- He has just started at a new nursery, and you have concerns that he has picked it from there.
- You are unsure if it is contagious. You also have a 9-month-old daughter – she and her brother are very close and share everything.
- You have a homeopathic cream that you would like to use, since you do not believe in antibiotics.
- You are concerned about the rash scarring.

CHAPTER 24: ONCOLOGICAL EMERGENCIES

SCENARIO 24.1: CAUDA EQUINA SYNDROME IN MALIGNANCY

- You are an 89-year-old retired architect
- You were diagnosed with prostate cancer 2 years ago and had an operation.
- You have been doing some gardening and thought that you had pulled a muscle in your back.
- You have been told that the cancer has spread to the bone.
- You have weakness in your left leg. You have noticed that you cannot control your bladder and have had a couple of accidents, which you find very embarrassing.
- You live alone and have a carer who comes in twice a day.
- You are otherwise well, but take tablets for high blood pressure and osteoarthritis.

SCENARIO 24.2: HYPERCALCAEMIA IN MALIGNANCY

Patient

- You are a 65-year-old cab driver.
- You were diagnosed with lung cancer and have been treated with radiotherapy.
- Over the last 3 days, you have noticed a deep boring pain in your left hip.
- You have come because you are finding it difficult to drive.
- You have also been very thirsty and have been drinking more water, which is inconvenient because you are in the cab all day.
- You are also forgetting your way around town, which is unusual since you have been a black-cab driver for over 40 years.
- You are otherwise well, but have had some abdominal pain, which you put down to a poor diet.
- You are concerned that you have diabetes, since you are drinking so much water.

F2

You may ask questions such as:

- What are the ECG findings in hypercalcaemia?
- How can the calcium be correct?
- What are the clinical features and management of hypercalcaemia?

CHAPTER 25: RHEUMATOLOGICAL EMERGENCIES

SCENARIO 25.2: BACK PAIN AND 'RED FLAGS'

- You are a 62-year-old landscape gardener.
- You have had a 3-day episode of lower back pain after sneezing.
- You took ibuprofen, which has not helped.
- You are now unable to walk, and have had to lie in bed for the last 2 days.
- You have had one episode where you wet yourself.
- There has been no change in your bowel habits.
- You are otherwise well, but are having investigations for prostate problems.

CHAPTER 26: PAEDIATRIC EMERGENCIES

SCENARIO 26.1: FEBRILE CONVULSION

- Your 2-year-old son has been brought to the emergency department after having an episode where he became unresponsive, his eyes rolled back and he was shaking for about 2 minutes.
- He has been unwell for 2 days and has had a cough and a high temperature, for which you have given him paracetamol.
- He has been off his food but drinking his juice.
- His urine has been dark and his stools have been a bit runny.
- He is otherwise well and has no other medical problems.
- He has an elder sister who is 6 and has had a cold; she had febrile convulsions when she was 14 months old.
- He is up to date with his vaccinations.
- You offer the 'red book' if the candidate forgets to ask for it.
- You are very worried about your son being an epileptic. You would like him to have a brain scan to see if he has brain damage, because you had a forceps delivery.
- You are not happy to take him home, since you are worried that he will have another fit.

SCENARIO 26.2: NON-ACCIDENTAL INJURY

- You have brought your 7-month-old son for an X-ray after seeing your GP.
- The child has been dragging his right leg for a week and has been refusing to stand on it when you make him stand.
- You have also noticed that he has cried a lot every time you touch his right leg – for example when you wash him or change his nappy.
- You noticed this 5 days ago and thought that he was playing up, but when he started to drag his leg, you went to the GP.
- He is otherwise well, but has missed some of his vaccinations because he had a cold.
- You have left his 'red book' at home.
- He is your second child. Your older child, who is now 8 years old, lives with your parents because you were unable to cope with him as he has cerebral palsy.
- You have been divorced for 2 years and have a new partner, who is the father of your 7-month-old child.
- You were the victim of domestic violence 9 months ago when your partner assaulted you, but you did not press charges, since he did it because he was drunk.
- You suffered from postnatal depression, but are now OK.
- You and your partner are planning to get married next month.

- You work as a healthcare assistant at the local hospital, and your partner, who is unemployed, looks after the child during the day.
- Your partner does not remember the child falling or hurting himself in the last couple of weeks.

SCENARIO 26.4: THE LIMPING CHILD

- You have brought your 5-year-old child to the emergency department because she has had a 2-day history of a painful limp
- She has mild learning difficulties, and is now refusing to walk and is complaining of pain in the right hip and knee.
- She had a cold last week, but is now well.
- She does not want to straighten her right leg.
- You have given her some paracetamol and ibuprofen.
- Today, you noticed that she had a high temperature and was off her food.
- She had a minor fall yesterday when she jumped off the bed, but was OK afterwards and did not complain of any pain.
- You are worried that she has been bullied at school because she has learning difficulties, and you are concerned about her teachers neglecting her.
- You have an older child, who is 8 and is otherwise well.

SCENARIO 26.5: UTI IN A CHILD

- You are 19 years old and have brought your 18-month-old brother to the hospital because your mother is in hospital having an operation for breast cancer.
- You have been looking after him while your mother is in hospital.
- Your father is at work and you have come home from university to help out.
- The child has been unwell for 2 days and has been vomiting and has had a fever.
- He has been off his food and he is not tolerating any fluids.
- You have noticed that his urine is strong and his nappies are rather smelly.
- You have not given him paracetamol, since you were not sure if you should.
- You are worried that you have done something wrong and given him food poisoning.
- You think that he has had antibiotics in the past for a urine infection and that he had to have a scan of his kidneys, but are unsure what the outcome was.

CHAPTER 27: PSYCHIATRIC EMERGENCIES

SCENARIO 27.1: ALCOHOL HISTORY

- You are a 48-year-old banker.
- You were told last week that you are going to be made redundant after your bank went into administration.
- You went out drinking last night and were found intoxicated in the street with a bruise on your forehead. You had your head scanned, and the scan was normal.
- You have been working in the finance industry for 10 years, and feel that drinking is a part of your job.
- You drink about 5 beers and maybe a couple of glasses of wine a day, which you do not think is too much. When you go out, this can be a lot more.
- You have been admitted to hospital twice before with intoxication, but you feel that this was because someone spiked your drinks.
- Your girlfriend keeps nagging you because she feels that you drink too much. This makes you feel angry, since you are only a 'social drinker'.
- You have tried to cut down, but you have had a lot of pressures at work.
- You do not feel guilty, since all of your work colleagues also drink when you go out.
- On occasions, you have had a drink in the morning before you go to work.

- You do not think that you have an alcohol problem, and could stop drinking completely if you wanted.
- You are worried about a tremor that you have had and are very anxious.
- You are otherwise well and not on any medications.
- You smoke 20 cigarettes a day and have taken cocaine in the past.
- You are willing to have help for your alcohol problems if the candidate offers it.

SCENARIO 27.2: DELIBERATE SELF-HARM HISTORY

- You are a 24-year-old graphic designer.
- You had an argument with your boyfriend because he feels that you are no longer interested in him.
- You tried to hang yourself with one of his ties in your flat.
- You left a note for him and texted him before you tried hanging yourself from the light fittings. The fittings broke, and your boyfriend found you in tears with the tie tight around your neck.
- You made your will last week, leaving everything to a local charity.
- You have been feeling down for the last couple of months, and you put this down to losing your job.
- You suffered from depression when you were a teenager, when you used to cut your wrists.
- You put this down to your parents, who were having a very messy divorce.
- Your mother committed suicide when you were 19.
- You found her after she had taken an overdose, and you blame yourself for not having found her sooner.
- You have had thoughts of killing yourself for 2 weeks. You have lost interest in sex and eating and you feel tired all the time.
- You saw your GP for some sleeping pills because you cannot sleep, but he declined because of your history of self-harm.
- You are otherwise medically well, with no serious illnesses.
- You do not drink or smoke, because your father was an alcoholic.
- You do not see any future and wish that you were dead.
- You are unhappy about being kept in hospital and demand to be discharged, since you know your rights.
- You refuse all treatment and assessment and are very tearful.

SCENARIO 27.3: MENTAL STATE EXAMINATION IN MANIA

- You are a 24-year-old man.
- You were on a busy dual carriageway.
- You were trying to help the police catch people who did not have their road tax so that you could bring them to justice.
- You have been employed to oversee traffic offences in your area.
- You are going to be the next commissioner of police and you have plans to manage crime and traffic in the area.
- You feel that you were wrongly arrested by the police and do not wish to be detained.
- You do not wish to sit down and you resist all attempts to sit in one place. You also speak continuously and ask for the head of MI5.
- You are also an undercover MI5 agent who is on a covert mission and are convinced that the cars on the dual carriageway were trying to run you over on purpose to thwart your mission.
- You have not been drinking, since you do not feel that you need alcohol.
- You are unable to concentrate on any of the tasks that you are set.
- You do not have any hallucinations.
- You have a history of bipolar disease, which you feel is a label to control your power.
- You have stopped taking your tablets (lithium) – 'kryptonite' – because they stop your special powers. You refer to yourself as 'Superman' and refer to your watch as the radar that can detect danger.
- You lived with your parents, but they have thrown you out because they cannot deal with your special powers.
- You have been sectioned twice before.

SCENARIO 27.4: ACUTE CONFUSIONAL STATE

Patient

- You are a 74-year-old man.
- You live alone and have been confused for 2 days.
- You are muddled about the time of day and ask for your breakfast repeatedly, and you think that the year is 2001.
- You cannot remember where you live, but know that you are in hospital.
- You know the dates of World War II and you describe how you fought on the beaches of Normandy.
- You cannot spell the word 'WORLD' backwards and find it difficult to remember the objects that you are asked to remember.
- You cannot remember any of the medications that you take or details of any illnesses.

Carer

- The patient has limited mobility and uses a Zimmer frame to get around his bungalow.
- The carers come in twice a day to help the patient with washing, dressing and grooming. He can feed himself but cannot cook.
- He has a long-term urinary catheter following an operation for prostate cancer. The district nurses change this regularly.
- You noticed that the urine looked rather dark and bloodstained 2 days ago.
- He is usually bright and chatty and, although forgetful, he can hold a conversation about current events.
- He suffers from high blood pressure and prostate cancer and had his right hip replaced 2 years ago. He often gets urinary tract infections.
- You have a list of his medications, including aspirin, ramipril, co-codamol and bendroflumethiazide.

CHAPTER 30: COMMUNICATION SKILLS

SCENARIO 30.1: THE ANGRY PATIENT

- You are a 54-year-old businessman who has a very important meeting today.
- You were late for the meeting and tripped as you got off the bus.
- Your right ankle is painful and swollen, but you can weight-bear.
- The bus driver called an ambulance, because you were in a lot of pain.
- You have waited for 2½ hours after being seen by a triage nurse, who said that your ankle was sprained and you would be seen by a doctor.
- You were seen by an emergency nurse practitioner, who examined you and confirmed that you have a soft tissue injury.
- You are angry because you have missed the meeting, you have been waiting for over 2½ hours, you have not been offered any painkillers and you have seen other people who came in after you see a doctor before you.
- You have planned a skiing trip, which you may have to cancel.
- You want to see a doctor and be X-rayed.
- You want to sue the bus company for negligence and have seen the TV adverts where you can claim financial compensation for an injury.
- You cannot believe the state of the NHS and feel that it is a poor service given what you pay for it.
- You calm down when you are offered analgesia and the doctor explains why an X-ray is not needed. You are willing to try conventional treatment when you are given crutches and the opportunity for follow-up with your GP and an X-ray if the pain does not improve.
- You are further pacified if the candidate offers to write you a letter on your behalf to the travel firm to see if you can have your trip refunded.

- You get angrier if the candidate is fixed in their views or becomes aggressive.
- If the candidate is aggressive and confrontational, you walk out of the scenario.

SCENARIO 30.2: BREAKING BAD NEWS

- You have been asked to come to the emergency department after being informed that your husband has been brought to hospital.
- You have been married for 5 years and are 14 weeks pregnant with your first child.
- Your husband is an avid motorcyclist and you have never been a fan of him riding a motorbike.
- At first, you cannot accept that he is dead and insist that there must be some mistake.
- You are shocked and stunned, since he only left for work a few hours ago.
- You would like to see him, but are scared.
- You want to know if he was in pain when he died.
- You are not keen on a post-mortem and would like a funeral as soon as possible because of your Islamic faith, and you ask if you can call an imam (priest). This is a major issue for you, and conflicts with the delay that may be caused by having a post-mortem.
- If the candidate does not raise the question of organ donation, you should ask if it is an option and how it works.

SCENARIO 30.3: THE DIFFICULT REFERRAL

- You are the orthopaedic registrar on call.
- The emergency department F2 tried to refer a patient to you earlier on, which you did not feel was appropriate, since the history that you were given did not suggest a significant injury.
- This has been your fifth emergency department referral since you started your shift.
- Your consultant has not been able to come in and your F2 has called in sick, so you are on your own.
- You are a bit grumpy because you are tired and stressed.
- You are about to start an emergency case and have been bleeped three times in quick succession from the emergency department.
- You ask the candidate if they have seen the patient and you suggest that the F2 had made an inappropriate referral and that the quality of emergency department referrals is poor.
- You are initially unwilling to see the patient until they have had a CT scan of their neck and have been seen by the neurologist for an opinion, but would compromise to see them after you finish your emergency case if the candidate arranges further imaging.
- You are aggressive and short with the candidate; if they become aggressive, you do not back down.
- You are more amenable if the candidate is calm and non-confrontational and offers a compromise.

SCENARIO 30.4: DEALING WITH A COMPLAINT

- You are a 60-year-old housewife who was given a prescription for co-amoxiclav despite telling the emergency department doctor you saw yesterday that you have a penicillin allergy.
- You had a bad reaction when you were younger, and luckily the pharmacist stopped the error before you took the tablets
- You have concerns about the doctor that you saw last night – they did not appear to be listening to you and were very dismissive.
- You request to make a formal complaint and want to know what the formal process is.
- You get cross if the candidate does not let you speak.
- Your husband died in the emergency department after having an abdominal aortic aneurysm rupture 4 months ago. He had presented to the emergency department two days in succession with abdominal pain and was sent home with constipation. You are in the process of suing the hospital and are still upset.
- You are worried that nothing will be done about the drug error and that the hospital will cover it up.
- You want to know what can be put in place to prevent further errors.

INDEX